W9-DGF-667

The nature of creativity

The nature of creativity

Contemporary psychological perspectives

Edited by
ROBERT J. STERNBERG
Department of Psychology
Yale University

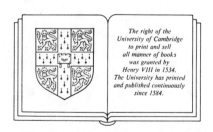

The right of the
University of Cambridge
to print and sell
all manner of books
was granted by
Henry VIII in 1534.
The University has printed
and published continuously
since 1584.

CAMBRIDGE UNIVERSITY PRESS

Cambridge
New York New Rochelle Melbourne Sydney

AL HARRIS LIBRARY
SOUTHWESTERN OKLA. STATE UNIV
WEATHERFORD, OK. 73096

Published by the Press Syndicate of the University of Cambridge
The Pitt Building, Trumpington Street, Cambridge CB2 1RP
32 East 57th Street, New York, NY 10022, USA
10 Stamford Road, Oakleigh, Melbourne 3166, Australia

© Cambridge University Press 1988

First published 1988

Printed in the United States of America

Library of Congress Cataloging-in-Publication Data
The nature of creativity.
Includes indexes.
1. Creative ability.   I. Sternberg, Robert J.
[DNLM: 1. Creativeness.   2. Psychology.   BF 408 N285]
BF408.N354   1988   153.3'5   87–20928

British Library Cataloguing in Publication Data
The Nature of creativity: contemporary
psychological perspectives.
1. Creative ability – Psychological aspects
I. Sternberg, Robert J.
153.3'5   BF410

ISBN 0 521 33036 X hard covers
ISBN 0 521 33892 1 paperback

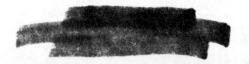

Contents

v

Part III   The role of the individual–environment interaction in creativity

The study of creative lives

The study of creative systems

Part IV   Integration and conclusions

Preface

Research in creativity has taken on the role of a prodigal stepbrother to research on intelligence. The work in creativity is a "stepbrother" because although it is in the same family, it never quite seemed, to many of those who follow it, to measure up. And indeed, it is the work in creativity that is continually compared to work in intelligence, rather than the other way around. The stepbrother never seems to be quite as good or quite as well accepted, regardless of what he does. The stepbrother is prodigal because of his tendency to go beyond accepted bounds, and even at times to be grandiose. Whereas intelligence has seemed like a problem that, with sufficient effort, could be resolved, creativity has sometimes seemed irresoluble, and some have even wondered if it exists as a single entity or class of entities, aside from in name. Various approaches have been taken to dealing with this prodigal stepbrother. Some, like J. P. Guilford, have tried to subsume creativity under the rubric of intelligence. Others, like Jack Getzels, have argued that creativity is an entity that is psychologically distinct from intelligence. Still others have simply ignored the connection between creativity and intelligence. The contributors to this book represent a diversity of perspectives, but all have in common that they have studied creativity for its own sake.

Creativity research, which had been stagnant for some time, received a new lease on life from J. P. Guilford's 1950 APA presidential address on the nature of creativity. Guilford brought back into the eye of the psychological public an entity that had long been languishing. During the 1950s there was a burst of research on creativity, and it seemed that at least some of the problems of creativity could be licked. Some of the major contributors during that era of research are represented in this book. Much of the research of that period was summarized in Philip Vernon's 1960 book entitled *Creativity*.

Some of the research on creativity continued into the 1960s and even 1970s, but other efforts faltered. It became clear by the end of the 1970s that the initial thrust would slow down and that only a few diehards, such as Howard Gruber and others, were continuing to study the field in a way that could make a difference. At least some researchers probably shared my attitude in the late 1970s, which was that few psychological issues are more interesting, but more intractable, than the issue of creativity. My remark to my colleagues was that there was no phenomenon that I would rather study, but that I just did not have any creative ideas regarding how to study it, and I was not sure how many other people were having creative ideas about it either.

By the early to middle 1980s, I became convinced that important work on creativity was once again being done from a number of different perspectives. As I surveyed the field, I became convinced that a not insubstantial number of the early investigators were continuing to study creativity in fruitful ways and that some new investigators were starting to have some genuinely penetrating insights into its nature. I then started to do a bit of research on creativity, although it did not become a major focus of my research. I became convinced that a lot of new contributions had been and were being made, but that they were not all as well known or as well integrated as they should be because these contributions were scattered into so many different outlets of publication. My conviction that the field was genuinely re-awakening and that there was a need to bring it together motivated this book. I decided to ask those individuals whom I considered to be the brightest lights in the field of creativity to contribute chapters to an edited book on the topic, and to my delight, almost all of them agreed to do so. Their efforts are represented in the chapters in this book.

I am grateful to the members of my research group who have influenced my thinking about creativity, particularly Janet Davidson, whose collaboration with me in studying insight has been particularly influential in my thinking. I am also grateful to Susan Milmoe, my editor at Cambridge University Press, who has seen me through yet another book. Most of all, I am grateful to the contributors to this book for taking time out from their busy schedules to write these chapters. This book is dedicated to J. P. Guilford, who showed how creativity could be understood as a part of intelligence, and to Jack Getzels, who showed how it could not be.

Robert J. Sternberg

Contributors

Teresa M. Amabile
Department of Psychology
Brandeis University
Waltham, MA 02254

Frank Barron
Department of Psychology
University of California
Santa Cruz, CA 95060

Mihaly Csikszentmihalyi
Department of Psychology
University of Chicago
Chicago, IL 60637

Sara N. Davis
Department of Psychology
City University of New York
New York, NY 10036

David Henry Feldman
Department of Child Study
Tufts University
Medford, MA 02155

Howard Gardner
Boston VA Hospital
Boston, MA 02130

Howard E. Gruber
Department of Psychology
University of Geneva
1121 Geneva 4 Switzerland

Beth A. Hennessey
Department of Psychology
Wellesley College
Wellesley, MA 02181

Philip N. Johnson-Laird
MRC Applied Psychology Unit
Cambridge, CB2 2EF England

Randolph Jones
Department of Computer Science
University of California
Irvine, CA 92664

Pat Langley
Department of Computer Science
University of California
Irvine, CA 92664

D. N. Perkins
School of Education
Harvard University
Cambridge, MA 02138

Roger C. Schank
Department of Computer Science
Yale University
New Haven, CT 06520

Dean Keith Simonton
Department of Psychology
University of California
Davis, CA 95616

Robert J. Sternberg
Department of Psychology
Yale University
New Haven, CT 06520

Twila Z. Tardif
Department of Psychology
Yale University
New Haven, CT 06520

Calvin W. Taylor
Department of Psychology
University of Utah
Salt Lake City, UT 84112

E. Paul Torrance
185 Riverhill Drive
Athens, GA 30606

Herbert J. Walberg
College of Education
University of Illinois
Chicago, IL 60680

Robert W. Weisberg
Department of Psychology
Temple University
Philadelphia, PA 19122

Introduction

Robert J. Sternberg

The goal of the chapters in this book is to explore the nature of creativity. The chapter authors take a wide variety of approaches in pursuit of this goal. The book is divided into four basic parts.

The first part, containing a single chapter, deals with the relationship between creativity and the external environment of the individual. In their chapter ''The Conditions of Creativity,'' Hennessey and Amabile describe what might be viewed as the necessary prerequisite conditions for creative performance. These conditions include things such as absence of external rewards and emphasis on intrinsic rather than extrinsic motivation and performance. Indeed, the authors formulate an intrinsic motivation principle of creativity: People will be most creative when they feel motivated primarily by interest, enjoyment, satisfaction, and challenge of the work itself – not by external pressures. This chapter is useful in setting the stage for the rest of the book because it specifies the environmental constraints that either facilitate or impede manifestation of the creative potential that lies within the individual.

The second part of the book deals with the relationship between creativity and the internal environment of the individual. This part of the book is divided into two sections, one focusing on the psychometric approach to creativity and the other focusing on cognitive approaches.

The psychometric approach is represented in the chapters by Torrance, Barron, and Taylor. Torrance describes creative thinking as a process of recognizing gaps and missing elements, formulating hypotheses about what is missing that creates these gaps, testing these hypotheses, revising and retesting the hypotheses, and, finally, communicating the results. He considers a number of formal definitions of creativity and also criteria for recognizing creative performance and then spends the bulk of his chapter reviewing the literature on the Torrance Tests of Creative Thinking. These tests measure skills such as fluency, flexibility, originality, elaboration, and so forth. The correlational data regarding the tests are impressive. They predict quite well, for a number of different groups, criteria such as quality and quantity of creative performance.

Barron, too, focuses his chapter on a test, but in his case the test is the Symbolic Equivalence Test. In this test, subjects are asked to think of metaphors, or symbolically equivalent images, for certain suggested stimulus images. Consider, for

1

example, "leaves being blown in the wind." Some possible symbolic equtivalences would be a civilian population fleeing chaotically in the face of armed aggression, or handkerchiefs being tossed about in an electric dryer. Different responses are given differing scores, depending on their quality. The test is scored for number of acceptable responses and for number of original responses. Barron has found that his test of creativity yields substantial positive correlations for creative performance in a variety of domains, including creative writing, architecture, art, and entrepreneurial pursuits.

Taylor focuses his chapter around psychometric conceptions of creativity that have evolved over a period of years. He describes his own and others' conceptions, focusing in particular on his "circular model." In contrast to Torrance and Barron, who focus on issues of assessment, Taylor brings the focus toward training, describing his "totem method" for developing creativity.

Whereas the psychometric approach concentrates on individual differences in creativity and their correlates, the cognitive approach concentrates on the mental processes and structures underlying creativity. The second section of the second part of the book opens with a chapter by Sternberg, who presents a "three-facet model of creativity." According to this model, there are three basic aspects that interact to generate creative performance. The first aspect is strictly cognitive, involving those aspects of intelligence having interface with creativity, for example, processes of insight. Sternberg draws this cognitive facet from his triarchic theory of human intelligence. The second aspect involves matters of intellectual style, in other words, how one uses one's intelligence. Drawing from his theory of intellectual styles as mental self-government, Sternberg describes, for example, how three different functions in the use of intelligence are the legislative, executive, and judicial. The legislative function concerns creation, the executive function involves acting on creation, and the judicial function has to do with evaluating creation. Although all three styles can play some role in creativity, Sternberg argues that the legislative function is the most important and that individuals with a primarily legislative style are more likely to express themselves creatively than are individuals with a primarily executive or judicial style. The last aspect of the model pertains to personality variables. Sternberg argues that certain personality attributes are more likely than others to lead to creative performance. In particular, individuals with high tolerance of ambiguity, willingness to surmount obstacles, willingness to grow, and so on, are more likely to be creative than are others. In sum, creativity is at the interface among the three aspects of the model.

In his chapter "Problem Solving and Creativity," Weisberg concentrates on what could be viewed as a central type of creativity, namely, insight. Perhaps the most widely held view of insight is what might be called the "special-process" view – that insight differs in kind from other problem-solving processes. Weisberg argues that it does not, that, in fact, insight processes are an extension of ordinary perceptual, memory, and problem-solving processes. He considers some of the great insights of history and how they can be accounted for in terms of ordinary rather than extraordinary information processing. He also recites the results of several experiments done in his laboratory that argue for his ''nothing-special'' view of insight. Weisberg's research shows, at minimum, that insights are not likely to happen in the absence of a great deal of task-relevant prior knowledge. Whatever they are, they do not come from nowhere, but rather from the presence and integration of the knowledge representation that is usable and useful in a given task.

Whereas the first two chapters in this section derive their theory and base their research on human subjects, the last three chapters base their theory on research more in the tradition of artificial intelligence. The first of these chapters, that by Langley and Jones, presents ''A Computational Model of Scientific Insight.'' Langley and Jones, like Weisberg, focus primarily on insight-related phenomena. Langley and Jones review three alternative computational models of insight and end up rejecting all three of them. Whereas the past theories relied primarily on the notion of a problem space, Langley and Jones, like Weisberg, emphasize memory phenomena. Also like Weisberg, they especially emphasize the role of analogy in memory. Insights are especially likely to occur when insightful problem solvers recognize analogies between new problems they are currently facing and problems they have solved before. The authors argue that insight is primarily dependent on analogical retrieval and that this retrieval occurs during the illumination stage of insightful problem solving. Moreover, the retrieval usually is cued by some external event. They suggest that a spreading activation model would account for how the external event touches off the analogy and hence the insight, and they build their theory of insight around the concept of spreading activation.

A related but somewhat different approach to the problem of creativity is taken by Johnson-Laird in his chapter ''Freedom and Constraint in Creativity.'' Johnson-Laird contends that creativity depends on arbitrary choices and on a mental device for producing such choices. He believes that a key to the processes of creativity is free will. Moreover, he likens creativity to a murder: Both depend on a motive, means, and opportunity! Johnson-Laird has devised a program that simulates creative performance in the domain of music. The program takes a chord sequence as input and delivers a bass line as output. To produce notes, it will generate a small step, a large step, or the same note again, according to the rules of the grammar for contours that Johnson-Laird has derived from the corpus of improvisation. Johnson-Laird notes that the program is quite competent, but that it lacks two abilities of jazz players: It makes no specific use of chromatic runs of several passing notes, and it makes no use of motifs. Johnson-Laird's chapter is a good example of how ideas about creative performance can be operationalized through computational mechanisms.

In his chapter ''Creativity as a Mechanical Process,'' Schank also bases his approach on artificial-intelligence notions, but applies these notions in a way quite different from that of Johnson-Laird. Schank, like Weisberg and like Langley and Jones, relies heavily on notions from human memory in his conceptualizing. Indeed, he draws heavily on his dynamic memory model of processing in order to understand creative performance. He believes that there are basically two subprocesses that characterize creativity. The first is a search process, which involves finding explanations. The second is an alteration process, which modifies and adapts the explanation in such a way as to allow an explanation originally derived from one situation to be relevant to another. Notice how this model, like that of Weisberg, draws heavily on analogy. Indeed, Schank notes that creativity results from applying old explanations in places where those explanations were never originally intended to apply. Thus, he believes that creativity depends on two primary factors: a set of methods for getting reminded, and a set of methods for adapting remindings in such a way as to fit a new situation. Schank shows how his notions can be used to generate creative behavior in a fairly wide variety of situations.

Part three of the book deals with the interaction between the internal and external environments of the individual. This part of the book is divided into two sections. The first section contains chapters that use the study of creative lives as a primary data base; the second section comprises chapters that are more generally historical in their orientation, using larger data bases rather than studies of small numbers of lives.

The first chapter in the first section of the third part of the book is by Gruber and Davis. Their chapter, which describes Gruber's "Evolving-Systems Approach to Creative Thinking," reviews Gruber's lifetime study of the creative enterprise, as well as Davis's dissertation work. According to the evolving-systems view, creativity bears virtually no resemblance to the flashes of creative insight that provide the basis for analysis in some of the earlier chapters. Rather, it is something that evolves over the course of a lifetime, combining manifold minor insights with some major ones and directed by a large-scale evolving enterprise. Gruber has intensively studied Darwin and the development of his theory of evolution and has shown how the theory of evolution was not a sudden major insight, but rather the culmination of scores of minor and major insights. Creativity is seen as a slowly evolving process of reflection and discovery rather than a sudden burst of enlightenment.

The next chapter is by Feldman, who has been heavily influenced by Gruber. Like Gruber, he describes the evolution of a set of creative ideas, but in Feldman's case, the creative ideas are his own. Whereas Gruber has focused in his research on adult creativity, Feldman has focused on child prodigies, and he reviews some of his work on prodigies in this chapter. He shows that some of our common conceptions about prodigious performance are incorrect. For example, many of us believe that prodigies are so outstanding that their prodigiousness would show under any environmental circumstances. Feldman shows, to the contrary, that prodigious performance in children results only because of a rare and complex coincidence of individual, family, societal, and cultural variables. Without just the right mix, the prodigious performance will never be achieved.

This aspect of prodigiousness distinguishes it from adult creativity, wherein some "bucking" of the environment is almost always necessary for creative performance to take place. One interesting aspect of prodigious performance is that it is by no means randomly distributed across fields. Whereas adult creativity can occur in almost any field, prodigious performance tends to be limited to a fairly small set of fields, particularly a field in which there is a constrained and clearly defined set of symbols to manipulate. Thus, chess, based on the manipulation of a small number of chessmen, is a more likely arena for prodigious performance than writing, which is based on the manipulation of tens of thousands of words and syntactic forms. Feldman's chapter provides a nice complement to Gruber's chapter in showing similarities and especially the differences between high levels of creative performance in adults and prodigious performance in children.

Like Gruber and Feldman, Gardner has chosen to study a small number of creative lives in his attempt to understand creativity through a "Synthetic Scientific Approach." Gardner concentrates on a single creative life, namely, that of Sigmund Freud. In his analysis of creativity, Gardner distinguishes among four levels of analysis. The subpersonal includes the biological subtraits and genetic endowments responsible for creative performance. The personal includes the cognitive processes and representations responsible for creative performance. It also includes factors of personality, motivation, and drive. The extrapersonal includes domain-specific factors responsible for the emergence of creative performance. Finally, the multipersonal includes the social context in which individuals make their creative contributions. Gardner analyzes Freud's performance in terms of each of these levels and helps us understand the multiplicity of factors that, in confluence, produced such a creative outpouring of work.

In the second section of the third part of this book, the focus shifts to the employment of historical data from many individuals in order to understand the antecedents and bases of creative performance.

The first chapter in this section is by Csikszentmihalyi, and it views the interactions of society, culture, and person to produce a systems view of creativity. According to Csikszentmihalyi, the creative individual takes information provided by the culture and transforms it, and if the changes are deemed valuable by society, they will be included in the domain in which the individual works, thus providing a new starting point for the next generation of persons. The actions of all three systems – person, domain (symbol system), and field (social organization of domain) – are necessary for creative performance to occur. Csikszentmihalyi reviews a variety of creative contributions and shows how his model can be applied to understand how they took place and how they came to be viewed as creative.

In his chapter "Creativity and Talent as Learning," Walberg suggests a novel theory of creativity called "human-capital theory." According to Walberg, "human capital" refers to the quality of work or the motivation, skills, and creativity of the worker. Human capital can be general or specialized. General capital includes knowledge and skills acquired in early life, mastery of the liberal arts and sciences, and so on. Specialized capital includes more specific skills and knowledge acquired only by the few, rather than the many. Using notions such as these, Walberg proceeds to an essentially economic analysis of creativity that is rather different from any of the other analyses in this book. For example, he notes the relevance of Merton's "Matthew effect" for understanding creativity. The basic idea behind the Matthew effect is that the rich get richer and the poor get poorer. The relevance of this notion is that individuals who have shown creative performance are likely to create and encounter the kinds of circumstances that will lead to further creative performance, whereas those individuals who thus far have not displayed creative performance are less likely to encounter or create such conditions. Walberg shows that economic analysis can account for certain aspects of creative performance that could be accounted for only with great difficulty through a standard psychological analysis.

The next chapter in this section, by Perkins, discusses "The Possibility of Invention." It bears a certain resemblance to Johnson-Laird's chapter in its heavy emphasis on philosophical analysis, and indeed Perkins is a philosopher by training. Perkins opens with a consideration of the *ex nihilo* problem, namely, how something can come out of nothing. His main mission in this chapter is to offer some broad answers to this question. He considers some standard answers to the question and rejects them. He then proceeds to construct his own answer, which is an evolutionary one: The main mechanisms of creative invention, according to Perkins, are generation, selection, and preservation. In essence, Perkins proposes that natural selection can be viewed as applying to the evolution of creative thought as well as to the evolution of species. At the same time, Perkins recognizes that the selection process for human creativity is much more strategic than what he refers to as nature's rolling of the genetic dice. Perkins devotes considerable attention in his chapter to the concept of boundaries, precisely because creativity involves going beyond boundaries. He also describes some of the cognitive heuristic processes people can use in order to achieve creative performance. Creative solutions rarely involve considering all possible solutions to a problem, and hence a creative individual needs a set of heuristics for deciding how to avoid combinatorial explosion in seeking solutions to problems. Perkins describes some of the methods for doing this, such as hill climbing and parallel processing.

The last chapter in this section, and indeed the last of the main chapters in the book, is by Simonton. Simonton opens his chapter with two major propositions concerning creativity. The first is that creativity is a form of leadership in that it entails personal influence over others, and the second is that creativity involves the participation of chance processes both in the origination of new ideas and in the social acceptance of those ideas by others. Simonton builds his chance-configuration theory around these two propositions. This theory, like that of Perkins, involves evolutionary thinking. Simonton proposes that solutions to novel problems require some means of generating ideational variation, that these heterogeneous variations must be subjected to a consistent selection process that deletes all but those solutions that feature adaptive fit, and that the variations that have been selected must be preserved and reproduced by mechanisms of retention. Simonton shows mathematically as well as psychologically how these factors combine to produce, and render effective, creative performance. Simonton also summarizes his innovative historiometric method, in which historical variables serve as bases for predicting when and where creativity is more and less likely to take place.

The fourth and last part of the book contains an overview and integration by Tardif and Sternberg. The goal of this chapter is to organize the main themes in the theorists' various views of creativity and to suggest a variety of commonalities that hold together their various points of view. The commonalities are prominent enough to suggest that a unified field of creativity may eventually be possible that will integrate the various perspectives advocated in this volume.

Part I

The role of the environment in creativity

1 The conditions of creativity

Beth A. Hennessey and Teresa M. Amabile

What is the origin of creative production? Can it be entirely attributed to a specific ability or constellation of personality traits possessed by the creator? Or are there other ingredients equally essential to this process? Our research demonstrates that social and environmental factors play major roles in creative performance. We have found that there exists a strong and positive link between a person's motivational state – motivational orientation, if you will – and the creativity of the person's performance. And in large part it is the social environment, or at least certain aspects of that environment, that determines this orientation. Guiding our investigations is what we have termed the *intrinsic motivation principle of creativity*:

People will be most creative when they feel motivated primarily by the interest, enjoyment, satisfaction, and challenge of the work itself – not by external pressures.

In essence, we are saying that the love people feel for their work has a great deal to do with the creativity of their performances. This proposition is clearly supported by accounts of the phenomenology of creativity. Most reports from and about creative individuals are filled with notions of an intense involvement in and un-rivaled love for their work. Thomas Mann, for example, described in one of his letters his passion for writing (John-Steiner, 1985), and physicists who were close to Albert Einstein saw in him a similar kind of intensity. In the words of the Nobel Prize–winning inventor Dennis Gabor, "no one has ever enjoyed science as much as Einstein" (John-Steiner, 1985, p. 67).

Similar references to the sustaining delights of creative endeavor are found throughout the letters, biographies, and autobiographies of a great many creative individuals (Amabile, 1983; Rosner & Abt, 1970). As cinematic director Henry Jaglom describes it, the joy of creating is like "being on a bicycle going down hill" (John-Steiner, 1985, p. 67), and Csikszentmihalyi (1975) describes the "flow state" experienced by many individuals at the peak of creative insight. Yet this exhilaration is in no way automatic. In our research we have found that the love felt for one's craft can be quite delicate and easily overshadowed by pressures in the environment.

As early as 1954, Carl Rogers talked about the "conditions for creativity" and the importance of setting up situations of psychological safety and freedom, of

11

providing an environment in which external evaluation is absent. It was Rogers's contention that creativity can flourish only in a climate in which the motivation to produce comes from within, and an examination of creative individuals' first-person accounts of their work supports this viewpoint. Over and over again, reference is made to the delicate balance needed between the desire for attention, praise, and support from friends, supervisors, editors, or colleagues, on the one hand, and, on the other hand, the necessity to maintain a certain protective distance from the opinions of these very same people (Hughes & McCullough, 1982; Steinbeck, 1969). A concern with evaluation expectation and actual evaluation, a focus on competition and external reward, a desire for external recognition, the difficulty of withstanding harsh criticism, a rebellion against time pressures, and a deliberate rejection of society's demands – paradoxically, all are recurrent themes in the phenomenology of outstandingly creative persons.

It is clear from case studies that an environment conducive to creative production is not easily established, and once achieved, it must be constantly reshaped and controlled. Love is not enough. The creative individual, often with great difficulty, must work to construct the personal environment that will offer the fullest opportunity for maintaining that love, that intrinsic motivational orientation so necessary for creative expression (Wallace, 1985, p. 371).

Some definitions

Having presented and briefly discussed the intrinsic motivation principle, we shall now define our terms a bit more precisely. Intrinsic motivation, which for the purposes of this discussion will also be referred to as intrinsic interest, has been variously described by a number of theorists. Harlow (1950) used this term to describe the interest shown by monkeys in puzzle manipulation. Taylor (1960), in an "information processing theory of motivation," suggests an inherent interest in cognitively engaging in tasks, and a similar construct has been developed by Hunt (1965).

More recently, some social psychologists (Lepper, Greene, & Nisbett, 1973) have defined intrinsic motivation from a cognitive perspective: Individuals are intrinsically motivated if they perceive themselves as engaging in activities primarily because of their own interest in those activities; they are extrinsically motivated if they perceive their engagement as a means to achieve extrinsic goals. Kruglanski (1975) expands on this notion with the addition of an endogenous/exogenous framework. According to this model, an actor's inference of intrinsic motivation follows whenever performance of a task appears to be a goal in itself. In this endogenous attribution, the implication of enjoyment, interest, and so on, derives from the fulfillment of the actor's desire. To the extent that this individual attributes the action to something outside of (exogenous to) the task, however, it implies the individual's negative affect – that is, the activity was a means rather than an end, and an exogenous attribution results.

Other theorists conceptualize intrinsic motivation more organismically. White (1959) and Harter (1978) believe that intrinsic motivation is based on the innate human need for competence in meeting optimal challenges, and deCharms (1968) proposes that intrinsically motivated behaviors stem from a desire to experience personal causation (also referred to as self-determination). In the models proposed by Deci and Ryan and their colleagues (Deci, 1971; Deci, 1975; Deci & Porac, 1978; Deci & Ryan, 1985), both a competence component and a self-determination component are included, but self-determination is highlighted as especially essential.

All of these definitions share the same fundamental elements: Persons who engage in activities because of their *own* interest or personal sense of satisfaction and fulfillment are intrinsically motivated, whereas persons who engage in activities to achieve some goal *external* to task engagement are extrinsically motivated. The intrinsic motivation principle on which we base our work contends that it is these differences in motivation that can lead to significant differences in creative performance.

The work of other psychological theorists suggests that creativity will most likely result from an intrinsically motivated state. Crutchfield (1962) proposes that "task-involved," intrinsic motivation will lead to higher levels of creativity than "ego-involved," extrinsic motivation, and in fact, personality data collected by Crutchfield (1961) indicate that high levels of intrinsic motivation accompany the work of notably creative persons. McGraw (1978) also suggests that performance on heuristic tasks (creativity tasks) should be adversely affected by increases in extrinsic motivation, whereas performance on algorithmic tasks should be enhanced. In an effort to explain this relationship between motivational state and creativity of performance, Lepper and Greene (1978) suggest that the intrinsically motivated person, as opposed to the extrinsically motivated person, should feel freer to take risks because those risks carry virtually no liability, save any that is self-imposed.

Finally, Deci and Ryan (1985) state that when people are intrinsically motivated, they will seek situations that interest them and that require the use of their creativity and resourcefulness.

But what do we mean by creativity? Psychologists have approached this problem of definition from a variety of angles and in the past have tended to center their discussions around either the creative person or the creative process. Although many contemporary theorists think of creativity as a process and look for evidence of it in persons (Stein, 1974–1975), their definitions most frequently use characteristics of the *product* as the distinguishing signs of creativity. Bruner (1962), for instance, views the creative product as anything that produces "effective surprise" in the observer, as well as a "shock of recognition" that the product or response, though novel, is entirely appropriate.

This combination of novelty and appropriateness is found in most conceptual definitions of creativity. An emphasis on the product is today widely regarded as the most useful for creativity research. Most assessment methods, however, use quite narrowly restricted "products" (Check, 1969; McGraw & McCullers, 1979; Sanders, Tedford, & Hardy, 1977). In the majority of creativity studies, performance on creativity tests is used as the criterion, and most creativity tests are constructed and scored similarly to tests of verbal and mathematical intelligence.

There does exist one small group of measures that entail the rating of actual products that were made in response to open-ended instructions (Getzels & Csikszentmihalyi, 1976; Simonton, 1980; Sobel & Rothenberg, 1980). Yet most of these measures present problems too, when the needs of the social-psychological researcher are considered. If we are to examine the effects of social-environmental factors on task motivation and creativity, the influence of domain-relevant skills must be carefully controlled so that the environmental effects will be detectable above individual differences in talent or experience. However, most of these assessment procedures that have judges rate actual single products (such as artworks) have proved too sensitive to large and stable differences in performance, thus threatening to swamp the more subtle (but no less important) influence of social environment. This problem of most assessment techniques in current usage is specific to social-psychological investigations. There is another large problem, however: Most creativity investigators, whether relying on creativity tests or on subjective assessments of products, have conducted their research in the absence of clear operational definitions.

The consensual assessment technique

Like most creativity researchers, we rely on a product definition: A product is viewed as creative to the extent that it is both a novel response and an appropriate, useful, correct, or valuable response to an open-ended task. What differentiates our approach is that we have gone on to formulate a specific operational definition of creativity that relies on a consensus of experts: A product or idea is creative to the extent that expert observers agree it is creative (Amabile, 1982b).

In the application of this operational definition and consensual assessment procedure, several important assumptions are made about the nature of creativity and creativity judgment. First, of course, we assume that products or observable responses must be the ultimate hallmarks of creativity and that it is not possible a priori to specify which objective features of new products will, in fact, be considered "creative." Rather, as is the case with most concepts tied to social-psychological research (Gergen, 1982), criteria for creativity require a historically bound social context.

Another assumption guiding our operational definition is that although creativity in a product may be difficult to characterize in terms of specific features, and although it is difficult to precisely characterize the phenomenology of observers' labeling of certain products as creative (Feldman, 1980), creativity is something that people can recognize and often agree on, even when they are given neither a guiding definition nor a list of specific features to be considered (Barron, 1965). In addition, in accord with previous theorists (Simon, 1967), we propose that there is one basic form of creativity, one basic quality of products that observers are responding to when they label something "creative," regardless of whether they are considering works produced in the scientific or artistic domain.

Finally, we assume that there are degrees of creativity, that observers can say with an acceptable level of agreement that some products are more or less creative than others. This assumed existence of a continuous underlying dimension is not new to psychological theorizing on creativity. Cattell and Butcher (1968), for example, stated that creativity "may be manifested . . . at widely differing levels, from discovering the structure of the atom to laying out a garden" (p. 279). And Nicholls (1972), while arguing against the assumption of a normally distributed personality trait of creativity, does concede that the assumption of continuity in judgments of creative *products* is a reasonable one.

In our own investigations, this consensual assessment procedure is implemented as follows: Subjects are asked to complete some task in a specific domain (such as poetry), and then experts in that domain (such as poets) independently rate the creativity of the products. The level of interjudge agreement is assessed, and if it is acceptable (generally above .70), the mean across-judge creativity ratings are used as our dependent measures of creativity. Before presenting studies that have employed this technique, it is necessary to describe the major features of our assessment method in more detail.

In selecting an appropriate creativity task, there are three requirements that must be met. First, the task must be one that leads to some product or clearly observable response that can be made available to appropriate judges for assessment. Second, the task should be open-ended enough to permit considerable flexibility and novelty in responses. Third, because it is desirable for social-psychological research that there not be large individual differences in baseline performances on the task, it should be one that does not depend heavily on special skills – such as drawing ability or verbal fluency – that some individuals have undoubtedly developed more fully than others. Certainly, for tasks that do depend heavily on special skills, it is possible to reduce extreme interindividual variability by choosing only individuals with a uniform level of baseline performance. However, this solution is impractical for most social-psychological studies of creativity. Whereas it is probably advisable in any case to eliminate subjects with deviantly high or low levels within the domain being explored, preliminary studies of a laboratory-based nature should use tasks that virtually all members of the population can perform adequately, without evidence of large variability in individual differences.

A number of requirements concerning the assessment procedure also deserve mention. First, judges should all have experience with the domain in question, although the levels of experience for all judges need not be identical. Basically, the consensual assessment technique requires that all judges be familiar enough with the domain to have developed, over a period of time, some implicit criteria for creativity, technical goodness, and so on.

The second procedural requirement is that judges make their assessments independently. The essence of the consensual definition is that experts can recognize creativity when they see it and that they can agree with one another in this assessment. If experts in a domain say (reliably) that something is highly creative, we must accept it as such. The integrity of the assessment technique depends on agreement being reached without attempts by the experimenter to impose particular criteria or attempts by the judges to influence each other. Thus, the judges should not be trained by the experimenter to agree with one another, they should not be given specific criteria for assessing creativity, and they should not have the opportunity to confer while making their assessments.

Third, in preliminary work on developing the technique for a given task, judges should make assessments on other dimensions in addition to creativity. Minimally, they should make ratings of the technical aspects of the products in question and, if appropriate, their aesthetic appeal as well. This will then make it possible to determine whether, in subjective assessments, creativity is related to or independent of those dimensions. Assessments of these other aspects of the work also make it possible to compare social-environmental effects on these aspects with social-environmental effects on creativity. This is of particular theoretical importance because, theoretically, there might be reasons to predict that a given social factor will have differential effects on creativity and on technical performance.

Fourth, judges should be instructed to rate the products relative to one another, rather than rating them against some absolute standard they might hold for work in their domain. This is important because, for most investigations, the levels of creativity produced by the "ordinary" subjects who participate will be low in comparison with the greatest works ever produced in that domain.

Finally, each judge should view the products in a different random order, and each judge should consider the various dimensions of judgment in a different random order. If this procedure were not followed and all judgments were made in the same order by all judges, high levels of interjudge reliability might reflect method artifacts.

Once the judgments are obtained, ratings on each dimension should be analyzed for interjudge reliability. In addition, if several subjective dimensions of judgment have been obtained, these should be factor-analyzed to determine the degree of independence between creativity and the other dimensions. Finally, if the products lend themselves to a straightforward identification of specific objective features, these features may be recorded and correlated with creativity judgments.

As implied by the consensual definition of creativity, the most important criterion for this assessment procedure is that the ratings be reliable. By definition, interjudge reliability in this method is equivalent to construct validity. If appropriate judges independently agree that a given product is highly creative, then it can and must be accepted as such. In addition, it should be possible to separate subjective judgments of creativity from judgments of technical goodness, aesthetic appeal, and so forth.

In an effort to firmly establish the utility of the consensual assessment technique, we have carried out a program of research using the technique for assessment of both verbal and artistic creativity. In over 30 separate investigations, judges have been asked to assess collages, stories, and poems produced by both children and adults – all with the same results. Interjudge reliability on ratings is consistently high, and ratings of creativity generally are separable from ratings of product technical goodness, clarity, and so forth. (See Amabile, 1982b, for more details on the use of the consensual assessment technique.)

The hypothesis guiding most of our research is that persons assigned to conditions of social and/or environmental constraint will perform with an extrinsic motivational orientation, and their products will, on the average, be significantly less creative than those of subjects assigned to control (no-constraint) groups. The sources of evidence relevant to this hypothesis include studies of the effects of constraint on subjects' intrinsic motivation and studies of the effects of constraint on subjects' creativity and other related qualitative aspects of performance.

Social and environmental influences

Intrinsic motivation

The number of studies investigating the impact of social-environmental constraints on motivation is substantial, and researchers continue to contribute to our understanding of this subject at a steady rate. The first published studies designed to consider this issue (Deci, 1971, 1972; Lepper et al., 1973) often involved a one-session paradigm. Experimental subjects generally worked for 1 hr at a task such as the Soma or hidden-figures puzzles under some condition of reward, feedback, or constraint, whereas control subjects performed in the absence of such constraint. In order to obtain the dependent measure of intrinsic motivation, the experimenter then left the subject for a period of 8 to 10 min under some credible pretext, such as needing to use the computer or having to get additional evaluation forms. The experimenter's absence created the free-choice period in which subjects were alone and had no extrinsic reasons for working on the activity. Because subjects were unaware that they were being observed, and because they had a variety of interesting things to do, the time they spent with the target activity was used as the measure of their intrinsic motivation.

Employing this and similar paradigms, researchers have successfully demonstrated the undermining effects of a variety of constraints. The impact of monetary rewards has received the greatest amount of attention, and the evidence is clear. The experience of performing a task for money significantly decreases subjects' intrinsic motivation for that activity (Calder & Staw, 1975; Deci, 1972; Pinder, 1976; Pritchard, Campbell, & Campbell, 1977). Yet monetary payment is not the only type of reward that has been observed to have such deleterious effects. Widely ranging varieties of reward forms have now been tested, with everything from good-player awards to marshmallows producing the expected decrements in intrinsic motivation (Greene & Lepper, 1974; Harackiewicz, 1979; Kernoodle-Loveland & Olley, 1979; Ross, 1975). Finally, a situation devised by Lepper, Sagotsky, Dafoe, and Greene (1982) was designed to determine whether or not one activity presented as a means to doing another activity would undermine subsequent intrinsic motivation, regardless of which activity was the means and which was the end. It was found that regardless of the specific task used, intrinsic motivation was undermined for the task that had been presented as the means.

It is important to note that other widely varying external constraints, in addition to reward, have also been found to decrease intrinsic motivation. Lepper and Greene (1975), for example, investigated the effects of surveillance on the intrinsic interest of preschoolers. The knowledge that they were being watched via video cameras had a significant undermining effect on the children's intrinsic motivation for solving puzzles. A 1980 investigation conducted by Thane Pittman and his colleagues has since extended these findings with the demonstration that direct surveillance by another individual will also decrease children's intrinsic motivation for a play activity.

One of our own early investigations examined the effect of deadlines. In this study (Amabile, DeJong, & Lepper, 1976), college students given deadlines while working on interesting word games demonstrated less subsequent intrinsic motivation in the experimental task than did their control (no-deadline) counterparts.

Detrimental effects of expected evaluation on intrinsic interest have been reported by Smith (1974). In an expansion of this paradigm, Karniol and Ross (1977) examined the effects of both informative and noninformative rewards. They found that although performance-contingent rewards (rewards delivered only if task performance meets some predetermined standard) did not significantly increase the intrinsic motivation of children above the level shown by nonrewarded controls, such informative rewards did at least maintain motivation relative to a task-contingent reward group (where rewards were noninformative). Thus, unless rewards contain explicit information about competence, they tend quite consistently to undermine intrinsic motivation.

These studies and others like them illustrate how extrinsic constraints can undermine subjects' motivation. The evidence is most convincing, even overwhelming. (For in-depth reviews of this literature, see Bates, 1979; Condry, 1977; Deci & Ryan, 1980, 1985; Kruglanski, 1978.) The fundamental question that has guided our program of research is whether or not these same factors can also affect subjects' creativity. Although relatively few other investigators have addressed this problem directly, there has been research on aspects of performance related to creativity.

Effects of constraints on creativity-relevant aspects of performance

Each of the studies to be described in this section relied on a modified version of the standard overjustification paradigm (Deci, 1972), with one important distinction.

Here, in addition to intrinsic motivation, qualitative aspects of subject performance are also assessed. In order to be appropriate for testing hypotheses about the social psychology of creativity, the experimental task not only must be intrinsically interesting but also must meet a number of criteria: (1) The task must be an open-ended (heuristic) task, (2) it must not depend heavily on specialized skills, and (3) it must be a task in which subjects produce an observable product or response that can be recorded and later presented to experts to be judged on creativity.

In a study of the effect of reward on children's artistic creativity, Lepper et al. (1973) found that for preschoolers who initially displayed a high level of intrinsic interest in drawing with felt-tip markers, working for an expected "Good Player Award" decreased their interest in the task. When compared with an unexpected-reward group and a control (no-reward) group, the subjects who had made their drawings in order to receive a Good Player Award spent significantly less time using the markers during free-play periods, and this decrement in interest persisted for at least a week beyond the initial experimental session. Furthermore, the globally assessed *quality* (as rated by teachers) of drawings made by children expecting a reward was lower than that for the unexpected-reward group or the control group.

Taking a somewhat similar approach, Greene and Lepper (1974) again offered rewards to preschoolers under one of two conditions: For one group of children, receipt of the Good Player Award was contingent only on task performance, whereas for the second group the reward was contingent on the "quality" of performance. Once again, children working under the reward conditions produced drawings of lower quality than their nonrewarded counterparts. The reduction in intrinsic interest in the drawing task was also replicated.

In a 1979 study, Kernoodle-Loveland and Olley also examined the effect of expected reward on preschoolers' drawings. Subjects were first observed during free-play periods and rated for initial interest in the target activity. During the main experimental session, one-half of the children were rewarded for their participation, whereas for the control group no reward expectation was established. Measures of time spent drawing during free periods and drawing quality were then collected 1 and 7 weeks later. Children with a high level of initial motivation for the drawing task lost interest when rewarded, whereas the same reward contingency caused children with initially low levels of motivation to gain interest. Further, at the time of reward, high-interest subjects drew more products than did their high-interest nonreward peers, yet their pictures were judged to be of poorer quality. Low-interest subjects, when rewarded, also drew more than did their low-interest non-rewarded counterparts, but for this group the quality of performance was not affected. This study raises interesting questions about the interaction between environmental factors and the individual's baseline level of interest, an issue that we shall pursue later in this chapter. For the purpose of our present discussion, however, it is important to note that decrements in interest were accompanied by decrements in drawing quality.

Employing a very different experimental task, Garbarino (1975) asked fifth- and sixth-grade girls to teach a matching task to girls in the first and second grades. The older children who served as teachers either were promised a reward (a free movie ticket) or were told nothing of reward. Two raters then observed the tutoring sessions and made independent assessments across an especially broad range of qualitative performance dimensions. These dependent variables included the following: the tutors' use of evaluation, hints, and demands; the learners' performances; the emotional tone of the interaction, including instances of laughter between the children during a session; the efficiency of the tutoring (learning per unit of time spent).

Overall, rewarded tutors conducted sessions that were high-pressured and businesslike, whereas nonrewarded tutors held sessions that were relaxed and yet highly efficient. The subjective ratings made by the two observers characterized the rewarded sessions as tense and hostile, and the nonrewarded sessions as warm and relaxed. In addition, the rewarded sessions were marked by more demands from the tutors, more negative evaluative statements by the tutors, less laughter, and poorer learning by the younger students.

Finally, Pittman, Emery, and Boggiano (1982) found that nonrewarded subjects showed a strong subsequent preference for complex versions of a game, whereas rewarded subjects chose simpler versions. And Shapira (1976) reported that subjects expecting payment for success chose to work on relatively easy puzzles, whereas subjects expecting no payment preferred much more challenging puzzles.

Each of these investigations points to the same conclusions as do the original findings of Lepper et al. (1973). For subjects who initially display a high level of interest in a task, working for an expected reward decreases their motivation and undermines the globally assessed quality of their performance.

Negative effects of constraints on creativity

More recently, several studies have focused specifically on creative aspects of subjects' performances. One of the earliest investigations of this type was conceived by Kruglanski, Friedman, and Zeevi (1971). Israeli high school students who either had or had not been promised a reward (a tour of the Tel Aviv University Psychology Department) were given two open-ended creativity tasks. These tasks, adapted from Barron (1968), required subjects to list as many titles as possible for a literary paragraph and to use as many words as possible from a 50-word list in writing their own story.

Product originality was assessed by two independent judges, with good interjudge reliability, and a clear and statistically significant superiority for nonrewarded subjects emerged. In addition, nearly significant differences were found between the two groups on two intrinsic measures: subjects' expressed enjoyment of the activities and their willingness to volunteer for further participation.

Like the majority of studies that have examined the effect of reward on intrinsic motivation, these investigators used a paradigm whereby subjects were promised some tangible reward before engaging in an activity, but the reward itself was not delivered until after that activity had been completed. Critics of overjustification research (Reiss & Sushinsky, 1975) have suggested that this procedure allows for alternative explanations of subsequent declines in task engagement. They suggest, for example, that subjects are so distracted by the anticipation of reward during the initial task engagement that their enjoyment of the activity is hampered. Thus, according to this explanation, later lack of interest in the activity occurs not because subjects have come to see it only as a means to some external goal but because their intrinsic enjoyment of the activity is directly blocked by the "competing response" of reward anticipation.

In one of our investigations of the effect of reward (Amabile, Hennessey, & Grossman, 1986, Study 1), we used a paradigm that renders the competing-response hypothesis untenable. The reward offered to children before task engagement was not a tangible gift to be delivered afterward. Instead, it was an attractive activity – playing with a Polaroid camera – that the children were allowed to engage in *before* completing the target task. In other words, children assigned to the reward condition promised to do the target activity in order to first have a chance to use the camera. Children in the no-reward condition were simply allowed to use the camera and then were presented with the target task; there was no contingency established between the two. Thus, because children in both conditions had already enjoyed the "reward" before the experimental activity began, it is unlikely that any reward-related competing responses were operating.

In a broad attempt to examine the mechanism behind this undermining of creativity, we also included a number of other manipulations and measures in our design. Subjects' levels of intrinsic interest were assessed through self-report and behavioral observation during a free-play period. And in addition to the offer of reward, task labeling (as work or play) was introduced as a second dependent variable. This was done in order to test the possibility that an affective response such as simply viewing activities as "work" can lead to the same undermining effects on intrinsic motivation and creativity as being placed under extrinsic constraints.

Finally, we tried to test the proposition that the undermining effect arises from a discounting of intrinsic interest when salient extrinsic forces are present (Bem, 1972; Lepper et al., 1973). To do this, we assessed the discounting capabilities of each of the children and set out to determine whether or not the reward contingency had different effects on subjects not yet capable of this cognitive process.

In order to examine the impact of reward expectation on children's verbal creativity, the elementary school subjects in this study were asked to tell a story to accompany a set of illustrations in a book with no words. They did this by saying "one thing" about each page into a tape recorder. Like all the creativity tasks used in our research, this storytelling activity was specifically designed with two goals in mind. First, it was necessary that the importance of individual differences in domain-relevant skills be minimized, because these could lead to high variability in baseline performances. In the storytelling task, for example, differences in children's verbal fluency were minimized by restricting their responses to one sentence per page. Second, in order to be appropriate for testing hypotheses about creativity, the task had to allow for a wide variety of responses. In other words, the target activity had to be an open-ended activity (Amabile, 1982b; McGraw, 1978).

At the beginning of the experimental session, children in grades 1 through 5 were given the opportunity to take two pictures with an "instant" camera. In order to have a chance to use the camera first, subjects in the reward condition promised to tell the story later. So that this contingency would be especially salient, children in this condition were asked to write their names on a piece of paper, a contract also signed by the experimenter. Subjects in the no-reward condition simply took the pictures and then told the story; there was no contingency established between the two tasks. In an application of the consensual creativity assessment technique (Amabile, 1982b), elementary school teachers familiar with children's writing later rated the stories for creativity, with a high level of interjudge reliability. Results indicated that, overall, children in the no-reward conditions told more creative stories than did children in the reward conditions. This main effect of reward was, in fact, statistically significant.

The results indicated that the work–play task labels had no effect on children's creativity or self-reported affect, nor did we find any differential effects of the reward manipulation on the creativity or intrinsic interest of subjects not yet able to discount. This study does, however, contribute to our understanding of the undermining effect of reward in one important respect. It is significant that this undermining effect occurs even when nonrewarded subjects also experience the "reward" and even when the reward is delivered *before* the target activity. The only difference in the experiences of the rewarded and nonrewarded children in this paradigm was their *perception* of the reward as contingent or not contingent on the target activity. It appears that the perception of a task as the means to an end is the crucial element for creativity decrements in task engagement.

Another of our investigations (Amabile, 1982a) also examined the effect of expected reward, but in this case the experimental task involved artistic creativity, and the reward was introduced in a competitive setting (incorporating an evaluative element). Girls whose ages ranged from 7 to 11 years made paper collages during one of two parties held in the common room of their apartment complex. Subjects in the experimental group competed for prizes, whereas those in the control group expected that the prizes would be raffled off.

Artist-judges later rated each collage on creativity, with a high interjudge reliability. The control group was judged significantly higher than the experimental group on creativity of collages. Once again, these results are consistent with the proposition that intrinsic motivation is conducive to creativity, whereas extrinsic motivation is detrimental.

Several intrinsic motivation theoriests have proposed that in order to undermine intrinsic interest, a reward must be salient (Ross, 1975) and must be perceived as a means to an extrinsic end (Calder & Staw, 1975; Deci, 1975; Kruglanski et al., 1971; Lepper et al., 1973). One method of demonstrating the crucial role of perceiving a task as a means to an end is to offer subjects a choice concerning task engagement. Although choice should influence motivation in a manner similar to that for other social-environmental variables, there are important differences between choice and other factors such as expectation of reward or evaluation. If subjects perceive themselves as freely choosing to perform an activity for which a reward is offered (or an evaluation promised), they may well adopt an extrinsic motivational orientation toward that activity – viewing the task as work, and their own engagement as motivated by external pressures. On the other hand, if subjects are simply presented with a task and told that they will be paid or evaluated, with no choice in the matter, we should not expect to observe this same detrimental effect. This phenomenon has in fact been demonstrated in a study conducted by Folger, Rosenfield, and Hays (1978).

Some of our investigations have also examined the role of choice. In a preliminary test of the effect of choice on creativity (Amabile & Gitomer, 1984), nursery school children were asked to make paper collages. Children assigned to the choice condition were allowed to choose any 5 out of 10 boxes of materials to use in this task. For children in the no-choice condition, however, the experimenter made the box selections – yoking the two conditions in a matched-pairs design. All subjects then completed their collages, which were later rated for creativity by artists.

Two weeks after this initial session had ended, a behavioral measure of subsequent intrinsic interest in the collage activity was obtained. Over a 3-day span, leftover materials were made available, and each child's engagement in the collage activity during free-choice periods was timed. As predicted, there was a substantial difference in collage creativity between the conditions. Subjects in the choice condition made collages that were significantly more creative than those made by subjects in the no-choice condition. In addition, children in the choice condition spent somewhat more time with collage materials during free play than did children in the no-choice condition.

In an investigation of the interactive effects of reward and choice on children's verbal creativity (Amabile et al., 1986, Study 2), the meaning of "reward" was directly manipulated by varying its method of presentation. We employed a 2 × 2 factorial design in which the presence or absence of choice was completely crossed with the presence or absence of reward. We predicted that creativity would be undermined only in those children who explicitly contracted with the experimenter to make the collage in order to obtain the reward.

Subjects in this investigation were 80 students in grades 3, 4, and 5. All children participated in the experimental session individually. Subjects in the choice–reward condition were told that either they could go back to their classrooms or, if they signed a contract promising to make a collage and tell a story, they could first take two pictures with an instant camera as a reward. Importantly, it was made clear that some children did in fact decide to leave.

In the choice–no-reward condition, the children were told that they could do the things described or go back to their classroom, and again it was made clear that the decision to go back to class was an acceptable response. In the no-choice–reward condition, subjects were told that because they were going to do things for the experimenter, they would first be allowed to take two pictures with the camera. And in the no-choice–no-reward condition, the picture taking was simply introduced as one in a series of tasks to be completed. The two tasks that followed, collage making and storytelling, were presented in different counterbalanced orders.

After they had completed each of these activities, all children were asked to answer two questions. Using a continuum of circles representing a range of responses from "I liked it a lot" to "I didn't like it at all," subjects each marked the circle that best described how they felt about making the design or telling the story. They were also asked, "If you were to tell another kid about what you did here, would you say you worked or you played?"

A 2 × 2 ANOVA on the creativity scores for both the stories and the collages revealed the predicted interaction between reward and choice. Subjects in the choice–reward condition produced stories lower in creativity than did subjects in the other three groups. The creativity of children who had been given a choice about their participation had been seriously undermined by the reward manipulation, whereas for the children who did not perceive that the decision to complete the task was under their control, no such deleterious effects were observed. (Analyses of the self-report measures of affect and the work–play distinction revealed no significant effects.) Thus, this study demonstrated that it is not reward per se but rather the functional significance of reward as controlling the performance that undermines creativity.

In an effort to conceptually replicate these findings, a second investigation (Amabile et al., 1986, Study 2) was carried out in which reward and choice were again crossed in a 2 × 2 factorial design. This study differed from its predecessor in a number of respects, however. The most important difference was that the subjects were adult women, rather than young boys and girls. In addition, a monetary reward was employed, and the money (though shown to rewarded subjects before task engagement) was awarded only after the task had been completed. The creativity task used here was the same collage-making activity as that presented to the children in the original investigation.

The results here provide a close replication of the results in Study 2. A 2 × 2 ANOVA again revealed a significant reward × choice interaction, resulting largely from the low creativity of subjects in the contracted-for reward group (choice–reward). As predicted, and as in Study 2, the lowest level of creativity was found in this condition.

None of the items on a post-task questionnaire designed to assess subjects' interest in and feelings toward the collage activity revealed significant main effects or interactions of the independent variables. However, correlational analyses do suggest a relation among intrinsic interest in the activity, enjoyment, and creativity.

Having established the deleterious effects of reward and conditions of restricted choice, what other extrinsic constraints might also have a negative impact on subjects' creativity? Our research has consistently demonstrated that the expectation of evaluation produces similar decrements in subjects' interest and task performance. The initial study of evaluation expectation (Amabile, 1979) was designed to test the hypothesis that such constraint will undermine creative performances on heuristic tasks. The task we used was a collage-making activity, and it was predicted that subjects placed under constraint (evaluation expectation) would show lower levels of both creativity and intrinsic interest in the task than would no-constraint controls. The subjects in this study were 95 women enrolled in an introductory psychology course at Stanford University. As a cover story, the experimenter explained that this investigation was actually a pretest for another experiment to be done the following quarter. The alleged purpose of this pretest was to identify activities that would affect most individuals' moods in predictable ways. Subjects assigned to the control condition were told also that their designs would not be used as sources of data – that the only information of interest was the mood they reported on a questionnaire. In contrast, subjects in the evaluation condition were told that their finished designs would be rated by graduate artists from the Stanford Art Department and would serve as important sources of information.

In introducing the art task, the experimenter stressed that subjects had complete freedom in using the materials to form a design, but that only the materials provided should be used. In addition, each subject was asked to make a design that conveyed a feeling of "silliness," as when a child is acting and feeling silly. In order to further reduce extraneous sources of variability, subjects with significant levels of experience in artistic or collage work were eliminated.

Each subject was left alone for 15 min to work on her collage. At the end of the session, the experimenter presented the subject with a Mood Questionnaire (in keeping with the cover story) and an Art Activity Questionnaire that included a number of questions designed to assess subjects' interest in and attitude toward the collage task. The 95 collages were rated by 15 artist-judges following the same consensual assessment techniques used in our other studies (Amabile, 1982b). The results supported the hypothesis that evaluation expectation is detrimental to creativity, with control (nonevaluation) subjects producing significantly more creative products than experimental (evaluation) subjects. In addition, control subjects scored higher in self-rated interest than did experimental subjects.

In order to firmly establish this finding that an expected evaluation has negative effects on an adult's creativity, two further investigations were undertaken.

In both studies, a replication with an artistic activity (Amabile, Golfarb, &

Brackfield, 1982, Study 2) and a replication with a verbal activity (Amabile et al., 1982, Study 1), there was a significant main effect of evaluation expectation on the creativity ratings. Nonevaluation subjects made collages and wrote poems that were judged significantly more creative than those produced by evaluation subjects.

In a study done with a group of colleagues (Berglas, Amabile, & Handel, 1981), we set out to examine the effects of prior evaluation on children's subsequent creativity. We predicted that highly salient evaluation on one task would lead children to expect evaluation on a later task with the same experimenter and, as a consequence, would lower their creativity on the later task. All subjects, boys and girls in grades 2–6, made two artworks. The first involved painting with a spinning disk, and the second (which was the target task) involved making a paper collage. Experimental-group children were positively evaluated by the experimenter on their "spin art" before they did the collage. Control-group subjects simply made the two artworks, with no evaluation. Creativity results indicated a clear superiority of the control group over the experimental group. In other words, we observed an overall negative impact of prior evaluation on creativity of performance – even though that evaluation had been positive.

Finally, Koestner, Ryan, Bernieri, and Holt (1984) set out to determine if the functional significance of another extrinsic constraint – behavioral limits – affects children's motivation and creativity. In this study, 5- and 7-year-old children were asked to engage in an intrinsically interesting painting activity under three limit-setting conditions that varied along an information/control dimension. In the controlling-limits group, restrictions pertaining to task neatness were stated in terms of "should" and "must." The informational group was presented with a verbal communication conveying the same behavioral constraints in the absence of external pressure, but with an acknowledgment of possible conflicting feelings about the imposed limits. For the control (no-limits) group, no mention was made of these constraints.

Following the period during which the children made their paintings, they were left alone for a free-play session. The amount of time spent during this period was used as a measure of intrinsic motivation. Finally, the children were asked to rate how much they enjoyed the painting activity. Paintings made during the main session were assessed by artist-judges for creativity, using our (Amabile, 1982a) consensual assessment technique. Results indicated a main effect for condition. This effect supports the main experimental prediction, in that subjects in the no-limits and informational-limits groups spent more free-choice time painting than did controlling-limits subjects. Thus, intrinsic motivation was significantly greater for children in the nolimitational and informational conditions than for children in the controlling condition. In addition, a marginal effect for limit-setting style emerged on the self-report measure of enjoyment. Effects for limit-setting style were also found for creativity, with the no-limits group significantly more creative than the controlling-limits group. The informational-limits group was intermediate.

A more positive approach: maintaining creativity by maintaining intrinsic motivation

In our attempt to demonstrate a definitive link between creativity and intrinsic motivation, it is just as important to demonstrate that creativity will be maintained when intrinsic motivation is maintained as it is to demonstrate that creativity will be undermined when intrinsic motivation is undermined. In a recent study with Barbara Grossman (in preparation), we set out to determine if special training sessions designed to directly address motivational orientation could "immunize" children against the usually deleterious effects of reward on intrinsic motivation and creativity of performance. In the first phase of this experiment, students in grades 3, 4, and 5 were randomly assigned to one of two conditions: intrinsic motivation training or control, both of which were run by the same female experimenter.

In the crucial intrinsic motivation training condition, subjects were shown videotapes depicting two attractive 11-year-old children talking with an adult about various aspects of their schoolwork. The scripts for these tapes had been specifically designed so that the boy and girl on the tape would serve as models of highly intrinsically motivated individuals. There were two primary messages conveyed by these intrinsic motivation training tapes. Our first goal was to get the children to focus on intrinsic reasons for doing work in school and to concentrate on those aspects for maximal enjoyment. The following is an example of a tape segment that addresses this issue:

Adult: Tommy, of all the things your teacher gives you to do in school, think about the one thing you like to do best and tell me about it.
Tommy: Well, I like social studies the best. I like learning about how other people live in different parts of the world. It's also fun because you get to do lots of projects and reports. I like doing projects because you can learn a lot about something on your own. I work hard on my projects, and when I come up with good ideas, I feel good. When you are working on something that you thought of, and that's interesting to you, it's more fun to do.
Adult: So, one of the reasons you like social studies so much is because you get to learn about things on your own. And it makes you feel good when you do things for yourself; it makes it more interesting. That's great!

The second issue addressed in the intrinsic motivation training tapes was the practice of cognitively distancing oneself from socially imposed extrinsic constraints – focusing instead on the inherently enjoyable aspects of a task in an effort to maintain intrinsic motivation in the face of such factors as reward or evaluation. An example:

Adult: It sounds like both of you do the work in school because you like it, but what about getting good grades from your teacher or presents from your parents for doing well. Do you think about those things?
Tommy: Well, I like to get good grades, and when I bring home a good report card, my parents always give me money. But that's not what's really important. I like to learn a lot.

There are a lot of things that interest me, and I want to learn about them, so I work hard because I enjoy it.

Sarah: Sometimes when I know my teacher is going to give me a grade on something I am doing, I think about that. But then I remember that it's more important that I like what I'm doing, that I really enjoy it, and then I don't think about grades as much.

Adult: That's good. Both of you like to get good grades, but you both know that what's really important is how you feel about your work, and that you enjoy what you are doing.

In small groups of 3 to 5 members, subjects met with the experimenter for two 20-min training periods on 2 consecutive days. Each intrinsic motivation training session consisted of showing segments of the videotape, interspersed with directed discussion. During these discussions, the children were asked to relate what they had seen on the tape, to answer for themselves the questions the adult had posed, and to give their own reactions to the content of Tommy's and Sarah's responses. Throughout, the experimenter offered interpretations of the tape and of the children's commentary and shared her own ideas, all with the aim of making them more aware of intrinsic motivation and methods of coping with extrinsic constraints. At the close of each of these brief meetings, the children were asked to complete a series of short exercises in which they indicated their preferences for a variety of school activities and described their feelings when performing their favorite tasks.

Subjects assigned to the control group also met in small groups over a 2-day period for the purpose of viewing videotapes. In this case, however, the discussion centered around their favorite things: foods, movies, animals, and so forth. In summary, then, all subjects participated in some form of group activity. All met with the experimenter, saw videotapes, and participated in group discussions. What differentiated the conditions was the focus of these sessions: intrinsic motivation or issues irrelevant to intrinsic motivation.

In the second phase of this experiment, after the training sessions had been completed, each child met individually with a different experimenter for testing. (The children's teachers and the experimenters were careful to avoid mentioning any connection between the training and testing sessions, and they denied a connection if any of the children inquired.) The Harter Scale of Intrinsic versus Extrinsic Orientation in the Classroom (Harter, 1981) was administered, and two dimensions of classroom motivation were assessed. These two dimensions, each having an intrinsic pole and an extrinsic pole, were (1) Curiosity/Interest versus Pleasing the Teacher/Getting Good Grades and (2) Independent Mastery versus Dependence on the Teacher.

After this administration, a reward manipulation was introduced. Following a procedure used in an earlier study (Amabile et al., 1986, Study 1), half of the children in each of the three training conditions were told that they could take two pictures with an instant camera if they promised that later they would tell a story for the experimenter. For the remaining children, this picture taking was presented simply as the first in a series of "things to do."

The major dependent measure – creativity on a storytelling activity – also paralleled that employed in a previous investigation (Amabile et al., 1986, Study 1). As a final task, the Unusual Uses Test of the Torrance Tests of Creative Thinking (Torrance, 1966) was administered.

We predicted that for subjects who had been trained to deal effectively with extrinsic constraints and to focus on intrinsic reasons for doing work in school, overall intrinsic motivation would be increased. Significant differences were, in fact, found between the scores on the Harter Curiosity scale for children in the two treatment conditions. Children receiving intrinsic motivation training scored higher than subjects in the control condition.

In addition, an examination of story creativity revealed the predicted interaction between training condition and reward manipulation. Although no main effects were found, expectation of reward did produce the predicted decrement in creativity for subjects assigned to the control group. By contrast, students in the intrinsic motivation condition who were rewarded for their participation told stories that were judged significantly more creative than those told by the no-reward intrinsic motivation subjects. It would seem that as a result of their training, these children had learned to treat reward not as an element that detracts from intrinsic interest but as something that can add to overall motivation. They had learned to overcome the deleterious effects of reward – so much so that their levels of intrinsic motivation (and therefore their levels of creativity) seem to have increased.

Mechanisms for the conditions of creativity

The results of our training study are at the same time extremely exciting and somewhat puzzling. How can we explain the fact that those children who had received intrinsic motivation training exhibited higher creativity when rewarded than when not rewarded? Perhaps the answer lies in their interpretation of the reward manipulation and storytelling activity. Perhaps our intrinsic motivation training sessions had caused these young subjects to perceive their situation differently in some crucial way than did the control group.

This possibility is, in fact, not without both theoretical and empirical support. In their recent book *Intrinsic Motivation and Self-determination in Human Behavior* (1985), Deci and Ryan observe that previous research has tended to focus primarily on the outward experimental events themselves: the presence or absence of surveillance and the nature of the reward structure, for example, and their *average* effects on people's motivation and related variables such as creativity (Deci & Ryan, 1985, p. 87). It is the belief of Deci and Ryan, however, that the impact of an event on motivational processes is determined not by the objective characteristics of the event but rather by "its psychological meaning for the individual" (p. 85).

According to their cognitive evaluation theory, all external events can be viewed as informational, controlling, or amotivating. An environmental event that is perceived as controlling is one that is interpreted by the perceiver as pressure to attain a given behavioral outcome – pressure that is interpreted to induce or coerce the recipient to perform in a specific manner. When this aspect is salient, the perception of an external locus of causality is facilitated, and intrinsic motivation tends to be undermined. An environmental event that is perceived as informational is one that provides the recipient with behaviorally relevant information in the absence of pressure to attain a particular outcome. A salient informational event increases intrinsic motivation if it signifies competence and decreases intrinsic motivation if it signifies incompetence. Finally, according to cognitive evaluation theory, it is also sometimes possible to classify some events as internally amotivating. These would be events occurring within a person, such as self-deprecation or hopelessness, that signify one's inability to master certain situations. Whether an event will be perceived as informational, controlling, or amotivating, Deci and Ryan believe, is an issue of the relative salience of these three aspects for the perceiver and is affected by one's sensitivities and past experiences as well as by the actual configuration of the event itself (p. 85).

How might this analysis be applied to the specific case of our intrinsic motivation training group? The message conveyed by our videotapes and guided discussions was that external rewards such as receiving good grades or money from parents are nice, but what is really important is that one truly enjoy what one is doing. In essence, what we had attempted, and evidently accomplished, was to develop a salient intrinsic orientation, or a more solidly internal locus of control, in our subjects. Thus, whereas the nontrained subjects perceived the reward manipulation as strongly controlling, the trained subjects most likely did not.

In our study, we attempted to *create* individual differences in motivational orientation between subjects. Other researchers have taken the route of examining differences that already exist. In one of the few investigations that have examined differences in the perceiver as possible mediators of the effects of extrinsic constraints on intrinsic motivation, Lonky and Reihman (1980) studied the impact of verbal praise on the intrinsic motivation of children scoring high and low on internal locus of control. They found that when children high on internal locus of control were praised, they showed an increase in intrinsic motivation over pretreatment assessments; but children scoring at the low end of the internal locus scale showed decreases in intrinsic motivation levels after being praised. These authors conclude that persons high on internal locus of control believe themselves to be more in control of outcomes and are more likely to interpret rewards and communications as informational, whereas persons low on internal control will be more likely to interpret these same elements as controlling.

Another study with a focus on individual differences was carried out by Boggiano and Barrett (1984). In this investigation, the effects of positive and negative feedback on the intrinsic motivation and performance of children who differed in their initial motivational orientation were assessed. It was found that success feedback increased the intrinsic motivation of intrinsically oriented children, but not that of extrinsically oriented children. Negative feedback also was observed to significantly increase the motivation of the intrinsically oriented subjects. For this group, it was apparently viewed as a challenge. However, for the extrinsically oriented children, the same negative message seemed to represent evidence of their incompetence, decreasing their intrinsic motivation even further and creating feelings of amotivation and helplessness.

In summary, the research outlined here demonstrates that characteristics of the perceiver (or recipient) of an environmental constraint, such as reward, have a great deal to do with how that constraint is received and interpreted. As Deci and Ryan point out, most situations are ambiguous enough that the relative salience of informational, controlling, and amotivational aspects of a situation can be unique for each individual. The same event can be perceived very differently, depending on the orientations of the persons involved. It would seem that in our training study, the intrinsic motivation training sessions sufficiently altered the children's perceptions of the reward manipulation so that they counteracted the usual undermining effects on motivation and creativity. Rather than passively receiving the parameters of the reward situation, it appears that these children actively constructed them. They seem to have tailored the environment to meet their needs. (Interestingly, this same ability to shape one's environment is something that Sternberg, 1985, has linked to gifted individuals.)

What we are really addressing here are questions that go far beyond the specific case of our intrinsic motivation training sessions to the broader issue of individual differences in general. For us, as well as for others, this is a relatively new area for theorizing and research on the linkage among environmental conditions, motivation, and creativity. Up until this point, we have been concerned primarily with global effects – with the general effects of extrinsic constraint on motivation and creativity across a variety of situations and subject populations. Ours has been a hydraulic model, not unlike that used by most early intrinsic motivation theorists (Lepper & Greene, 1978): Intrinsic motivation is conducive to creativity, and extrinsic motivation is detrimental; as extrinsic constraints increase, intrinsic motivation and creativity must decrease. Yet, as our research and that of others has begun to demonstrate, perhaps this formula does not accurately describe all situations. Perhaps, under certain circumstances or with certain individuals, intrinsic and extrinsic forces can combine in an additive fashion. Certainly this appears to be what happened in the training study. Rather than detracting from the children's performances, the offer of reward augmented the curiosity and the creativity of performance of the intrinsic motivation group. Apart from the internal–external distinction in locus of control and the related intrinsic–extrinsic orientation distinction, might there be other naturally occurring individual differences that would make some people less vulnerable to the negative effects of extrinsic constraint on their intrinsic motivation and creativity?

Our observations of and interviews with people in the workplace lead us to believe that this is so. In a recent interview study (Amabile & Gryskiewicz, in press), we discovered that research and development scientists working within the same laboratory sometimes perceive the same extrinsic constraints quite differently.

There are two interesting subgroups in the sample, exemplifying opposite extremes around the usual "modal" response to constraints: those who feel constantly suppressed by the constraints in their environment, and those who have somehow managed to rise above these constraints (or at least manage to view them in a perspective that does not interfere with creative production). Although we do not have detailed individual difference measures on these scientists, we can speculate on what might be the crucial distinguishing characteristics between these two types of workers.

One dimension that may be relevant is that of self-esteem. In fact, an examination of the literature reveals that this personality construct may play a significant role where intrinsic motivation and creativity are concerned. A study conducted by Deci, Nezlek, and Sheinman (1981) revealed, for example, that children in public school classrooms run by teachers who were oriented toward supporting autonomy had higher self-esteem and more intrinsic motivation than children assigned to classrooms where teachers were oriented toward controlling behavior. Similar findings were reported by Harter (1982). Ryan and Grolnick (1984) also found strong positive correlations between intrinsic motivation and self-esteem in children, and Deci and Ryan (1985) presented data indicating that "strong and stable self-esteem seems to emanate from a strong sense of self, which motivationally means intrinsic motivation and more integrated internalization of extrinsic motivation" (p. 142). The more internalized one's extrinsic motivation, the more likely it is to contribute to a sense of positive self-esteem.

The evidence does not stop here. As early as the 1950s, researchers were pointing to the tendency of creative individuals to display strong self-acceptance and positive self-evaluation behavior (Fromm, 1959; Guilford, 1950). In a detailed treatise on the antecedents of self-esteem, Coopersmith (1967) observes:

There thus appears to be an underlying similarity in the processes involved in creative innovation and social independence, with common traits and postures required for expression of both behaviors. The difference is one of product – literary, musical, artistic, theoretical products on the one hand, opinions on the other – rather than one of process. In both instances the individual must believe that his perceptions are meaningful and valid and be willing to rely upon his own interpretations. He must trust himself sufficiently that even when persons express opinions counter to his own he can proceed on the basis of his own perceptions and convictions. (p. 58)

The importance of self-esteem for creative expression appears to be almost beyond disproof. Without a high regard for himself the individual who is working in the frontiers of his field cannot trust himself to discriminate between the trivial and the significant. Without trust in his own powers the person seeking improved solutions or alternative theories has no basis for distinguishing the significant and profound innovation from one that is merely different. . . . An essential component of the creative process, whether it be analysis, synthesis, or the development of a new perspective or more comprehensive theory, is the conviction that one's judgment in interpreting the events is to be trusted. (p. 59)

Despite this conviction that self-esteem is an essential prerequisite for creative expression, Coopersmith could find no studies that had directly investigated this relationship. Recognizing this gap in the literature, he set out to test this hypothesis and administered three tests to a group of adolescents: Unusual Uses, Circles, and Draw a Person (Torrance, 1966). His results were especially revealing. Groups high in subjective self-esteem performed in the most creative fashion on all three batteries, whereas groups low in self-esteem were significantly less original and innovating. Coopersmith observed these differences across the variety of conceptual, linguistic, and artistic skills required in the several tasks and suggested that this consistency indicates that persons high in self-esteem are likely to be more assertive, independent, and creative than persons with lower self-esteem – the conclusion being that individuals with high self-esteem listen to themselves more and are far more likely to trust their own judgments and reactions (Coopersmith, 1967).

In a similar investigation conducted by Garwood (1964), these predicted relationships between personality factors and creativity were again examined, this time within a population of young scientists. Using the Self-Acceptance scale of the California Psychological Inventory (CPI) as an index of self-esteem, creative subjects were observed, as a group, to score significantly higher than their not-so-creative colleagues.

Although both of these investigations are highly suggestive, they offer only observational evidence of the connection between creative expression and high levels of self-esteem. Equally essential to the support of this relationship are data of a more experimental nature. If it could be shown, for example, that interventions designed to increase subjects' creativity can also have a positive effect on their self-esteem, or that conditions affecting self-esteem also affect creativity, our case would be strengthened considerably. Three recent studies have accomplished this end.

The first (Stasinos, 1984) employed a pretest–posttest control-group design. As a pretest, the verbal and figural subtests from the Torrance Tests of Creative Thinking (TTCT) (1968 revised) and two self-esteem instruments designed by Coopersmith (1967) were first administered to a group of 90 middle and upper school mentally handicapped Greek children. Subjects assigned to the treatment condition then received 16 weeks of exposure to the Mark 1, New Directions in Creativity (NDC) program (Renzulli, 1973). Subjects assigned to the control-group classes continued regular activities during this time. At the end of this training period, the same examinations and instruments used in pretesting were again employed. Analyses of variance yielded the predicted results. As a result of their training, the experimental group scored significantly higher than did the control group on five of the seven indices of creativity employed. In addition, the two groups differed greatly in terms of subjective self-esteem measures, with the experimental group attaining the higher score, probably as a result of the creativity training program.

Taking a very different approach, Brockner and Hulton (1978) also present strong evidence of a substantial link between creativity and high levels of self-esteem. Recognizing a suggestion in the literature that persons low in self-esteem (low SEs) are more self-conscious than persons high in self-esteem (high SEs) (Ickes, Wicklund, & Ferris, 1973; Turner, Scheier, Carver, & Ickes, 1978), they went on to predict that it is self-consciousness that can impair task performance. It was reasoned that if low SEs could be led to focus their attention away from themselves and onto the task, performance would improve relative to high SEs. Subjects high and low in chronic self-esteem performed a concept formation task under three conditions: (1) in the presence of an audience, where self-focused attention is presumed to be high; (2) in a control group, in which attention was not manipulated; and (3) with instructions to concentrate diligently on the task itself. In this, a 2×3 between-subjects factorial design, a significant effect was in fact obtained. Low SEs performed worse than high SEs in the audience condition, no differently in the control condition, and better than the high SEs when instructed to concentrate on the task. Brockner and Hulton conclude that the attentional state of low SEs makes them more susceptible or prone to be adversely affected by certain environmental factors. In the face of failure, for example, they suggest that low SEs will become preoccupied with their deficiencies. In a related study, Cheek and Stahl (1986) found that the poetry-writing creativity of nonshy women was unaffected by expected external evaluation, but the creativity of shy women was significantly lower under evaluation than under nonevaluation conditions.

These results on the linkage among performance, environmental conditions, and self-esteem (or the related dimensions of self-consciousness and shyness) clearly suggest a mediation mechanism: Environmental conditions such as expected evaluation can be perceived quite differently by persons who vary in self-esteem, and as a result these environmental conditions can have quite disparate effects on the creativity of persons who differ along this dimension.

Beyond whatever might be said about self-esteem as a mediator among environment, motivation, and creativity, this line of inquiry suggests a new approach to creativity research in general. For most of the past four decades, creativity researchers have focused almost exclusively on individual differences – the qualities of talent, experience, and personality that distinguish highly creative persons from their less creative peers. Our own research, and that of a few colleagues, has taken the quite different approach of examining the influence of social-environmental factors on intrinsic motivation and creativity. Both lines of inquiry have produced interesting and useful information; both have contributed to theory and practice. But, as is clear from our recent research and from work on individual difference mediators of social effects, both lines of inquiry are incomplete.

There is no doubt that personal qualities of ability and personality have great impact on creative behavior. There is no doubt that salient factors of extrinsic constraint in the social environment can have a consistently negative impact on the intrinsic motivation and creativity of most people most of the time. What we must now develop are research paradigms acknowledging that neither class of factors, by itself, can carry the day. Fluctuations in any individual's level of creative output must be examined in light of environmental influences on motivation, and environmental effects must be examined in light of an individual person's *perceptions* of these influences. Only then can the "conditions of creativity" be understood as complex interactions between and among both internal and external conditions. We believe that this is the crucial next step.

References

Amabile, T. M. (1979). Effects of external evaluation on artistic creativity. *Journal of Personality and Social Psychology, 37*, 221–233.

Amabile, T. M. (1982a). Children's artistic creativity: Detrimental effects of competition in a field setting. *Personality and Social Psychology Bulletin, 8*, 573–578.

Amabile, T. M. (1982b). Social psychology of creativity: A consensual assessment technique. *Journal of Personality and Social Psychology, 43*, 997–1013.

Amabile, T. M. (1983). *The social psychology of creativity.* New York: Springer-Verlag.

Amabile, T. M., DeJong, W., & Lepper, M. R. (1976). Effects of externally imposed deadlines on subsequent intrinsic motivation. *Journal of Personality and Social Psychology, 34*, 92–98.

Amabile, T. M., & Gitomer, J. (1984). Children's artistic creativity: Effects of choice in task materials. *Personality and Social Psychology Bulletin, 10*, 209–215.

Amabile, T. M., Golfarb, P., & Brackfield, S. C. (1982). *Effects of social facilitation and evaluation on creativity.* Unpublished manuscript, Brandeis University, Waltham, MA.

Amabile, T. M., & Gryskiewicz, S. S. (in press). Creative environment and personality: Innovation in the R&D lab. In R. L. Kuhn (Ed.), *Handbook for creative and innovative managers.* New York: McGraw-Hill.

Amabile, T. M., Hennessey, B. A., & Grossman, B. S. (1986). Social influences on creativity: The effects of contracted-for reward. *Journal of Personality and Social Psychology, 50*, 14–23.

Barron, F. (1965). The psychology of creativity. In T. Newcomb (Ed.), *New directions in psychology* (Vol. 2, pp. 3–134). New York: Holt, Rinehart & Winston.

Barron, F. (1968). *Creativity and personal freedom.* New York: Van Nostrand.

Bates, J. (1979). Extrinsic reward and intrinsic motivation: A review with implications for the classroom. *Review of Educational Research, 49*, 557–576.

Bem, D. (1972). Self-perception theory. In L. Berkowitz (Ed.), *Advances in experimental social psychology* (Vol. 6, pp. 1–62). New York: Academic Press.

Berglas, S., Amabile, T. M., & Handel, M. (1981). *Effects of evaluation on children's artistic creativity.* Unpublished manuscript, Brandeis University, Waltham, MA.

Boggiano, A. K., & Barrett, M. (1984). *Performance and motivational deficits of helplessness: The role of motivational orientations.* Unpublished manuscript, University of Colorado, Boulder.

Brockner, J., & Hulton, A. J. (1978). How to reverse the vicious cycle of low self-esteem: The importance of attentional focus. *Journal of Experimental Social Psychology, 14*, 564–578.

Bruner, J. (1962). The conditions of creativity. In H. Gruber, G. Terrell, & M. Wertheimer (Eds.), *Contemporary approaches to creative thinking* (pp. 1–30). New York: Atherton.

Calder, B., & Staw, B. (1975). Self-perception of intrinsic and extrinsic motivation. *Journal of Personality and Social Psychology, 31*, 599–605.

Cattell, R. B., & Butcher, H. J. (1968). *The prediction of achievement and creativity.* New York: Bobbs-Merrill.

Check, J. F. (1969). *An analysis of differences in creative ability between white and negro students, public and parochial, three different grade levels, and males and females. Final report.* Washington, DC: Office of Education.

Cheek, J. M., & Stahl, S. S. (1986). Shyness and verbal creativity. *Journal of Research in Personality, 20*, 51–61.

Condry, J. (1977). Enemies of exploration: Self-initiated versus other-initiated learning. *Journal of Personality and Social Psychology, 35*, 459–477.

Coopersmith, S. (1967). *The antecedents of self-esteem*. San Francisco: Freeman.

Crutchfield, R. (1961). The creative process. In *Proceedings of the conference on "the creative person"* (pp. VI-1–VI-16). Lake Tahoe: University of California Alumni Center.

Crutchfield, R. (1962). Conformity and creative thinking. In H. Gruber, G. Terrell, & M. Wertheimer (Eds.), *Contemporary approaches to creative thinking* (pp. 120–140). New York: Atherton.

Csikszentmihalyi, M. (1975). *Beyond boredom and anxiety*. San Francisco: Jossey-Bass.

deCharms, R. (1968). *Personal causation*. New York: Academic Press.

Deci, E. (1971). Effects of externally mediated rewards on intrinsic motivation. *Journal of Personality and Social Psychology, 18*, 105–115.

Deci, E. (1972). Intrinsic motivation, extrinsic reinforcement, and inequity. *Journal of Personality and Social Psychology, 22*, 113–120.

Deci, E. (1975). *Intrinsic motivation*. New York: Plenum.

Deci, E., Nezlek, J., & Sheinman, L. (1981). Characteristics of the rewarder and intrinsic motivation of the rewardee. *Journal of Personality and Social Psychology, 40*, 1–10.

Deci, E., & Porac, J. (1978). Cognitive evaluation theory and the study of human motivation. In M. Lepper & D. Greene (Eds.), *The hidden costs of reward*. Hillsdale, NJ: Lawrence Erlbaum.

Deci, E., & Ryan, R. (1980). The empirical exploration of intrinsic motivational processes. In L. Berkowitz (Ed.), *Advances in experimental social psychology*. New York: Academic Press.

Deci, E., & Ryan, R. (1985). *Intrinsic motivation and self-determination in human behavior*. New York: Plenum.

Feldman, D. (1980). *Beyond universals in cognitive development*. Norwood, NJ: Ablex.

Folger, R., Rosenfield, D., & Hays, R. P. (1978). Equity and intrinsic motivation: The role of choice. *Journal of Personality and Social Psychology, 36*, 557–564.

Fromm, E. (1959). The creative attitude. In H. H. Anderson (Ed.), *Creativity and its cultivation*. New York: Harper & Row.

Garbarino, J. (1975). The impact of anticipated reward upon cross-age tutoring. *Journal of Personality and Social Psychology, 32*, 421–428.

Garwood, D. (1964). Personality factors related to creativity in young scientists. *Journal of Abnormal and Social Psychology, 68*, 413–419.

Gergen, K. J. (1982). *Toward transformation in social knowledge*. New York: Springer-Verlag.

Getzels, J. W., & Csikszentmihalyi, M. (1976). *The creative vision: A longitudinal study of problem-finding in art*. New York: Wiley-Interscience.

Greene, D., & Lepper, M. (1974). Effects of extrinsic rewards on children's subsequent interest. *Child Development, 45*, 1141–1145.

Guilford, J. P. (1950). Creativity. *American Psychologist, 5*, 444–454.

Harackiewicz, J. (1979). The effects of reward contingency and performance feedback on intrinsic motivation. *Journal of Personality and Social Psychology, 37*, 1352–1363.

Harlow, H. (1950). Learning and satiation of response in intrinsically motivated complex puzzle performance by monkeys. *Journal of Comparative Physiological Psychology, 43*, 289–294.

Harter, S. (1978). Effectance motivation reconsidered: Toward a developmental model. *Human Development, 21*, 34–64.

Harter, S. (1981). A new self-report scale of intrinsic versus extrinsic orientation in the classroom. *Developmental Psychology, 17*, 300–312.

Harter, S. (1982). The Perceived Competence Scale for Children. *Child Development, 53*, 87–97.

Hughes, T., & McCullough, F. (Eds.). (1982). *The journals of Sylvia Plath*. New York: Dial.

Hunt, J. (1965). Intrinsic motivation and its role in psychological development. In D. Levine (Ed.), *Nebraska Symposium on Motivation* (Vol. 13). Lincoln: University of Nebraska Press.

Ickes, W. J., Wicklund, R. A., & Ferris, C. B. (1973). Objective self-awareness and self-esteem. *Journal of Experimental Social Psychology, 9*, 202–219.

John-Steiner, V. (1985). *Notebooks of the mind*. Albuquerque: University of New Mexico Press.

Karniol, R., & Ross, M. (1977). The effects of performance irrelevant rewards on children's intrinsic motivation. *Child Development, 48*, 482–487.

Kernoodle-Loveland, K., & Olley, J. (1979). The effect of external reward on interest and quality of task performance in children of high and low intrinsic motivation. *Child Development, 50,* 1207–1210.

Koestner, R., Ryan, R., Bernieri, F., & Holt, K. (1984). Setting limits on children's behavior: The differential effects of controlling vs. informational styles on intrinsic motivation and creativity. *Journal of Personality, 52,* 233–248.

Kruglanski, A. (1975). The endogenous-exogenous partition in attribution theory. *Psychological Review, 82,* 387–406.

Kruglanski, A. (1978). Endogenous attribution and intrinsic motivation. In M. Lepper & D. Greene (Eds.), *The hidden costs of reward.* Hillsdale, NJ: Lawrence Erlbaum.

Kruglanski, A., Friedman, I., & Zeevi, G. (1971). The effects of extrinsic incentive on some qualitative aspects of task performance. *Journal of Personality, 39,* 606–617.

Lepper, M., & Greene, D. (1975). Turning play into work: Effects of adult surveillance and extrinsic rewards on children's intrinsic motivation. *Journal of Personality and Social Psychology, 31,* 479–486.

Lepper, M., & Greene, D. (1978). *The hidden costs of reward.* Hillsdale, NJ: Lawrence Erlbaum.

Lepper, M., Greene, D., & Nisbett, R. (1973). Undermining children's intrinsic interest with extrinsic rewards: A test of the "overjustification" hypothesis. *Journal of Personality and Social Psychology, 28,* 129–137.

Lepper, M., Sagotsky, G., Dafoe, J., & Greene, D. (1982). Consequences of superfluous social constraints: Effects on young children's social inferences and subsequent intrinsic interest. *Journal of Personality and Social Psychology, 42,* 51–65.

Lonky, E., & Reihman, J. (1980, September). *Cognitive evaluation theory, locus of control, and positive verbal feedback.* Paper presented at a meeting of the American Psychological Association, Montreal.

McGraw, K. (1978). The detrimental effects of reward on performance: A literature review and prediction model. In M. Lepper & D. Greene (Eds.), *The hidden costs of reward.* Hillsdale, NJ: Lawrence Erlbaum.

McGraw, K., & McCullers, J. (1979). Evidence of a detrimental effect of extrinsic incentives on breaking a mental set. *Journal of Experimental Social Psychology, 15,* 285–294.

Nicholls, J. G. (1972). Creativity in the person who will never produce anything original and useful: The concept of creativity as a normally distributed trait. *American Psychologist, 27,* 717–727.

Pinder, C. C. (1976). Additivity versus non-additivity of intrinsic and extrinsic incentives: Implications for theory and practice. *Journal of Applied Psychology, 61,* 693–700.

Pittman, T. S., Davey, M. E., Alafat, K. A., Wetherill, K. V., & Kramer, N. A. (1980). Informational versus controlling verbal rewards. *Personality and Social Psychology Bulletin, 6,* 228–233.

Pittman, T. S., Emery, J., & Boggiano, A. K. (1982). Intrinsic and extrinsic motivational orientations: Reward-induced changes in preference for complexity. *Journal of Personality and Social Psychology, 42,* 789–797.

Pritchard, R. D., Campbell, K. M., & Campbell, D. J. (1977). Effects of extrinsic financial rewards on intrinsic motivation. *Journal of Applied Psychology, 62,* 9–15.

Reiss, S., & Sushinsky, L. (1975). Overjustification, competing responses, and acquisition of intrinsic interest. *Journal of Personality and Social Psychology, 31,* 1116–1125.

Renzulli, J. S. (1973). *New Directions in Creativity: Mark 1.* New York: Harper & Row.

Rogers, C. (1954). Towards a theory of creativity. *ETC: A Review of General Semantics, 11,* 249–260.

Rosner, S., & Abt, L. (Eds.). (1970). *The creative experience.* New York: Grossman.

Ross, M. (1975). Salience of reward and intrinsic motivation. *Journal of Personality and Social Psychology, 32,* 245–254.

Ryan, R. M., & Grolnick, W. S. (1984). *Origins and pawns in the classroom: Self-report and projective assessments of individual differences in children's perceptions.* Unpublished manuscript, University of Rochester, Rochester, NY.

Sanders, S. J., Tedford, W. H., & Hardy, B. W. (1977). Effects of musical stimuli on creativity. *Psychological Record, 27,* 463–471.

Shapira, Z. (1976). Expectancy determinants of intrinsically motivated behavior. *Journal of Personality and Social Psychology, 34,* 1235–1244.

Simon, H. (1967). Understanding creativity. In J. C. Gowan, G. D. Demos, & E. P. Torrance (Eds.), *Creativity: Its educational implications.* New York: Wiley.

Simonton, D. K. (1980). Thematic frame, originality, and musical Zeitgeist: A biographical and trans-historical content analysis. *Journal of Personality and Social Psychology, 38,* 972–983.

Smith, W. E. (1974). *The effects of social and monetary rewards on intrinsic motivation.* Unpublished doctoral dissertation, Cornell University, Ithaca, NY.

Sobel, R. S., & Rothenberg, A. (1980). Artistic creation as stimulated by superimposed versus separate visual images. *Journal of Personality and Social Psychology, 39,* 953–961.

Stasinos, D. (1984). Enhancing the creative potential and self-esteem of mentally handicapped Greek children. *Journal of Creative Behavior, 18,* 117–132.

Stein, M. (1974–1975). *Stimulating creativity* (Vols. 1–2). New York: Academic Press.

Steinbeck, J. (1969). *Journal of a novel.* New York: Viking.

Sternberg, R. J. (1985). Cognitive development in the gifted and talented. In F. D. Horowitz & M. O'Brien (Eds.), *The gifted and talented: A developmental perspective.* Washington, DC: American Psychological Association.

Taylor, D. (1960). Toward an information processing theory of motivation. In D. Jones (Ed.), *Nebraska Symposium on Motivation: 1960.* Lincoln: University of Nebraska Press.

Torrance, E. (1966). *The Torrance Tests of Creative Thinking: Technical-norms manual.* Princeton, NJ: Personnel Press.

Torrance, E. P. (1968). *Torrance Tests of Creative Thinking: Directions manual and scoring guide.* Princeton, NJ: Personnel Press.

Turner, R. G., Scheier, M. F., Carver, C. S., & Ickes, W. J. (1978). Correlates of self-consciousness. *Journal of Personality Assessment, 42,* 285–289.

Wallace, D. (1985). Giftedness and the construction of a creative life. In F. D. Horowitz & M. O'Brien (Eds.), *The gifted and talented: Developmental perspectives.* Washington, DC: American Psychological Association.

White, R. (1959). Motivation reconsidered: The concept of competence. *Psychological Review, 66,* 297–323.

Part II

The role of the individual in creativity

Psychometric approaches

2　The nature of creativity as manifest in its testing

E. Paul Torrance

Creativity defies definition

Creativity defies precise definition. This conclusion does not bother me at all. In fact, I am quite happy with it. Creativity is almost infinite. It involves every sense – sight, smell, hearing, feeling, taste, and even perhaps the extrasensory. Much of it is unseen, nonverbal, and unconscious. Therefore, even if we had a precise conception of creativity, I am certain we would have difficulty putting it into words.

However, if we are to study it scientifically, we must have some approximate definition. There have been many attempts to define creativity. They all seem to have something in common, and yet each is slightly different. Some are more inclusive than others. Some are more precise, but no more approximate – perhaps less. Some of them are boring and uninteresting, whereas others excite the imagination and the senses. I would like to review a few of my attempts.

Attempts at definition

When I began my formal study of creativity at the University of Minnesota in 1958, I realized that I must have a definition. I carefully reviewed the many existing definitions and my own observations of creative behavior as I knew it. I found several approaches, and I saw value in each.

Newness as a criterion

The production of something new is included in almost all of the definitions I found, either explicitly or implicitly. Thurstone (1952) argued that it does not make any difference whether or not society regards an idea as novel. He maintained that an act is creative if the thinker reaches the solution in a sudden closure that necessarily implies some novelty to the thinker. To Thurstone, the idea might be artistic, mechanical, or theoretical. It might be administrative if it solves an organizational problem. It might be a new football play, a clever chess move, or a new slogan. Stewart (1950) shared Thurstone's view on this issue, maintaining that creative thinking may occur even though the idea produced may have been produced by someone else at an earlier time. By this definition, creative thinking may take place

43

in the mind of the humblest woman or in the mind of the most distinguished statesman, artist, or scientist.

Stein (1953), contrary to Thurstone and Stewart, insisted that creativity must be defined in terms of the culture in which it appears. To him, "novelty" or "newness" meant that the creative product did not exist previously in the same form. Stein also believed that to be creative the novel work had to be accepted as tenable and useful or satisfying by a group in time (Stein, 1953, p. 322). He hypothesized that studies of creative persons may reveal a sensitivity to the gaps in knowledge that exist in their own culture and that their creativity may be manifest in calling attention to these gaps.

Creativity versus conformity

A number of investigators (Crutchfield, 1962; Wilson, 1956) have defined creativity by contrasting it with conformity. In general, creativity has been seen as contributing original ideas, different points of view, and new ways of looking at problems. Conformity has been seen as doing what is expected, not disturbing or causing trouble for others. Perhaps another way of viewing this phenomenon is best expressed in Lefrancois's definition: ". . . just as very low intelligence is stupidity, so very low creativity is ordinariness" (1982, p. 264).

However, Starkweather (1976) saw the creative person as being neither conforming nor nonconforming, but as being free to conform or not conform, depending on what is true, pleasing, good, or beautiful. My observations and research confirm Starkweather's conclusions.

True, generalizable, and surprising

Selye (1962), in his definition, requires that basic discoveries or creative contributions possess to a high degree and simultaneously three qualities: "They are true not merely as facts but also in the way they are interpreted, they are generalizable, and they are surprising in the light of what was known at the time of the discovery" (1962, p. 402).

H. H. Anderson (1959) also emphasized the search for the truth in his definition of creativity. He was especially insistent that the creative environment provide freedom for one to respond truthfully with one's whole person as one sees and understands the truth.

Bartlett (1958) employed the term "adventurous thinking," which he defined as "getting away from the main track, breaking out of the mold, being open to experience, and permitting one thing to lead to another" (1958, p. 103).

Definitions involving process

Spearman (1930) saw creative thinking basically as a process of seeing or creating relationships, with both conscious and subconscious processes operating. According to one of his principles, when two or more percepts or ideas are given, a person may perceive them to be in various relations (near, far, the cause of, the result of, a part of, etc.). Another principle held that when any item and a relation to it are cognized, then the mind can generate in itself another item so related.

Ribot (1906) and others after him have emphasized the capacity of thinking by analogy as the essential, fundamental element of creative thinking. He maintained that the process of analogizing gives rise to the most unforeseen and novel combinations, but he warned that it produces in equal measure absurd combinations and very original inventions. Recognizing the nonrational aspects of creative thinking, several investigators have called attention to the exercise of discrimination or choice as a part of the creative process. Barchillon (1961), for example, says that the thinking processes involved in creation are of two kinds: *cogito,* to shake and throw things together; and *intelligo,* to choose and discriminate from many different alternative possibilities and then synthesize and bind together elements in new and original ways. What he has in mind by *cogito* is apparently similar to what Kubie (1958) conceptualizes as taking place in the preconscious system. The preconscious is able to scan experiences and memories, to condense, to join opposites, and to find relationships at speeds impossible to achieve in the conscious system. The resulting intuitions, however, are not very precise and are subject to the primary process type of thinking.

Wallas (1926) identified four steps in the creative process: preparation, incubation, illumination, and revision. Apparently the process flows somewhat as follows: First, there is the sensing of a need or deficiency, random exploration, and a clarification or "pinning down" of the problem. Then ensues a period of preparation accompanied by reading, discussing, exploring, and formulating many possible solutions, and then critically analyzing these solutions for advantages and disadvantages. Out of all this comes the birth of a new idea – a flash of insight, illumination. Finally, there is experimentation to evaluate the most promising solution for eventual selection and perfection of the idea. Such an idea might find embodiment in inventions, designs, scientific theories, improved products or methods, novels, musical compositions, paintings, or sculptures.

Among those who have elaborated and refined Wallas's conceptualization are Osborn (1948), Patrick (1955), Parnes (1962), de Bono (1967), Parnes, Noller, and Biondi (1977). In fact, one can detect the "Wallas process" as the basis for almost all of the systematic, disciplined methods of training in existence throughout the world today.

Mental abilities approach

J. P. Guilford (1956, 1959, 1960, 1986) has conceptualized creativity in terms of the mental abilities involved in creative achievement. In his well-known structure of intellect, he sees creative thinking as clearly involving what he categorizes as divergent production. He defines divergent production as the generation of information from given information, where the emphasis is on variety of output from the same source (innovation, originality, unusual synthesis or perspective). Included in the divergent thinking category are the factors of fluency, flexibility, originality, and elaboration. He concludes, however, that creative thinking cannot be equated with divergent thinking. He believes that sensitivity to problems and redefinition abilities are also important in creativity. The redefinition abilities involve transformations of thought, reinterpretations, and freedom from functional fixedness in deriving unique solutions. Sensitivity to problems seems to be essential in getting the creative thinking process in motion.

Levels of creativity

A few investigators have contended that it is necessary to consider levels of creativity. I. R. Taylor (1959) sought to reconcile some of the apparent differences in opinion concerning creativity by suggesting that we think of creativity in terms of levels. He suggested the following five levels:

1. Expressive creativity, as in the spontaneous drawings of children.
2. Productive creativity, as in artistic or scientific products where there are restrictions and controlled free play.
3. Inventive creativity, where ingenuity is displayed with materials, methods, and techniques.
4. Innovative creativity, where there is improvement through modification involving conceptualizing skills.
5. Emergenative creativity, where there is an entirely new principle or assumption around which new schools, movements, and the like can flourish.

Taylor pointed out that many people have the fifth level in mind when they talk about creativity. Because this fifth level is so rare, the lower levels usually have been involved in most investigations regarding creative behavior. Taylor also objected to the frequent confusion of creativity and prevalent interpretations of traditional logic, scientific method, and intelligence. He maintained that fantasy associations and relaxation for unconscious play are so essential for creative thought that creativity cannot be subjected to the same interpretations as logic and scientific method.

Inventive creativity has perhaps been subjected to more systematic definition and specification of criteria than any other level. U.S. Patent Office criteria have been spelled out, and manuals have been developed for evaluators (Cochran, 1955). Newness itself is not enough. The thing must not have been known before and must be useful. In general, one is considered to have invented something if one has originated something of merit that others skilled in the art or science to which it relates would not have thought of or would not have achieved if they had thought of it. The invention should overcome some prior failure or some special difficulty, offer something remarkable or surprising, overcome prior skepticism about possible success, or meet an unfulfilled need.

Choice of a definition

At the initiation of my formal research on creativity I had to choose a research definition. As my research got under way I added some "artistic" definitions that illuminated my research definition and enabled me to communicate some of the things I discovered that I could not communicate with words. Prior to my formal research I had been engaged in research concerning U.S. Air Force survival training. The Survival School was training men to respond creatively in emergencies and extreme conditions. I now refer to the definition I used then as my "survival definition." Before proceeding to what I have learned from testing creativity, I would like to review these definitions.

My research definition

I chose a process definition of creativity for research purposes. I thought that if I chose process as a focus, I could then ask what kind of person one must be to engage in the process successfully, what kinds of environments will facilitate it, and what kind of products will result from successful operation of the process (Torrance, 1965).

I tried to describe creative thinking as the process of sensing difficulties, problems, gaps in information, missing elements, something askew; making guesses and formulating hypotheses about these deficiencies; evaluating and testing these guesses and hypotheses; possibly revising and retesting them; and finally communicating the results.

I like this definition because it describes such a natural process. Strong human needs appear to be at the basis of each of its stages. If we sense an incompleteness, something missing or out of place, tension is aroused. We are uncomfortable and want to do something to relieve the tension. As a result, we begin investigating, asking questions, manipulating things, making guesses or hypotheses, and the like. Until these hypotheses have been tested, modified, and retested, we are still uncomfortable. Then, even when this is done, the tension is unrelieved until we tell someone what we have discovered or produced. Throughout the process there is an element of responding constructively to existing or new situations, rather than merely adapting to them. Such a definition places creativity in the realm of everyday living and does not reserve it for ethereal and rarely achieved heights of creation.

To illustrate the process, I sometimes give an audience as it assembles one of the tests we have developed for assessing the creative thinking abilities, such as the Incomplete Figures Test. After a while I check with the audience to find out what has happened. Most of them will admit that the incompleteness or some other quality of the figures made them uncomfortable. Usually some of them went ahead and completed the figures in some way, either by actually drawing lines or imaginatively by thinking of completing the figures. I then ask them to go ahead and complete the figures in some way that will be satisfying. There is then an obvious atmosphere of relief, increased liveliness, even smiles and laughter. There is also spontaneous interest in communicating the results and seeing what others have created.

If the thinking of the audience is bound to some specific curricular content, such as reading, art, science, or language arts, I try to show how the process operates with that specific curricular content. For example, take the problem of reading creatively. When one reads creatively, one must first of all become sensitive to the problems and possible gaps in whatever one reads. One makes oneself aware of the gaps in information, unsolved problems, missing elements, and things that are incomplete or out of focus. To resolve this tension, the creative reader sees new relationships, creates new combinations, synthesizes relatively unrelated elements into coherent wholes, and redefines or transforms certain pieces of information to discover new uses and build onto what is known. In this search, the creative reader produces a variety of possibilities, uses many approaches, looks at the information from many perspectives, breaks away from commonplace solutions into bold new ways, and develops ideas by filling in the details and making these ideas attractive or exciting to others.

If I want to communicate something about the qualities of the creative product, I ask my audience to discuss the qualities of the products they have just produced. In addition to divergent thinking qualities (fluency or number of ideas, flexibility or shifts in approaches, originality or unusualness, and elaboration or amount of detail or completeness manifested), we talk about such qualities as humor, fantasy, color-fulness and richness of imagery, unusual visualization, internal visualization, boundary pushing, movement, articulateness in telling a story, and the like.

To develop an understanding of the importance of the "press" or environment, I have on several occasions conducted a tape-recorded exercise created by Cunnington and myself (1962, 1965) called "Sounds and Images." It has built into it several "presses," applications of research findings that have been shown to facilitate originality and other qualities of creative thinking. The tape recording consists of four different sound effects, ranging from an easily recognizable familiar sound having few "missing elements" to a strange effect made up of six relatively unrelated sounds. This set of four sound effects is presented with a slight pause between each, with instructions to the listener to write down a word picture of the image generated by each sound effect. The sound effects are then repeated, with instructions to let the imagination roam more widely and depart from the most obvious images. After this, the sound effects are repeated a third time, with instructions to let the imagination swing free. An attempt is made to free the audience from threats of evaluation and to encourage them to have fun. An attempt is also made to break the "set" between each of the repetitions of the sound effects. Finally, the audience is asked to select its favorite images and translate them into a picture. I then ask members of the audience to describe what they have experienced, trying to identify what features of the environment (the taped exercise, the situation, the other members of the audience, etc.) facilitated or hindered their efforts to produce

CREATIVITY IS...

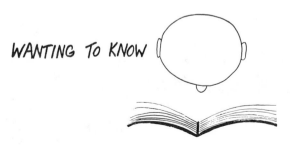

WANTING TO KNOW

Figure 2.1.

original images. They quickly identify such things as the built-in warm-up process, going from easy to difficult, going from simple to complex, the legitimacy of thinking divergently, freedom from evaluation, and the like (Torrance, 1965).

If I want to develop understandings about the importance of the person, I identify built-in environmental features and then ask the audience to identify those forces in themselves that facilitated or inhibited them in making use of these built-in helps. This usually results in a rather long list of personality factors (most of which have been found through research to be related to creative behavior), and hopefully in an increased awareness by the audience of their own creative potential and an increased understanding of the forces in individual personalities that influence their creative functioning and that of their associates.

My "artistic" definition

Perhaps even more useful than my research definition has been my "artistic" definition. It has been especially useful in generating hypotheses, suggesting ideas, theorizing, organizing my thinking, and communicating the nature of creativity. It was given to me in 1964 by Karl Anderson, a student of mine at the University of California at Berkeley. It consisted of simple line drawings and simple sentences. I long ago lost the original, but several artists have attempted to interpret the verbal part of the definition. Most of their productions have been more elaborate than those of Karl Anderson, and most of them have been more colorful, but none of them have been more meaningful.

To make them really meaningful, one has to look on them as analogies. I suggest that instead of saying of each, "Creativity is . . . ," one say, "Creativity is like. . . ." Beginning with this as an analogy, one can play with it, as in the "synectics" (Gordon, 1961) approach to creative problem solving, and elaborate it. The drawings made by Nancy Martin in 1985 are more like the originals than any of the others, and so I present them (Figures 2.1–2.14). I like the simple line draw-

CREATIVITY IS...

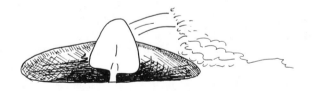

DIGGING DEEPER

Figure 2.2.

CREATIVITY IS...

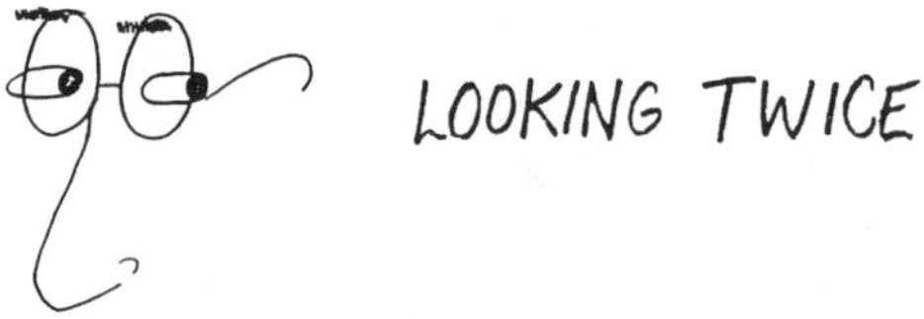

LOOKING TWICE

Figure 2.3.

CREATIVITY IS...

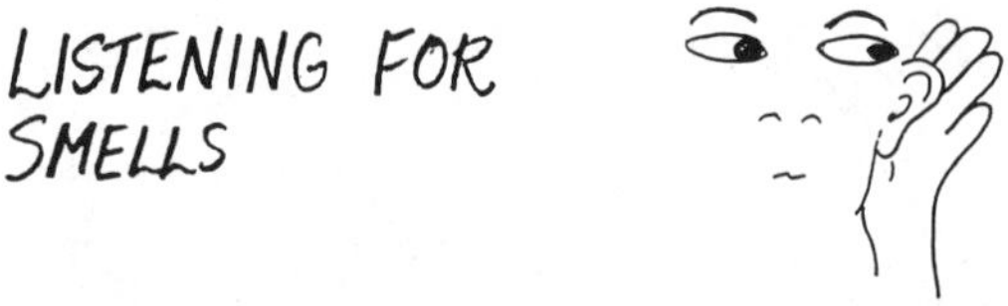

LISTENING FOR
SMELLS

Figure 2.4.

CREATIVITY IS...

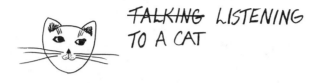

~~TALKING~~ LISTENING TO A CAT

CROSSING OUT MISTAKES

Figure 2.5.

CREATIVITY IS...

GETTING IN

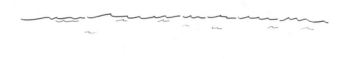

Figure 2.6.

CREATIVITY IS...

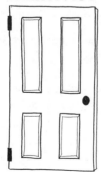

GETTING OUT

Figure 2.7.

CREATIVITY IS...

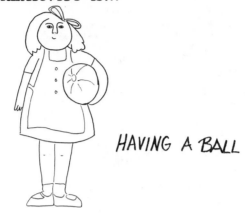

HAVING A BALL

Figure 2.8.

CREATIVITY IS...

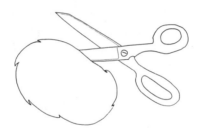

CUTTING HOLES TO SEE THROUGH

Figure 2.9.

ings. Just enough detail is given to inspire an infinity (almost) of meaning and ideas. Some of the other illustrations give more detail and are better for transmitting information. For example, Matt Daly of Palmyra, New York, did an excellent set of illustrations (Goetzmann, 1979) that communicate more information than those of Karl Anderson and Nancy Martin. Consider Figure 2.15, which parallels Figure 2.11 (plugging into the sun). Figure 2.11 is very simple. It is not too difficult to "discover" the meaning, but it is difficult enough to elicit "Aha!" from most people, at least a small one. One does not find that in Figure 2.15. The analogy is quite direct, saying "plug in for more energy," and suggests seven sources. Of course, a teacher or leader might say that these are only seven examples of sources

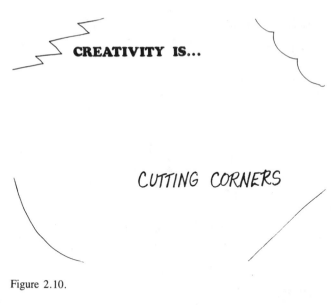

Figure 2.10.

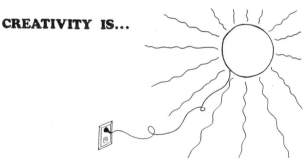

Figure 2.11.

of energy or information. The viewer has already been limited. There is not the infinity of sources suggested by Figure 2.11, which uses the sun as the analogy. What about religion, the home, music, art, exercise, ocean waves, the ocean's roar, and so forth, as sources of energy?

Let us also examine Figure 2.16, which parallels Figure 2.2 (digging deeper). It is much more difficult to attribute meaning to Figure 2.16 than to Figure 2.2, and when we do, we cannot be certain it is what the artist intended. Figure 2.16 was drawn by Earl Ginter (1980) as a part of his creative self-exploration, trying to

CREATIVITY IS...

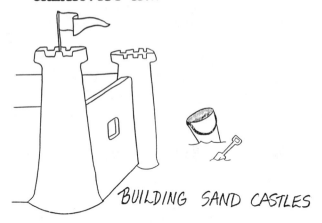

BUILDING SAND CASTLES

Figure 2.12.

CREATIVITY IS...

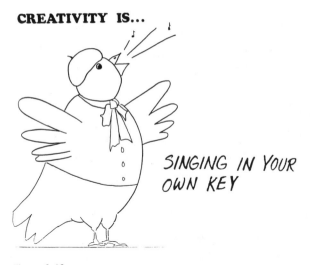

SINGING IN YOUR OWN KEY

Figure 2.13.

recapture some of the skill and some of the love he had once had for art. Its potential for generating ideas and concepts is great, but the risk is also great.

I like Figure 2.17, Matt Daly's illustration for this analogy (Goetzmann, 1979). He pictures several shallow holes that have been abandoned, and the digger now has hit "pay dirt" (diamonds) by digging deeper. This analogy, however, has the opposite result from that used by Edward de Bono (1967) in trying to communicate his concept of lateral thinking (what I define as "creative thinking"). He explains that vertical (logical) thinking digs the same hole deeper, whereas lateral thinking is concerned with digging a hole in a different place. Young Matt Daly's analogy

CREATIVITY IS...

SHAKING HANDS WITH TOMORROW

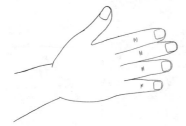

Figure 2.14.

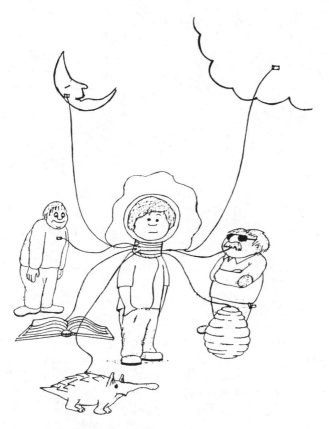

Figure 2.15. Plug in for more energy.

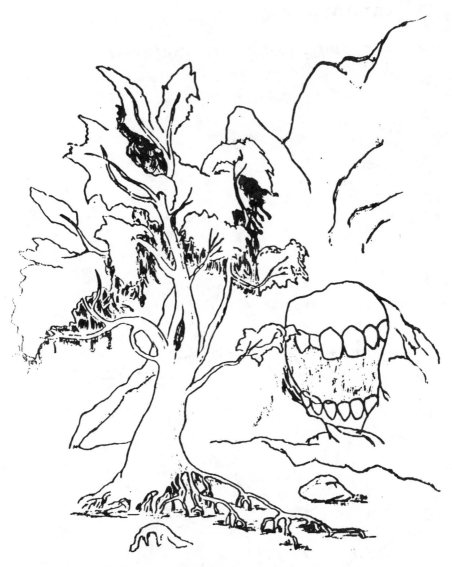

Figure 2.16. Creativity is digging deeper.

suggests that we may have to dig several or many holes before we settle on one place and dig deeper.

I have for a long time particularly liked the following analogical definition of creativity, in spite of the fact that it is entirely verbal:

Creativity: an arbitrary harmony, an expected astonishment, a habitual revelation, a familiar surprise, a generous selfishness, an unexpected certainty, a formable stubbornness, a vital triviality, a disciplined freedom, an intoxicating steadiness, a repeated initiation, a difficult

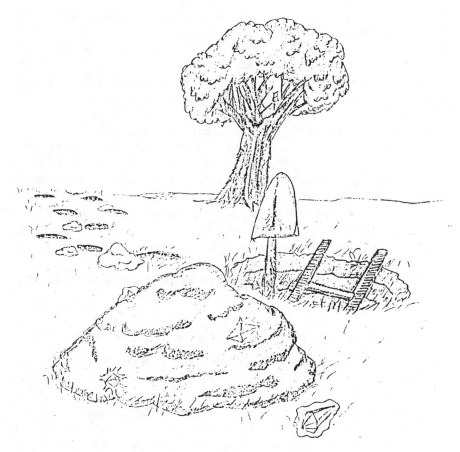

Figure 2.17. Dig deeper.

delight, a predictable gamble, an ephemeral solidity, a unifying difference, a demanding satisfier, a miraculous expectation, an accustomed amazement. (Prince, 1970, p. xiii)

This definition is difficult or puzzling enough to bring forth some ''Ahas'' as insights begin to be discovered. In teaching, it is useful to ask students to think of examples of each analogy from their own lives or observations. Notice how difficult it is to transform them into words once insights have occurred.

My ''survival'' definition

My briefest and in some ways most satisfactory definition of creativity is what I refer to as my survival definition: When a person has no learned or practiced solution to a problem, some degree of creativity is required. I spent 7 years directing a program of research in support of U.S. Air Force survival training (1951–1957).

The air force was training its aircrewmen to survive emergencies and extreme conditions (cold, heat, lack of food and/or water, lack of shelter, lost at sea or in the jungle, down in enemy territory, etc.). They were given information about how they might deal with all these environmental conditions. They were given information about how others had escaped from POW camps and successfully evaded the enemy. In survival training, crews were also practiced in simulated situations. However, in the actual emergency and extreme conditions, the aircrewman was facing a new situation for which he had no learned and practiced solution.

The truly creative is always that which cannot be taught. Yet creativity cannot come from the untaught. Creative solutions to aircrew survival situations required imaginatively gifted recombination of old elements (information about how the American Indians had lived off the land, how the early explorers survived in the Arctic, how men had survived shipwreck, how airmen in World Wars I and II had escaped and evaded, etc.) into new configurations – what is required now. The elements of a creative solution can be taught, but the creativity itself must be self-discovered and self-disciplined. Thus, an important part of survival training involved practicing means of self-discovery and self-discipline and use of the imagination (Torrance, 1957a).

The case for learning about the nature of creativity from testing

My chief way of learning about the nature of creativity has been through testing and teaching creative behavior. I believe that these are valid ways of knowing and that testing and teaching creative behavior have analogues in real-life creative achievements. The strongest evidence of a relationship between test behavior and real-life creative achievement comes from two longitudinal studies: one involving high school students tested in 1959 and followed up 7 and 12 years later and the other involving elementary school pupils tested in 1958 and for 5 subsequent years and followed up 22 years later (Torrance, 1972a, 1972b, 1981).

The criteria of creative adult behavior consisted of the following indices (Torrance, 1981):

1. Quantity of publicly recognized and acknowledged creative achievements (patents and inventions; novels; plays that were publicly produced; musical compositions that were publicly performed; awards for artworks in a juried exhibition; founding a business; founding a journal or professional organization; developing an innovative technique in medicine, surgery, science, business, teaching, etc.).
2. Quality of creative achievements. Subjects were asked to identify what they considered their three most creative achievements; these data, plus responses to the checklist of achievements, were judged by three judges.
3. Quality of creative achievement implied by future career image. Three judges assessed this primarily by responses to the following two questions in the follow-up: (1) What are your career ambitions? For example, what position, responsibility, or reward do you wish to attain? What do you hope to accomplish? (2) If you could do or be whatever you choose in the next 10 years, what would it be?
4. Quantity of high school creative achievements (used only in elementary school study) (similar to item 1, but limited to achievements during the high school years).
5. Quantity of creative style of life achievements, not publicly recognized (such as

Table 2.1. *Product-moment coefficients of correlation between creativity predictors established in 1959 and the criterion measures established in 1966 and 1971*

	Criterion variables					
Predictions	Quality 1966 $N = 46$	Quality 1971 $N = 52$	Quantity 1966 $N = 46$	Quantity 1971 $N = 52$	Aspiration 1966 $N = 46$	Aspiration 1971 $N = 52$
Fluency (TTCT)[a]	.39[b]	.53[b]	.44[b]	.54[b]	.34	.49[b]
Flexibility (TTCT)	.48[b]	.59[b]	.44[b]	.58[b]	.46[b]	.54[b]
Originality (TTCT)	.43[b]	.49[b]	.40[b]	.54[b]	.42[b]	.51[b]
Elaboration (TTCT)	.32	.40[b]	.37[b]	.43[b]	.25	.41[b]

[a]Torrance Tests of Creative Thinking.
[b]Coefficient of correlation is significant at the .01 level.

Table 2.2. *Product-moment coefficients of correlation between predictor and criterion measures of total high school sample*

Predictors	Number	Quantity	Quality	Aspiration
Fluency	254	.30[a]	.30[a]	.27[a]
Flexibility	254	.28[a]	.29[a]	.24[a]
Inventiveness	254	.36[a]	.41[a]	.35[a]
Total (1959)	254	.32[a]	.36[a]	.32[a]
Originality	254	.40[a]	.43[a]	.39[a]
Intelligence	254	.21[a]	.38[a]	.39[a]
Achievement	254	.27[a]	.47[a]	.43[a]

[a]r is significant at better than the .01 level.

organizing an action-oriented group, designing a house, designing a garden, initiating a new educational venture, painting that was not exhibited, musical composition not publicly performed, etc.) (used only in elementary school study).

In the high school group, follow-up data were obtained from the seniors in 1966 and 1971 ($N = 46$ in 1966 and 52 in 1971). In 1971, criterion data were obtained for 254 altogether. In 1980, criterion data were obtained from a total of 211.

Table 2.1 shows the results obtained from the seniors in the high school study who supplied follow-up data in 1966 and 1971 (Torrance, 1972a). It will be observed that the creativity test predictors successfully predicted the criterion measures (judged quality of three most creative achievements, number of publicly acknowledged and recognized creative achievements, and judged quality of creative achievements projected for the future) in 1966 and 1971. It is interesting to note that the predictions are somewhat higher in 1971 than in 1966.

Table 2.3. *Predictive validity of the Torrance Tests of Creative Thinking for males, females, and total sample for five criteria of creative achievement in 22-year follow-up*

Criteria of creative achievement	Males (N = 95)	Females (N = 116)	Total (N = 211)
Number of High School Creative Achievements	.33	.44	.38
Number of Post-High-School Creative Achievements	.58	.42	.46
Number of Creative Style-of-Living Achievements	.42	.48	.47
Quality of Highest Creative Achievements (ratings)	.59	.57	.58
Quality of Future Career Images	.62	.54	.57

Note: All coefficients of correlation are significant at the .001 level.

The predictive validity for the entire high school sample (N = 254) supplying follow-up data is shown in Table 2.2 (Torrance, 1972a, 1972b). Again, it is seen that all of the creativity test predictors are statistically significant at the .01 level. The combined predictor correlates with the combined criterion at .51 (.59 for males and .46 for females).

From these studies (Torrance, 1972a, 1972b) the following conclusions were drawn:

1. Young people identified as creative on the basis of creativity tests during the high school years tend to become productive, creative adults.
2. At least 12 years after high school graduation appears to be a more advantageous time than 7 years as the time for a follow-up of creative adults.

For the 22-year follow-up of the elementary school students first pretested in 1958, the predictive validity is shown in Table 2.3. Again, all the creativity test predictors correlate with all of the creativity achievement criteria at the .001 level or higher. When all of the predictors are combined to predict the combined criterion, a correlation of .63 is attained. For males, the overall validity coefficient was .62; for females, it was .57. Although the creativity test predictors leave considerable unexplained variance, it is unusual to find higher predictive validity for intelligence and achievement tests or other predictor variables in similar studies. In the present study, validity coefficients for measures of intelligence ranged from −.02 to .34 and averaged .17. In the present study it was found that additional variance could be explained by such things as having certain teachers known for encouraging creativity, having a mentor, having a future career image during the elementary school years, and having experiences with foreign study and living. Thus, I believe that the predictive validity is as good as we have any right to expect for almost any kind of predictor of adult achievements (Torrance, 1981).

Although there have been several predictive validity studies with the Torrance Tests of Creative Thinking (TTCT), as well as with other creativity predictors,

Table 2.4. *Product-moment coefficients of correlation between Sounds and Images scores in 1961 and criteria of creative achievement in 1980* (N = 92)

Scoring variable	Quality	Quantity	Future	Style
Originality of images	.31[a]	.35[a]	.39[a]	.40[a]
Strangeness, fantasy	.32[a]	.31[a]	.28[a]	.33[a]
Unusual sensory images	.25[a]	.27[a]	.26[b]	.25[b]
Synthesis into coherent whole	.35[a]	.38[a]	.29[a]	.45[a]
Colorful image, rich detail, appealing	.40[a]	.44[a]	.34[a]	.31[a]
Movement and action images	.25[b]	.25[b]	.17	.14
Number of correct sounds as images	−.14	−.21[b]	−.09	−.14[a]
Number of common images	−.30[a]	−.27[a]	−.40[a]	−.32[a]

[a]Significant at .01 level.
[b]Significant at .05 level.

except for two by Howieson (1981, 1984), all of them have been for relatively short periods (usually about 5 years). Howieson (1981) reported a 10-year follow-up study covering the period from 1965 to 1975 in Australia. Her subjects were 400 seventh graders, and the criterion data consisted of responses to the Wallach and Wing (1969) checklist of creative achievements outside of the school curriculum. The total score on the TTCT correlated .30 with the total criterion score. As in the Torrance studies, the predictions were more accurate for the males than for the females. Howieson (1984) completed a 23-year follow-up study using predictor data collected in 1960 by Torrance in Western Australia. Although the verbal measures derived from the TTCT failed to predict adult creative achievements at a satisfactory level for the 306 subjects who returned their questionnaires, the figural measures fared rather well. For her measure of quality of publicly recognized creative achievements, Howieson obtained a multiple correlation coefficient of .51; for quantity of personal (not publicly recognized) creative achievements, a multiple coefficient of correlation of .33; and for quality of personal creative achievements, one of .44.

Sounds and Images (Khatena & Torrance, 1973), another of the TTCT, was also used as a predictor in the elementary follow-up study. Sounds and Images was administered in 1961 to 92 of the subjects who supplied follow-up data. The results of this study are shown in Table 2.4 (Torrance, 1984). From the data presented in Table 2.4 it will be observed that almost all of the hypothesized relationships were statistically significant. Originality in images, strangeness, unusual sensory images, coherent syntheses, colorful images, and movement and action images were positively related to the criteria of young adult creative achievement. Only two of the coefficients of correlation, for movement and action images (Future Career Image and Creative Style-of-Living Achievements), failed to meet the criterion of statistical significance ($p < .05$). The number of common images (zero scores) was consistently correlated negatively with the criteria. A similar trend was found for a number of specific sounds correctly identified and reported as images, but only the correlations for Quantity of Creative Achievements and Number of Creative Style-of-Living Achievements reached statistical significance.

Although several hundred studies have dealt with the validity of creativity tests, these longitudinal studies with real-life criteria seem to offer the strongest link to test behavior of creative achievement. We seem to be justified in assuming analogies between test behavior and school or training behavior and "real-life" creative behavior.

Manifestations of the nature of creativity through creativity testing

I believe that I have learned some useful things about the nature of creativity by studying variations in testing conditions, the skills involved in creative thinking, the characteristics of the creative person, and group factors that facilitate or interfere with creative function. I shall review briefly each of these areas.

Variations in test conditions

Creativity tests, especially the TTCT, have been subjected to more experimentation regarding ways of administering them than any other educational or psychological tests in the history of testing. This has been good. From it, we have learned a great deal about what procedures enhance, facilitate, or hinder creative thinking in general. One conclusion is clear: How a creativity test is administered, and under what conditions, can influence performance. Also, rather consistently, such experiments have shown that the test administration instructions given in the manual do give the most reliable and valid results.

Even before publication of the TTCT, I had performed numerous experiments concerning the wording of the instructions for these tests and had made systematic observations regarding various conditions. For example, we found that addition of the words "Try to think of something no one else will think of" decreased the amount of copying from one another and increased the originality of responses. I observed that children in an overheated, stuffy classroom were poorly motivated and did not perform as well as children in a comfortable and well-ventilated room. I also observed that children in late May did not perform as well as they had performed earlier, despite training and motivation of high quality.

After publication of the tests in 1966, I was able to locate 16 experiments that had been published between 1968 and 1972 involving variations in testing conditions. They are summarized Table 2.5 (Torrance, 1972c). In 1982, I made a similar survey of studies that had been published between 1972 and 1982. Twenty such experiments were identified and are summarized in Table 2.6. A detailed analysis of these results indicates that for 70% of the measures, the experimental testing condition did result in statistically significant increases. From them, we learn much that is useful about maintaining classroom conditions favorable to learning and creativity. Some of them might be incorporated in standard testing conditions. Some are

Table 2.5. *Summary of experiments involving variations in testing conditions prior to 1972 survey*

Investigator	Grade level	Nature of treatment	Significant (.05) differences
Aliotti (1969)	1	Movement and verbal warm-up day prior to testing	TTCT differences not significant
Boersman & O'Bryan (1968)	4	Standard vs. relaxed	Relaxed: TTCT
Elkind *et al.* (1970)	5–12 years	Interruption of interesting vs. uninteresting task	Uninteresting tasks significantly higher on Wallach-Kogan test
Feldhusen *et al.* (1971)	5, 8	Standard, incubation, take-home, game-like	Highest TTCT r's with achievement on standard and lowest on game-like
Hooper & Powell (1971)	1, 3	Absolute music vs. program music	Absolute music, TTCT
Khatena (1971)	10, 12	Variations in time limits for response	Increased time for incubation, increased originality, TTCT
Kogan & Morgan (1969)	5	Test-like and game-like	Game-like, higher fluency and (timed) unique responses Wallach tests
Mohan (1970)	4	Cue-rich and cue-poor testing room	TTCT variables; helped high creatives more than lows
Nash (1971)	1	Warm-up immediately prior to testing	TTCT Figural increased significantly
Norton (1971)	6	Music	No significant differences TTCT
Roweton & Spencer (1972)	Intermediate	Practice	Significant effect only on Figural A, TTCT
Torrance (1969)	6 (gifted)	Take-home after timed administration	Take-home more valid for teacher curiosity nominations, TTCT
Towell (1972)	4	Untimed	No significant increment, TTCT
Van Mondfrans *et al.* (1971)	5, 8	Standard, incubation, take-home, game-like	Standard, highest verbal means; take-home, scores that fit best concept of creativity as unitary factor orthogonal to intelligence, TTCT
Ward (1969)	Nursery	Cue-poor, cue-rich environment	No significant environment effect Wallach-Kogan measures
Ward (1969)	7–8 years	Successive time periods	Increased uncommonness with time

Source: Data from Torrance (1972c, pp. 131–132).

Table 2.6. *Summary of experiments involving variations in testing conditions reported between 1972 and 1982*

Investigator	Grade level	Nature of treatment	Significant (.05) differences
Aliotti (1973)	1	Individual administration, verbal warm-up, physical warm-up	TTCT Verbal, no difference
Belcher (1975)	4, 5	(1) Saw film of model giving original; (2) same model giving unoriginal responses; (3) read book designed to stimulate ideation	Both film groups better on TTCT Verbal fluency & Originality; group 1 excelled group 2
Carroll (1980)	2, 4, 6	Warm-up, peer evaluation, teacher evaluation	TTCT no difference in 2 and 4; warm-up group significantly better in 6
Dixon (1973)	5, 6	Evaluation vs. unevaluation atmosphere	TTCT Verbal, no difference
Friedman, Raymond, Feldhusen (1978)		(1) Barren room, (2) enriched room, (3) look around for cues, (4) enriched room + look around for cues each 5 min	TTCT (2 Figural, 1 Verbal), significantly higher for enriched room + instructor to keep looking
Frost (1976)	5	Frustrating and non-frustrating conditions	TTCT, no significant difference
Frost (1976)	11, 12	Three levels of frustration	TTCT Figural, no difference
Gakhar (1974)	7–9	Standard conditions, encouraged to be more original, untimed	TTCT significantly higher, encouraged & untimed
Hattie (1980)	6	(1) Untimed, game-like, (2) timed, test-like, (3) test-like, 2 consecutive days	TTCT, generally higher on both test-like conditions
Hudgins (1974)	HS	High and low structure	TTCT Lines and Circles, significantly higher synthesis for low structure
Johnson (1974)	3, 5	Immediate reward, delayed reward, no reward	TTCT Figural, reward conditions consistently significantly higher
Kaltsounis (1973)	5	Sound, speech, music, silence	TTCT Figural, music group significantly higher except for elaboration
Kandil (1980)	1–5 (EH)	Positive verbal reinforcement vs. no verbal reinforcement, individual administration	TTCT Verbal, consistent significant differences on all measures in favor of positive verbal reinforcement

Table 2.6 (*Continued*)

Investigator	Grade level	Nature of treatment	Significant (.05) differences
Kerns (1979)	6, 10	Unisensory vs. bisensory stimulation	TTCT Figural, significantly higher on all measures for unisensory
Landreneau & Halpin (1978)	6	Modeling of response to unusual uses, varying levels of flexibility and originality	TTCT (Just Suppose & Unusual Uses), positive effect only on Fluency
Lero (1974)	5	Timed vs. untimed	TTCT Lines and Circles, untimed group significantly higher on Fluency and Originality
McCormack (1975)	3	Nonverbal vs. verbal directions	TTCT Figural B, significantly higher Fluency & Elaboration for nonverbal
Peters & Torrance (1972)	2–6 years	Same-sex dyads vs. individual administration & then same-sex dyads	Construction task with blocks, dyads enhanced performance of 6-year-olds; no effects on 2–5
White & Torrance (1978)	2	Warm-up with song *How Many Ways* vs. no warm-up	TTCT Circles, significantly higher for warm-up
Ziv (1976)	10	Humor (played record of comedian) vs. standard conditions	TTCT Unusual Uses & Just Suppose, significant difference in favor of humor

impractical insofar as tests go; yet they certainly can be used as a part of teaching. For example, it might not be practical and fair as a test administration practice to give creativity tests as take-home tests. Yet we try to keep the incubation processes going in every lesson.

Although the results of these two surveys seem to show some inconsistencies, there also are some clear and consistent trends. Generally, psychological warm-up given before testing results in small but consistent and statistically significant gains over standard conditions. Warm-up that is too long or that is given too far in advance of the testing does not help. Doing something to set the incubation processes to work ahead of time can be helpful.

Take-home testing results in greater variability. In most instances, scores are no higher than under timed conditions. However, if one is successful in motivating students and in setting up conditions for incubation, take-home tests are bound to produce superior results.

Both relaxed and stressful conditions can produce increased performance. Some arousal is necessary for creativity, but too much stress is detrimental. In the same way, conditions may become too playful, so that no work is accomplished, and making creative productions is "work." Students need to be made comfortable, physically and psychologically, so that they can focus on the creative task.

It is important, however, to give some reason for the testing. It should make sense. The subjects should be told why they are being tested. Some creativity tests do not do this; subjects are deliberately not told what they are being tested for. If we wanted to measure the jumping ability of the children in our school or the young people in a college, we would not measure how high they just happened to be jumping. We would do something to get them jumping. We would also tell them if we wanted to see how high they could jump, how far they could jump, and so forth. It is necessary to do the same thing to get a valid measure of creative thinking ability. For this reason, subjects are motivated on the TTCT to fluency, flexibility originality, elaboration, and so forth.

The experiments on providing cue-rich and cue-poor environments for testing also proved to be productive. Mohan (1971) found that children scored higher in a room rich in cues (a variety of objects in view in the room) than did those in a barren room. However, he found that this difference came almost entirely from the high creatives. The cue-rich environment did not help the low creatives; apparently they were not accustomed to scanning the environment for cues to ideas for transformation, combinations, and the like. However, Friedman, Raymond, and Feldhusen (1978) found that by suggesting every 5 min that the subjects look around, higher scores could be achieved. Deliberate training of low creatives to scan the environment and instruction in how to use environmental cues might be used to improve their creative functioning.

Skills involved in creative thinking

Edward de Bono (1975) sees thinking as a skill like reading, writing, riding a bicycle, swimming, playing tennis, cooking, or skiing. Improvement in thinking skills requires practice with the right tools and in the right environment. The problem then becomes one of what component skills underlie creative thinking and how these can best be trained.

On the TTCT (Torrance, 1979, 1984) we have identified a variety of skills that seem to be important in producing creative responses. They are mentioned frequently in studies of the creative giants, in personality studies of creative persons, in training guides, and in other creativity literature. The responses to both the verbal and figural tests, Sounds and Images, and other creativity tests give evidence of these abilities, which can be scored (Torrance, 1981, 1984; Wechsler, 1982). We have also shown that they are valid predictors of creative achievement.

For example, we have identified the following abilities in the figural forms of the TTCT (Torrance, 1979; Torrance & Ball, 1984):

1. Fluency, number of responses.
2. Flexibility, number of ways circles or lines were used.
3. Originality, unusualness, or rarity of the response.

4. Elaboration, number of details that contribute to the "story" told by the response.
5. Abstractness of the title, level of abstraction of the response.
6. Resistance to closure on the incomplete figures or the ability to "keep open."
7. Emotional expressiveness of the response.
8. Articulateness of storytelling, putting the response in context, giving it an environment.
9. Movement or action shown in the response.
10. Expressiveness of the titles, ability to transform from the figural to the verbal and give expression.
11. Synthesis or combination, joining together two or more figures and making it into a coherent response.
12. Unusual visualization, seeing and putting the figure in a visual perspective different from the usual.
13. Internal visualization, seeing objects from the inside.
14. Extending or breaking the boundaries, getting outside the expected.
15. Humor, juxtaposition of two or more incongruities.
16. Richness of imagery, showing variety, vividness, liveliness, and intensity.
17. Colorfulness of imagery, exciting, appeal to the senses, flavorful, earthy, emotionally appealing.
18. Fantasy, unreal figures, magic, fanciful fairy tale characters, science fiction characters.

In order to validate these skills as represented by test scores, I had the test protocols of samples from my two longitudinal studies rescored by independent scorers according to the manual (Torrance & Ball, 1984) and correlated with two criteria: judged quality of creative achievements and number of publicly recognized and acknowledged creative achievements. In the high school study (Torrance & Ball, 1984), all of the correlations were statistically significant, ranging from .22 to .79 ($N = 162$) and averaging .53. An index made up of all the variables correlated .79 with the combined criteria. In the elementary school study with the criteria collected 22 years later, the total index correlated with the criterion .50 for tests taken in the third grade, .34 for the fourth grade, .46 for the fifth grade, and .42 for the sixth grade.

Characteristics of the creative person

I titled the volume containing a collection of my papers about the creative person *The Blazing Drive* (Torrance, 1987). This title sums up the essence of what I have learned about the nature of creativity and the creative person. The title was inspired by *Jonathan Livingston Seagull* (Bach, 1970), in which Jonathan says of his prize pupil, "He was strong and light and quick in the air, but far and away more important, he had a blazing drive to learn to fly" (p. 75). Teresa Amabile (1986) recently wrote that "extraordinary talent, personality, and cognitive ability do not seem to be enough – it's the 'labor of love' aspect that determines creativity" (p. 12). This conclusion comes from dozens of findings from testing for creativity, but especially from my longitudinal studies.

In my 22-year study of elementary school children first tested in 1958, I asked them each what they were in love with, what they wanted to become when they were adults (Torrance, 1981). Some of the children consistently responded "I don't know." Others were inconsistent, changing their future images every year. Most of these continued to change and are now in work different from any that they had mentioned as youngsters. Some gave responses in terms of what was expected or what they thought was expected of them. For example, one second grade boy's response was "physician or surgeon," the occupation of his mother and father. In the third and fourth grades his response was the same. All the time, however, musical symbols and objects were appearing on his figural creativity tests. For example, in third grade, he used the circles to draw the "Beatles," a drum, a horn, and the like. Finally, in the fifth grade he excelled so well in a summer music camp that he had the courage to turn away from the "games" others expected him to play and for the first time began considering a career in music. Some, of course, never reach this point, and the consequences are tragic.

Surprisingly, about half of my subjects were consistent in their choices and have persisted in careers consistent with the future career images they expressed as children. Using the five different sets of criteria already described in this chapter, having childhood future career images that they could stick with proved to be a statistically significant predictor of adult creative achievement. In fact, this indicator (having or not having future career images that they were in love with) was a better predictor of adult creative achievement than were indices of scholastic promise (IQ).

Since I reached the conclusion that the essence of the creative person is being in love with what one is doing, I have had a growing awareness that this characteristic makes possible all the other personality characteristics of the creative person: courage, independence of thought and judgment, honesty, perseverance, curiosity, willingness to take risks, and the like. For example, Roger Tory Peterson (Beebe, 1986) at a very young age was in love with nature, especially birds. He was a social outcast in his youth because of this. He still will not say what nicknames the taunting youngsters called him. "It wasn't very nice," he says. This has been a common experience of many of our most eminent inventors, scientists, artists, musicians, writers, and so on. To maintain an intense love for something and survive these kinds of pressures, one has to develop courage, independence, perseverance, and the like. On the basis of these and other insights, I developed a set of guides (Torrance, 1983) for creative youngsters that Morgan Henderson and Jack Presbury called a "Manifesto" and made it into a poster that carries these words:

"How to Grow Up Creatively Gifted"
E. Paul Torrance

1. Don't be afraid to "fall in love with" something and pursue it with intensity. (You will do best what you like to do most.)
2. Know, understand, take pride in, practice, develop, use, exploit, and enjoy your greatest strengths.
3. Learn to free yourself from the expectations of others and to walk away from the games they try to impose upon you.
4. Free yourself to "play your own game" in such a way as to make good use of your gifts.

5. Find a great teacher or mentor who will help you.
6. Don't waste a lot of expensive, unproductive energy trying to be well-rounded. (Don't try to do everything; do what you can do well and what you love.)
7. Learn the skills of interdependence. (Learn to depend upon one another, giving freely of your greatest strengths and most intense loves.)

Factors in groups

The focus in group research usually has been on decision making. However, in most instances what makes the decision making worth studying is the creativity that takes place in the process. I have engaged in at least four programs of research that investigated the group factors that facilitate or interfere with the creative process. Each of them involved a series of rather complex experiments and tests, and so it is possible to deal only with the highlights.

The first set of such experiments was conducted at the U.S. Air Force Advanced Survival Training School and involved both laboratory experiments and realistically simulated situations (Torrance, 1955). From 7 years of research and dozens of experiments and observational studies, I think that the most important finding affecting creativity in groups was that willingness to tolerate disagreement resulted in better decisions, higher creativity, and better combat performance. This finding was cross-validated by several experiments, observational studies, and combat studies in Korea (Torrance, 1957b). There were dozens of findings of factors that facilitated or inhibited the process, but they all went back to the question whether the factor identified facilitated or inhibited the group's willingness to disagree, to consider a wider range of alternatives, to listen to all members of the crew, and to introduce unusual solutions.

We also conducted a series of leadership studies (Torrance, 1957c). From these studies, the creative leader seems to be one who, in emergency and extreme conditions,

1. rapidly restructures the group and the situation,
2. uses the expertness (both air force and civilian) within the crew to get out of trouble,
3. is willing to take risks (trying new skills, trying new foods, etc.),
4. is willing to make decisions and take action, distributing responsibility, taking responsibility for decisions,
5. acts outside of his authority, taking care of his men, taking emergency actions not anticipated by standard operating procedures,
6. is willing to share the dangers and discomforts of the situation, sharing unpleasant tasks, being able "to take it" despite handicaps, and
7. develops a pattern of mutual support.

My second set of group dynamic studies involving creativity was with elementary school children in grades 3–6. Even by the third grade, children have adopted many of the strategies used by adults to limit the creative production of the group (Torrance, 1963, 1965). Among the strategies observed in the 5-person groups in one sixth grade class were these:

1. Assigning the most creative member to lead the group.
2. Assigning the most creative member to be the recorder.
3. The most creative member (a girl) began with a burst of creativity, but, sensing disapproval, she became the group clown.
4. The most creative member worked in isolation.
5. The most creative member became counteraggressive when he received pressure from his teammates.
6. The most creative member was silent and preoccupied, finally leaving the group.

Some excellent strategies were also exhibited. In fact, the most frequently used strategy was initiating structure, leading, and coordinating. The second most frequently employed was not leading at all, but filling in the gaps, offering ideas when no one else would do so.

It was in groups heterogeneously arranged according to creativity scores that stressful situations arose. In homogeneously arranged groups, a cooperative atmosphere and positive strategies prevailed. They were less active than the heterogeneous groups. In the groups arranged heterogeneously according to IQ, the group pressure was on the most intelligent member to produce ideas. Many of them, not being able to excel at this "game," were embarrassed that they were unable to meet the group's expectations. The homogeneous groups were more creatively productive than the heterogeneous groups (Torrance, 1965).

The subjects of the third set of experiments were graduate students arranged in 5-person groups designed to test specific parts of some group dynamic theories (field, T group, psychoanalytic, sociodramatic, creative problem solving, and synectics group theories). The limitations of this chapter make it impossible to discuss the creativity measures, the treatment procedures, and the theories involved. I shall only enumerate illustrative findings (Torrance, 1972d).

1. Groups whose members were acquainted with each other produced more original responses than the unacquainted groups.
2. After working on a problem in a group, "Aha" experiences were reported 5 days later as occurring during the process (32%), during feedback in class (4%), soon afterward, the same day (44%), delayed (on the second, third, or fourth day) (56%), and when they were given the follow-up questionnaire (14%). Fifty-four percent said that their new insights (ideas, "Ahas," etc.) occurred through group interaction.
3. Practice of a systematic, disciplined, creative problem-solving process, after 3 hr of training, brought few complaints from "freedom-oriented" groups, as determined by the Runner Studies of Attitude Pattern (Runner & Runner, 1965), whereas the "control-oriented" groups had significant numbers of such complaints (26% vs. 83%).
4. Freedom-oriented groups produced more original responses than control-oriented groups, but following an evaluative feedback the controlled groups made more gains in originality than freedom-oriented groups. Under creative feedback conditions, however, freedom-oriented groups made greater gains in originality.

The fourth set of experiments on group creativity involved preschool children. Again, the creativity tests involved in these experiments, the treatment procedures, and the results are far too varied and too complex to present here. The most important conclusion about the nature of creativity, in my opinion, was that so-cialization could be achieved without sacrificing creativity. In my opinion, the two can reinforce one another. By becoming more socialized, a child can become more creative, and vice versa (Torrance, 1970).

In one series of studies, I investigated the role of dyadic interaction with 5-year-olds in facilitating creativity. Twenty-four children were tested alone, and 22 of their randomly selected classmates were tested in dyads. Dyadic interaction facili-tated creative output, and the children persisted longer and seemed to have a more enjoyable experience.

Creative people are willing to attempt the difficult, and children, too, in order to learn and grow creatively, must be willing to tackle difficult tasks. To do this, teachers must create social and peer conditions conducive to attempting tasks of appropriate difficulty. In another experiment, I hypothesized that 5-year-olds placed in dyads would be more willing to attempt a difficult task than alone or in class. A target game (a wastepaper can and bean bags at varying distances) was used in this experiment. There were 22 children in each of three conditions. The results clearly supported the hypothesis that 5-year-old children are most willing to attempt a difficult task in dyads and least willing when performing before the entire class.

The ability to support curiosity by skill in asking questions is important for both socialization and creativity. In one experiment, I examined the effects of group size on the question-asking behavior of eight classes in preprimary education. In the test task, groups were asked to produce as many questions as they could in a 10-min period concerning a picture. It was required that questions be about things that could not be ascertained by looking at the picture. Groups of 24, 12, 6, and 4 were studied. Production was significantly higher in the small groups, although in most respects 4-child groups seemed to have no advantage over 6-child groups.

Many early childhood educators argue that any imposed structure discourages creativity, whereas others argue for its necessity. In one experiment with 5-year-old children, an attempt was made to improve the small-group behavior of children by increasing the task structure. The children were first asked to draw dream castles and then decide which member's dream castle to construct, using Lego blocks. In the second experiment, an attempt was made to improve this type of behavior through increasing the group structure by designating one member as leader. In the first experiment, there were twelve 6-child groups in each condition; in the second experiment, there were six 6-child groups in each condition. In the first experiment, the task structure resulted in increases in planning and cooperating behavior, de-creases in verbal and physical aggressiveness, and an increase in the judged creativity of the products produced. In the second experimental manipulation, the structure increased the planning behavior and the judged creativity of the products, but failed to decrease the verbal and physical aggressiveness.

In the socialization process, children find increasingly that they are forbidden to touch and to manipulate objects. In an earlier study (Torrance, 1963) I had found that the degree of manipulation of the toys used in the product-improvement task was highly related to fluency and originality scores. This suggested the hypothesis that provision of opportunities to manipulate stimulus objects would facilitate question asking among 5-year-old children. The 48 subjects were randomly assigned within the classrooms to eight 6-child groups. The manipulation and nonmanipulation were presented in an alternate-form design in the two classrooms. The stimulus objects were a plastic bee that made a buzzing sound when twirled and a toy musical instrument that made a variety of sounds when manipulated. The manipulation condition, when compared with the nonmanipulation condition, produced a statistically significantly larger number of questions and larger numbers of hypothesis-stating questions and questions about puzzling phenomena. The results suggest that previous findings concerning the facilitating effects of manipulation in the production of inventive ideas can be generalized to question-asking and hypothesis-making skills.

These are only examples of how testing children may add to our understanding of the nature of creativity.

Limitations

My understanding of the nature of creativity as manifest by testing creativity is limited because my efforts to assess creativity have thus far been limited largely to the rational-thinking view of creativity. Little attention has been given to assessment of the creativity that goes beyond the rational – the suprarational – not contrary to reason, but outside the province of reason. I have made some tentative forays into this domain, but my measures are not well enough developed to include in this chapter. Of course, my "artistic" definition and the work that extends it are in this direction. I have proposed that there are some practical abilities included in this domain and that it is important that we develop means of assessing them (Torrance & Hall, 1980). I have identified the following such abilities and made tentative suggestions for measuring them (Torrance & Hall, 1980):

1.   The ability to perform "miracles" – the ability to accomplish things that go beyond logical expectations.
2.   Empathy and superawareness of the needs of others.
3.   Charisma.
4.   The ability to solve collision conflicts for which there are no rational, logical solutions.
5.   A sense of the future.

Summary

I have discussed the nature of creativity as it has been manifested to me by testing for creativity. Creativity is a multifaceted phenomenon that defies precise definition. Many very useful definitions have been offered, but I have chosen three that have guided my research over the years: a research definition, an artistic definition, and a very simple survival definition. I have sought to translate these definitions into measurement devices that will then have analogues in learning and in "real life." My argument for testing as a legitimate way of learning about the nature of creativity is based on the fact that test behavior does have analogues in learning behavior and real life, supported by validity evidence linking test behavior and real-life creative achievements. Evidence of this link has been presented.

Examples have been given from my research and observations concerning what has been learned from testing for creativity, as well as what has been learned about the nature of conditions facilitating and inhibiting creativity, the skills involved in being creative, the characteristics of the creative person, and group factors that facilitate and inhibit creative behavior. I admit that these insights are derived only from tests that represent the rational view of creative behavior. Finally, I urge investigators to explore assessment of the further reaches of creativity, the suprarational. I identify what some of these abilities are and suggest ways of proceeding.

References

Amabile, T. (1986). The personality of creativity. *Creative Living, 15*(3), 12–16.

Anderson, H. H. (Ed.). (1959). *Creativity and its cultivation.* New York: Harper & Row.

Anderson, K. (1964). *Creativity is.* Unpublished manuscript, University of California, Berkeley.

Bach, R. (1970). *Jonathan Livingston Seagull.* New York: Macmillan.

Barchillon, J. (1961). Creativity and its inhibition in child prodigies. In *Personality dimensions of creativity.* New York: Lincoln Institute of Psychotherapy.

Bartlett, F. (1958). *Thinking.* New York: Basic Books.

Beebe, M. (1986, June 22). The birdman of Jamestown. *Buffalo Magazine,* pp. 10–16.

Cochran, W. W. (1955). Elementary patent law. In *Training manual for patent examiners.* Washington, DC: U.S. Patent Office, U.S. Department of Commerce.

Crutchfield, R. S. (1962). Conformity and creative thinking. In H. E. Gruber, G. Terrell, & M. Wertheimer (Eds.), *Contemporary approaches to creative thinking* (pp. 120–140). New York: Atherton Press.

Cunnington, B. F., & Torrance, E. P. (1962). *Sounds and images.* Minneapolis: Bureau of Educational Research, University of Minnesota.

Cunnington, B. F., & Torrance, E. P. (1965). *Sounds and images.* Boston: Ginn & Company.

de Bono, E. (1967). *New think: The use of lateral thinking in the generation of new ideas.* New York: Basic Books.

de Bono, E. (1975). *Think links.* Blandford, Dorset, UK: Direct Education Services.

Friedman, F., Raymond, B. A., & Feldhusen, J. F. (1978). The effects of environmental scanning on creativity. *Gifted Child Quarterly, 22,* 248–251.

Ginter, E. (1980). *Creativity self-experiment.* Unpublished manuscript, Department of Educational Psychology, University of Georgia, Athens.

Goetzmann, K. (1979). *Conquering a dragon.* Unpublished manuscript, Palmyra, NY.

Gordon, W. J. J. (1961). *Synectics.* New York: Harper & Row.

Guilford, J. P. (1956). Structure of intellect. *Psychological Bulletin, 53,* 267–293.

Guilford, J. P. (1959). *Personality.* New York: McGraw-Hill.

Guilford, J. P. (1960). Basic conceptual problems of the psychology of thinking. *Proceedings of the New York Academy of Sciences, 91,* 6–21.

Guilford, J. P. (1986). *Creative talents: Their nature, uses and development.* Buffalo, NY: Bearly Limited.

74 E. P. TORRANCE

Henderson, M., & Presbury, J. (1983). *A manifesto for children* (Poster). Staunton, VA: Full Circle Counseling.

Howieson, N. (1981). A longitudinal study of creativity: 1965–1975. *Journal of Creative Behavior, 15,* 117–135.

Howieson, N. (1984). *The prediction of creative achievement from childhood measures: A longitudinal study in Australia, 1960–1983.* Unpublished doctoral dissertation, University of Georgia, Athens.

Khatena, J., & Torrance, E. P. (1973). *Thinking creatively with sounds and words.* Bensenville, IL: Scholastic Testing Services.

Kubie, L. S. (1958). *The neurotic distortion of the creative process.* Lawrence: University of Kansas Press.

Lefrancois, G. R. (1982). *Psychology for teaching: A bear rarely faces the front.* Belmont, CA: Wadsworth.

Martin, N. (1985). *Creativity is* (Drawings). Unpublished drawings. Athens, GA: Georgia Studies of Creative Behavior.

Mohan M. (1971). *Interaction of physical environment with creativity and intelligence.* Unpublished doctoral dissertation, University of Alberta, Edmonton, Canada.

Osborn, A. F. (1948). *Your creative power.* New York: Charles Scribner's Sons.

Parnes, S. J. (1962). Can creativity be increased? In S. J. Parnes & H. F. Harding (Eds.), *A source book for creative thinking* (pp. 185–191). New York: Charles Scribner's Sons.

Parnes, S. J., Noller, R. B., & Biondi, A. M. (1971). *Guide to creative action.* New York: Charles Scribner's Sons.

Patrick, C. (1955). *What is creative thinking?* New York: Philosophical Library.

Prince, G. M. (1970). *The practice of creativity.* New York: Harper & Row.

Ribot, T. (1906). *Essays on the creative imagination.* London: Routledge & Kegan Paul.

Runner, K., & Runner, H. (1965). *Manual of interpretation for the interview form III of the Runner Studies of Attitude Patterns.* Golden, CO: Runner Associates.

Selye, H. (1962). The gift for basic research. In G. Z. F. Bereday & J. A. Lauwerys (Eds.), *The gifted child: The yearbook of education* (pp. 339–408). New York: Harcourt, Brace & World.

Spearman, C. E. (1930). *Creative mind.* Cambridge University Press.

Starkweather, E. K. (1976). Creativity research instruments designed for use with preschool children. In A. M. Biondi & S. J. Parnes (Eds.), *Assessing creative growth: The tests – book I* (pp. 79–90). Buffalo, NY: Creative Education Foundation.

Stein, M. I. (1953). Creativity and culture. *Journal of Psychology, 36,* 311–322.

Stewart, G. W. (1950). Can productive thinking be taught? *Journal of Higher Education, 21,* 411–414.

Taylor, I. A. (1959). The nature of the creative process. In P. Smith (Ed.), *Creativity* (pp. 51–82). New York: Hastings House.

Thurstone, L. L. (1952). Creative talent. In L. L. Thurstone (Ed.), *Applications of psychology* (pp. 18–37). New York: Harper & Row.

Torrance, E. P. (1955). Techniques for studying individual and group adaptation in emergencies and extreme conditions. In *Air Force human engineering personnel and training research* (pp. 286–297). Washington, DC: National Academy of Sciences/National Research Council.

Torrance, E. P. (1957a). Psychology of survival. Unpublished manuscript, Air Force Personnel Research Center, Lackland Air Force Base, TX.

Torrance, E. P. (1957b). Group decision-making and disagreement. *Social Forces, 35,* 314–318.

Torrance, E. P. (1957c). Leadership in the survival of small isolated groups. In *Symposium on preventive and social psychiatry* (pp. 309–327). Washington, DC: Walter Reed Army Institute of Research/NRC.

Torrance, E. P. (1963). *Education and the creative potential.* Minneapolis: University of Minnesota Press.

Torrance, E. P. (1965). *Rewarding creative behavior.* Englewood Cliffs, NJ: Prentice-Hall.

Torrance, E. P. (1966). *The Torrance Tests of Creative Thinking: Technical-norms manual* (research ed.). Princeton, NJ: Personnel Press.

Torrance, E. P. (1970). Achieving socialization without sacrificing creativity. *Journal of Creative Behavior, 4,* 183–189.

Torrance, E. P. (1972a). Career patterns and peak creative experiences of creative high school students 12 years later. *Gifted Child Quarterly, 16,* 75–88.

Torrance, E. P. (1972b). Predictive validity of the Torrance Test of Creative Thinking. *Journal of Creative Behavior, 6,* 236–252.

Torrance, E. P. (1972c). Can we teach children to think creatively? *Journal of Creative Behavior, 6,* 114–143.

Torrance, E. P. (1972d). Group dynamics and creativity. In C. W. Taylor (Ed.), *Climate for creativity* (pp. 75–96). New York: Pergamon Press.

Torrance, E. P. (1974). *The Torrance Tests of Creative Thinking: Technical-norms manual.* Bensenville, IL: Scholastic Testing Services.

Torrance, E. P. (1979). *The search for satori and creativity.* Buffalo, NY: Bearly Limited.

Torrance, E. P. (1981). Predicting the creativity of elementary school children (1958–1980) – and the teacher who made a "difference." *Gifted Child Quarterly, 25,* 55–62.

Torrance, E. P. (1983). The importance of falling in love with "something." *Creative Child and Adult Quarterly, 8,* 72–78.

Torrance, E. P. (1984). Sounds and images productions of elementary school pupils as predictors of the creative achievements of young adults. *Creative Child and Adult Quarterly, 7,* 8–14.

Torrance, E. P. (1987). *The blazing drive: The creative personality.* Buffalo, NY: Bearly Limited.

Torrance, E. P., & Arsan, K. (1963). Experimental studies of homogeneous and heterogeneous groups for creative scientific tasks. In W. W. Charters, Jr., & N. L. Gage (Eds.), *Readings in the social psychology of education* (pp. 133–140). Boston: Allyn & Bacon.

Torrance, E. P., & Ball, O. E. (1984). *Torrance Tests of Creative Thinking: Streamlined (revised) manual, Figural A and B.* Bensenville, IL: Scholastic Testing Services.

Torrance, E. P., & Hall, L. K. (1980). Assessing the further reaches of creative potential. *Journal of Creative Behavior, 14,* 1–19.

Wallach, M. A., & Wing, C. W., Jr. (1969). *The talented student.* New York: Holt, Rinehart & Winston.

Wallas, G. (1926). *The art of thought.* New York: Harcourt, Brace & World.

Wechsler, S. (1982). Identifying the creative strength in the responses to the verbal forms of the Torrance Tests of Creative Thinking. Doctoral dissertation, University of Georgia, 1981. *Dissertation Abstracts International, 43,* 3521A (University Microfilms No. 82-01588).

Wilson, R. C. (1956). The program for gifted children in the Portland, Oregon, schools. In C. W. Taylor (Ed.), *The 1955 University of Utah research conference on the identification of creative scientific talent* (pp. 14–22). Salt Lake City: University of Utah Press.

3   Putting creativity to work

Frank Barron

Is *applied creativity* a barbarous notion? What would an artist say, or a poet? Shall we have *applied poetry* next? And are we not all of us artists at heart, in our lives? Is not creativity a spark of the divine in us? Do we not reduce it, reduce ourselves, in fact, when we subordinate creativity to utility, when we make our creativity serve extrinsic ends? Is not this call, the call to create, nothing less than a call to give ourselves to the sacred in human life? Is it not the master, are we not its servitors? Put creativity to work, indeed!

With all due respect for that archetypically artistic point of view, in this chapter I urge that in fact we have reached such a point of development of our knowledge of creativity that it is ready for application and, further, that as a species we are at such a point of historical no return that it behooves us to muster all our powers, in the name of the Creator if necessary, to meet consciously the problems that our own evolution has set for us. So, the thesis of this chapter: Put creativity to work!

The research roots

It has become traditional in historical reviews of psychological research on creativity to cite J. P. Guilford's 1950 presidential address to the American Psychological Association as a sort of watershed, the beginning of serious empirical work on the topic. And 1969 is often cited as marking a decline in interest and activity. Actually, of course, as one might expect, the development began earlier, was more continuous and sustained, and has simply moved into a phase in which applications and evaluation are receiving more attention.

Still, there is some justice in the observation that 1950 marked a turning point. Earlier research usually had been directed to questions about originality and imagination. "Creativity" became a popular term that included a lot of earlier work identified under other names. As late as the mid-1950s, when *Scientific American* decided to publish a special issue on "Innovation in Science," imagination was still the more commonly recognized rubric. My own contribution to that issue was written to the title "The Psychology of Imagination" (Barron, 1958). Imagination somehow belonged to general psychology and was seen as a natural and universal function of mind, as well known to inner experience as to outer expression.

76

Creativity *is* in fact more of a social outcome, marked by certain kinds of behavior and having utilitarian value.

There is also some justice in the observation that interest in creativity began to wane as the decade of the 1960s drew to a close. But again, mass behavior and social values were the main factors in this waxing and waning. There had been a sort of self-conscious creativity in the way that social innovations and changes in style were embraced in the psychedelic sixties, and when it proved hollow, or at least not yet sound enough to endure in the face of practical problems, creativity itself got a bad name.

Meanwhile, however, a solid body of research, ready for a less obtrusive but pragmatically important role, continued to accumulate. The work in the 1950s and early 1960s had established a beachhead that would be ready for a breakout at a propitious time. I think the image appropriate; creativity was not at all unlike an invasion, resisted, or at least not altogether welcome, in conventional, mainstream psychology.

A look backward at that period of creative ferment seems very much in order, however, now that we can say with some assurance that it did lead on to a well-established body of knowledge and to excellent techniques of measurement and identification. That disciplined knowledge remains somewhat underused, as a matter of fact, considering the impressive validity of some of the measures and methods. But there has now been a resurgence of social interest in creativity, especially in the applied aspects of selection and training, as well as in idea production. This renewed interest is far from faddish, and it is not simply a late blooming that can be expected soon to fade. The first rapid growth of research got its impetus from the situation of nation and world in those wide-open days that followed World War II, when anything seemed possible to the intelligence and the technological aptitudes of humanity. This second growth comes from the sudden awareness, finally, that reality has indeed changed, that the problems of human beings are now threatening the well-being of the planet, and that the species itself is in really serious danger of extinction. There is no other way to read the world situation as we approach the end of the twentieth century. Creativity is needed more than ever before. New adaptations are necessary. The matter is urgent. If psychology can be of use, especially in the ways in which it has proved itself most conspicuously – measurement of abilities, identification of talent, selection for challenging assignments, intensive training, behavior change, and encouragement of new ways of thinking – then it should be at the ready and should make its readiness known.

The ingredients of creativity

Creativity as an applied discipline began for me in the decade of the 1980s when a vice-president of Chevron USA called me at my office to ask if I could "spotlight the ingredients of creativity." The image of a huge tank brimful of creativity, each element distinctly colored, leaped to my mind and stayed there as I heard the rest of the story: that Chevron was putting together a very large museum exhibit on the theme "Creativity: The Human Resource," and it was to be organized around a list of ingredients. I allowed as how I could oblige, and we soon agreed on a time and place for getting it on the road.

In the ensuing months I did literally hit the road from Santa Cruz every Saturday to get together in San Francisco with Bruce Burdick, head of the well-known environmental design company, the Burdick Group, which was in fact responsible for the entire exhibit. (I was chief psychological consultant, but I would not want to be seen as claiming more credit than is my due; this was Bruce Burdick's show, and Chevron's.)The ingredients, as we worked them out, were the following:

1. Recognizing patterns
2. Making connections
3. Taking risks
4. Challenging assumptions
5. Taking advantage of chance
6. Seeing in new ways

As it turned out, the exhibit *was* huge, weighing 60 tons when crated for shipment. We incorporated in it some of the psychological tests of metaphorical ability and contingent thinking I shall discuss here, putting them into an interactive computer terminal format that allowed visitors to play at the tests. We also developed a series of lessons in creativity, for use by schools, packaged with a film strip on the topic "Creativity, The Human Resource" (Elliot Eisner, professor of art and education at Stanford, was my coproducer on this). Some 12,000 copies of the film and instructor's manual were distributed free on request to schools in the urban areas in which the exhibit was shown.

Finally, one-third of the exhibit was organized around 18 creative careers of contemporary Americans. Documents and artifacts, supported by many photographs and videotaped interviews of the creative people whose achievements were thus celebrated, were organized in display units so that viewers could see contained within a small space the historical record of these achievements and the persons responsible for them.

In brief, the exhibit "Creativity: The Human Resource" put on display a coherent set of ideas, images, words, and persons as instruments of creativity. And this indeed is how creativity works: through a motivated, purposeful, acting *self* using imagination, reason, and the astonishing human ability to put experience into words. The exhibit traveled the nation as planned, entertaining and instructing more than 5 million people in 21 major cities, and it can be counted a great success. At this point down the road, "Creativity: The Human Resource" is parked permanently in the Pacific Science Center in Seattle, where it continues to be viewed by large numbers of visitors each year.

In spite of the joshing I took from my fellow academics, as well as from the Chevron USA people, who never failed to refer to me as "professor" and to make some remarks about the ivory tower when we met, I felt this to be a very worthwhile use of the knowledge I had gained from the preceding three decades of my research on creativity. As for the ivory tower, there was some justice in the jibes. The Social Sciences Building, now Clark Kerr Hall, at the University of California, Santa Cruz, cannot be seen from anywhere on campus until one is at the door. It is tucked safely into a grove of redwood trees, and the Performing Arts Building shelters it from passersby on the main road. Fortunately, there is some research on mapping going on on the fourth floor, in the cognitive psychology section, and indeed one needs a very good map to get to Social Sciences. Without belaboring the point, I think our tower in the redwoods an excellent metaphor for the social sciences vis-à-vis public policy, a virtual paradigm of the times.

A consensus about creativity

Although I had been amenable to the notion of analyzing creativity into its ingredients, I could be so easy about it because a lot of defining and spotlighting had already gone on. Creativity by 1980 had at last merited a 10-year review in the *Annual Review of Psychology* (Barron & Harrington, 1981). A full reading of research on the topic from 1970 to 1980 gave an impression of sustained activity in empirical psychological approaches to what by now was a field of psychology in itself. Consider these topics that had emerged as dominant: creativity in women; hemispheric specialization opposing right brain to left as the source of intuition, metaphor, and imagery; the contribution of altered states of consciousness to creative thinking; new methods of analysis of biographical material and a vigorous new approach to the study of genius and creativity by way of generational analysis and historiometry; the relationship of thought disorder to originality; the inheritance of intellectual and personal traits important to creativity; the enhancement of creativity by training; creativity and politics; creative environments. In the years from 1970 to 1980, publications in the field had been fairly constant in number, averaging about 250 per year. This variety naturally cost something in the way of uniformity, but in all of it a core of shared premises could be found. Creativity is central to all of psychology; it is general psychology, and it reaches out to philosophy, the arts and humanities, the natural sciences, and human affairs generally in its ramifications.

I myself had authored the first *Encyclopaedia Britannica* article on the subject (Barron, 1963a), and I was aware even then of a substantial consensus among scholars. When I reviewed the field again for an article in the *Encyclopedia Americana* some 10 years later (Barron, 1971), difficulties of interpretation of empirical results had become manifest, but the conceptual consensus was, if anything, stronger. The increasing appearance of contradictory findings noted in the most recent review, the *Social Sciences Encyclopedia* article on creativity (Barron & Harrington, 1985), was due at least in part to failures of cross-validation when unreliable measures and haphazardly chosen samples had been used by investigators who had only a sketchy knowledge of the now voluminous literature. It was due also, however, to an increasing maturity that has led to finer interpretations and questions. In spite of this appearance of diffusion, certain points of agreement are found again and again in journal articles, unpublished theses, and reviews of the literature:

1. Creativity is an ability to respond *adaptively* to the needs for new approaches and new products. It is essentially the ability to bring something new into existence purposefully, though the process may have unconscious, or subliminally conscious, as well as fully conscious components. Novel adaptation is seen to be in the service of increased flexibility and increased power to grow and/or to survive.

2. The "something new" is usually a *product* resulting from a *process* initiated by a *person*. These are therefore the three modes in which creativity may most easily be studied: as product, as process, as person.

3. The defining properties of these new products, processes, and persons are their originality, their aptness, their validity, their adequacy in meeting a need, and a rather subtle additional property that may be called, simply, *fitness* – esthetic fitness, ecological fitness. optimum form, being "right" as well as original at the moment. The emphasis is on whatever is fresh, novel, unusual, ingenious, clever, and apt.

4. Such creative products are quite various, of course: a novel solution to a problem in mathematics; an invention; the discovery of a new chemical process; the composition of a piece of music, or a poem, or a painting; the forming of a new philosophical or religious system; an innovation in law; a fresh way of thinking about social problems; a breakthrough in ways of treating or preventing a disease; the devising of new ways of controlling the minds of others; the invention of mighty new armaments, both of offense and defense; new ways of taxing the citizens of a country by its government; or simply a change in manners for multitudes of people in a specific period of time (a decade, for example, or a century, or, nowadays, half a decade, for things seem to be speeding up as we approach the millennium).

To these four points I would add these notes of qualification:

5. Many products are processes, and many processes are products. And a person is both a product and a process. Each is in a sense "a field within a field" – a field that never closes, for we are talking about open systems, mutually interdependent, with no hard and fast line dividing product from process from person.

6. Creativity is not just an ability, but a characteristic of evolving systems. Psychology, by asking how and under what conditions novelty appears in human psychological functioning, links itself to the general scientific enterprise of describing the evolution of forms in the natural world. The Greeks spoke of cosmogenesis, the cosmos itself being a system, or an ordered, all-inclusive whole, whose origins were steeped in mystery and lost in time. From chaos came cosmos; out of an infinite, undifferentiated darkness emerged material forms, which evolved continuously. (Furthermore, if one pushes chaos hard, one is likely to find a cosmos in it.)

7. Darkness and light, chaos and order, the unlimited and the limited; these are the terms in which the physical and natural creation were to be understood. And for each of these there is an analogous psychological state. Darkness is akin to the unconscious, light to consciousness.

8. Psychic creation, including the creation of the self, is a form of evolution. It is part of the evolution of consciousness. A new kind of person is potentially a step in evolution.

9. Psychic creation is also an analogue to sexual procreation. Its stages are conception (in a prepared matrix), gestation (through time, in intricately coordinated forms and sequences), parturition (the suffering to be born, the emergence to light of the new), and – let us not forget! – the bringing up of baby (a further period of realization and responsibility following the birth of the idea or image or new self).

10. Creation goes hand in hand with destruction. De-structuration often must precede the building of new structures. The strife between opposites is an important source of energy for an evolving new synthesis. In brief, there is a thorn to the rose: Watch out! Good, bad, or indifferent, creativity does not ask permission; it simply arrives. Change is incessant and inescapable, and most mutations are lethal. New needs will require new ways of looking at things – and often the unfamiliar is distasteful and upsetting.
11. Finally, and above all (for this is frequently overlooked in the psychology of creativity), innovations need to be entertained with criticism, wisdom, and responsibility if they are to serve human purposes and "the relief of man's estate." It is up to society to receive or to reject the gift (or sometimes just the imposed will) of the innovator. (The "new order" is not always what we need, and it may even take a lot of effort to defeat!)

The Berkeley studies of creativity, 1950–1970

Much has indeed been learned about creativity since 1950, when its empirical study by test and experiment may fairly be said to have begun in earnest. Wartime selection of combat crews for the U.S. Air Force and of men for irregular warfare assignments by the Office of Strategic Services (OSS) had led to a lot of practical knowledge about how to pick people for resourcefulness, flexibility, courage, and, yes, creativity. "Creativity" was not yet a word being used by the military, but in fact the men and women who had been recruited by the Manhattan Project for the making of the atomic bomb were chosen above all for their intellectual creativity, both theoretical and applied.

When the war ended, most of the gentleman-scholars who had rallied to the cause of fighting the fascist powers returned to the universities that had been the congenial settings for the development of the ways of thinking and the techniques of assessment they had applied so effectively in fighting the enemy. But they returned with a lot of leftover curiosity about just what they had been doing. Psychologists in particular had theoretical questions about the nature and measurement of creativity, questions about the validity of the techniques they had been pressed into using, and curiosity, even eagerness, about new, nonmilitary applications.

Many lines of inquiry began separately, in this or that university. It fell to my lot to become involved in the work initiated in 1949–50 at the University of California, Berkeley, under the leadership of Donald W. MacKinnon, who had headed the main station of the OSS Selection Service. Given the directorship of the newly established Institute of Personality Assessment and Research (IPAR), MacKinnon began to recruit for a rather different purpose and to launch a program of research into "effective functioning," a term that was made to embrace originality, personal soundness, and professional success.

The IPAR staff in 1949 was an unlikely assemblage of psychologists, particularly so in view of its high morale and its strong identity as a unit. It was enthusiastically pledged to new explorations in psychology; yet it represented perspectives somewhat alien to one another, even then. There were two psychoanalysts (Erik H.

Erikson and R. Nevitt Sanford), two clinical psychologists (Robert E. Harris and Harrison G. Gough), an experimental social psychologist grounded in the gestalt tradition in cognitive psychology (Richard S. Crutchfield), two more or less uncommitted graduate research assistants (Ronald Taft and myself), and the director of the institute, Professor MacKinnon, a personologist in the Harvard Psychological Clinic tradition, but with a strong interest also in the work of Kurt Lewin and "the life space."

MacKinnon, as noted, had come to Berkeley from the OSS, where he had played a key role in selecting men for behind-the-lines operations during World War II. Erikson was already known internationally as a leading psychoanalytic theorist of the life cycle, and he had also written one of the first published psychoanalytical interpretations of Hitler. Sanford was the leading figure in the Berkeley studies of racial prejudice, especially anti-Semitism, and authoritarianism. And all three had been intimately involved in the seminal work in American personology, Henry A. Murray's *Explorations in Personality*.

Crutchfield, too, had been prominent in American military psychology. He headed the U.S. Strategic Bombing Survey at the conclusion of the war, gathering and making sense of a mass of survey and interview data. Harris was chief psychologist at Langley Porter Clinic, doing research on stress and its psychosomatic consequences, as well as on prognosis in psychotherapy. Gough had just completed his doctoral work at the University of Minnesota, where he had worked closely with Paul Meehl and Herbert McCloskey on the measurement of sociopolitical attitudes as aspects of personality. Taft was an Australian, interested naturally enough in patterns of immigration and in the logic of prediction.

I had come to Berkeley psychology by way of Cambridge University and the University of Minnesota. I had brought with me the influences of Frederic C. Bartlett, whose seminar on thinking and remembering I had taken at Cambridge, and Richard M. Elliott, through a tutorial devoted to the concept of the self in the psychology of William James. Imagery, words, and schemata were the main topics in Bartlett's seminar, as they were in his classic book, *Remembering*. His seminar meshed for me with the Clark Lectures, given that year (1946) at Cambridge by the poet C. Day Lewis under the title *The Poetic Image* (Lewis, 1946).

The development of measures, experiments, interviews, and theoretical frameworks proceeded apace at IPAR. These new measures, experiments, and techniques, several dozen in all, were used through two decades of research with groups of subjects chosen for some special reason, usually related to creativity and/or personal effectiveness. The special reason often included also a declared career intention, or membership in a recognized profession. Thus, we studied groups as diverse as doctoral candidates in the natural and social sciences, flying officers in the military, psychological warfare officers, physicians, mathematicians, writers, architects, artists, engineers, businessmen, and mountain climbers.

It would be quite impossible for me in this brief space to give even a summary account of the results of the IPAR studies, which after all have found publication in several hundred professional journal articles and several books. I have elected therefore to limit myself to the development of measures arising from my own philosophic, literary, and esthetic interests. This allows me to focus on what I know best, while yet permitting a reasonable range in considering the more general aspects of creativity.

Berkeley as laboratory, Cambridge as catalyst

My first publications as a staff member of the Berkeley group dealt mainly with personality variables measured by verbal questionnaires: *basic religious beliefs, independence of judgment,* and a postulated personality dimension that I called *complexity of outlook.* This latter variable seemed to cut across the well-known conservative–liberal dimension in religion, politics, and social issues; I was thus led to construct a set of scales for inclusion in a comprehensive *inventory of personal philosophy.* But I had worked from the outset in developing quite another set of measures, cognitive in nature, with emphasis on visual images and words. The first of these was a measure of preferences among visual displays, in which *symmetry* and *asymmetry, simplicity* and *complexity,* were the chief dimensions. A second was an attempted simplification, both as to metric and stimulus complexity, of a scale for the dispositional tendency to give "human movement" responses to inkblots, introducing the concept of threshold and of precisely graded evocative power in the stimuli themselves. A third set of measures was concentrated on discernment of patterns within congeries of letters and words – from anagrams to jumbled sentences (word rearrangement) to compositional tasks in which the respondent was given a set of nouns, verbs, and adjectives to be woven into a story (with instructions to use the given words and as few others as possible to achieve coherence). The aim of all this psychometric effort was to study *the transformation of images,* in modes ranging from the literal to the highly symbolic.

Theory, at that point, certainly was taking a back seat to what was simply a frontal attack, with both barrels blazing, on the obvious fact that the ability to change things – to produce or even just to allow transformations – is central to the creative process. New forms do not come from nothing, not for us humans at any rate; they come from prior forms, through mutations, whether unsought or invited. In a fundamental sense, there are no theories of creation; there are only accounts of the development of new forms from earlier forms.

Granting this, one would, of course, like to know about the conditions under which novelty is most likely to emerge or can be most easily produced. In the human case, the study of lives, with special attention to periods of high creativity and to decisive events in the production of important innovations, offered itself as a difficult but most promising method. At the same time, transformations that could be produced in the laboratory, if not by precise experiment then at least in a standard format for observation, should be given special attention.

This was a point of view I had had impressed on me in the Psychological

Laboratory at Cambridge, where I had spent the Lent term in 1946 while still in service with the U.S. Army. The extraordinary vividness with which I still recall that brief term at Cambridge comes, in part, I am sure, because it succeeded so soon the war's ending. The intensity of the experience came, too, from the contrast between combat zone and quad, the disorder and sometimes near meaninglessness of the war and the tranquillity and hard-core reasonableness of the university. Suddenly it had become possible to reflect on events in the round: the actions in which I had taken part as a combat medic, the savagery of the bombing of cities, the shock of the concentration camps, and, finally, the birth and use of The Bomb, that startling announcement by unexampled violence of intellect's most awesome triumph. Reality had indeed changed; there was that fact to absorb, to think about. Creativity had taken on a new meaning. Humanity had a new image in its mind's eye: the mushroom cloud of the atomic bomb. It had a new word: Hiroshima.

Image and word, meaning and changes in meaning – these were the very themes in Bartlett's seminar. By chance, C. Day Lewis in the Clark Lectures (*The Poetic Image*) was focusing on the same themes, and because my interests were as much in literature as in psychology, I attended both. (It was not really by chance, of course, because Lewis was wrestling with new images and needed new words to express new meanings, as we all did.)

One evening, midway in the lecture series, the poet spoke to a point that was to become a central concern for me in the psychology of creativity. It was, though he had different words for it, the problem of gestalt transformation in memory. Later I was to deal with it as a productive thinking ability, *symbolic scope,* with emphasis on individual differences. Its elements are both images (in a variety of sensory modalities) and words. The process requires the recognition of patterns, and the genesis, spontaneous or sought, of one pattern from another.

Lewis began his lecture, "The Living Image," with two examples from his own experience:

A poet, lying half awake one night on the seacoast of North Devon, listened to the sound of a storm. The sound presently could be separated into three – a diapason roar, quite steady, which was the wind chiefly but augmented by a continuous growling of the sea; a higher, hissing note, variable in pitch and volume but no less intermittent, given off by the surf seething forward and then sucked back down the pebbles; and, behind these, a rhythmical, not quite regular throbbing – the beat of the waves on the beach. . . . He was suddenly transported to a day in childhood, when he stood on a platform at a London terminus beside an express engine. The sound this engine made was identical with the storm. There was a high irregular hiss of steam blowing off, the deep roar of the forced draught in the furnace, and the same rhythmical throbbing, all blended into one.

Another time, the poet was looking out of his bedroom window in blitzed London. A searchlight practice was on. The beams swung about the sky, then leaned together like the framework of a wigwam, and at the apex an aircraft could be seen, silver, moth-like, flying slowly, found, lost, found again by the searchlights. It was a common enough sight just then . . . but this time the poet saw it differently, as a dramatic paradox; it seemed to him that candle-beams were desirously searching for the moth. (Lewis, 1946)

Lewis had gone on to use these examples as point of departure for an inquiry into a more specific question. As he put it, "How far can the poet successfully make use of objects like aeroplanes and engines in metaphor?" But my own imagination had been attracted by the more general problem: first, the process of transformation of the presenting image, and then the originality, complexity, and aptness of the correlative image, whether produced or recalled (recognized, if you will).

This led directly to the first procedure I constructed for the IPAR studies of creativity. Though it goes under the name Symbolic Equivalence Test, it is not so much a test as an occasion for observing the process whereby a standard stimulus image is changed by design into a nonliteral or symbolic image that is recognizably another version of the original configuration.

The transformation of images

To study the process of transformation of images, I betook myself first to declared poets. I began by proposing rather complex images, similar to the two examples from C. Day Lewis. "A twig is floating down a stream, reaches a point in the flowing water where a log has been thrown across it, spins slowly in the swirls of water set up by the log, finally gets around the log and floats on." Or, "a single white car, parked all by itself at midnight on a black macadam parking lot, under a flashing neon sign."

Images like these proved too difficult, or at least unappealing to my subjects. Then I remembered a synopsis for children of Melville's *Moby Dick,* presented really as a good fishing story (which, after all, it is). The contrast between checkers and chess came to mind; children of age six can play checkers and have fun at it, and in fact they usually think they are playing very well; chess is closed to them, unless they can make checkers out of it. I wanted to construct a test that could be used through a wide age range and at quite different levels of ability. And so I discovered the important principle: Keep it simple, and let the respondent make it complex. In the lingo of test builders, do not put a ceiling on it, and make the floor as low as possible.

This is an important point in the psychology of creativity. For the creative solution is not known beforehand, and there is an immense range of possibility for new developments once we get deep into a problem. Not only are there no "right or wrong" answers, there really are no "answers" at all, until they have been tested in someone else's perception, or by external reality. And the criterion centers on qualities like "fitness," "surprise," "novelty," "ingenuity," and even "adequacy in meeting a need" (for something equivalent, of course; a common enough demand in life).

In this sense, the Symbolic Equivalence Test had in it the main requirements for both the creative process and the creative product. Though essentially a laboratory procedure, it condensed some of the most important practical features of conditions for creativity in life in the large. Think for a moment of these problems in psychological theory: (1) the specification of the properties of a pattern in determining *stimulus equivalence* and *response equivalence* for the study of generalization in learning; (2) the recognition in dreams and in neurotic symptom formation of the equivalence of images – traumatic events and their consequences, for example – or the mechanisms of substitution and displacement in dream figures, not to mention personages in one's "real" life who are chosen for love, hate, or indifference simply on the basis of their symbolic equivalence to someone else who had been there earlier; (3) the changes a scene may undergo in memory – the whole problem that set gestalt psychology afire, that is, the retention in memory of the transformed gestalt features rather than the more elementary or component features of the original stimulus pattern; (4) all the many personifications of Fate, the Soul, the Race, the Homeland, seasons and skies, and passages from birth to death – the images the Greeks named archetypes.

To give concreteness to some of these transformations, examples drawn from the Symbolic Equivalence Test procedure itself may be useful. The instructions to the respondent are as follows:

In this test, you will be asked to think of metaphors, or symbolically equivalent images, for certain suggested stimulus images. The task can best be made clear by an example.
EXAMPLE:
Suggested stimulus image:
        Leaves being blown in the wind.
Possible symbolic equivalents:
        A civilian population fleeing chaotically in the face of armed aggression.
        Handkerchiefs being tossed about inside an electric dryer.
        Chips of wood borne downstream by a swiftly eddying current.

The test example was not chosen with any particular poetic equivalent in mind. Shelley's "Ode to the West Wind," however, is an elegant, sustained example of "an equivalent." Recall the opening lines of that great poem, and the images that run through the five stanzas:

        Oh wild West Wind, thou breath of Autumn's being,
            Thou, from whose unseen presence the leaves dead
        Are driven, like ghosts from an enchanter fleeing,
            Yellow, and black, and pale, and hectic red.
        Pestilence-stricken multitudes . . .

What has Shelley done, if we imagine this to be an elaboration of an image of "leaves being blown in the wind"?

1. He has specified the wind, to make it the wind of autumn, and therefore the dying of the year.
2. He has made the presence of oncoming death unseen, save in its effects on the leaves – presumably once green, they have lost the sap of springtime and the vigorous hue of summer and are now pale, black, yellow, or hectic red, the last overwhelmed fling of impulse.
3. The leaves are driven like ghosts, fleeing from a tyrannical enchanter; they are scurrying, eager to get away.

4. The leaves are multitudes: frightened exiles, old folks and orphans, all homeless, driven by the onward rush of pestilence, an unchecked destructive power.

Interestingly enough, the possible answers suggested in the test example do have the idea in them of a chaos within a coherence (the tossed handkerchiefs, the bereft victims of the winds, of the pestilence, of war, the speed and the chance eddies of a current immensely stronger and deeper than the chips of wood; the chips are particles, like the leaves, and they are massed yet in disorder and subject to the whims of the greater natural power).

Shelley goes on to invoke the cycle of the seasons to offer hope:

> The winged seeds, where they lie cold and low,
> Each like a corpse within its grave, until
> Thine azure sister of the Spring shall blow
> Her clarion o'er the dreaming earth . . .

And then, rebirth from the ashes and the unextinguished creative spark:

> Drive my dead thoughts over the universe,
> Like wither'd leaves, to quicken a new birth;
>
> Scatter, as from an unextinguished hearth
> Ashes and sparks, my words among mankind.

Poems did come from some of our test stimulation, I might add, and although Shelley was not there, we did "assess" some famous writers and architects who have a claim to genius. A test response is not yet a poem, of course; the complex integral act is a very different matter, as we never forgot.

But back to the laboratory. Following the example, the test respondent is instructed to make up three possible equivalents for each of 10 images. A time limit of 20 min is used for this form of the test. The stimulus images are as follows: haystacks seen from an airplane; a train going into a tunnel; the sound of a foghorn; a candle burning low; a ship lost in fog; a floating feather; the increasing loud and steady sound of a drum; sitting alone in a dark room; empty bookcases; tall trees in the middle of a field.

The Symbolic Equivalence Test was scored for (1) number of acceptable or admissible, but not original, responses and (2) number of original responses. Admissible responses were in turn differentiated as to degree of aptness, scored as 1, 2, or 3; original responses were differentiated as to degree of originality, scored as 4 or 5. The total score on the test was simply the sum of the ratings of the individual responses. For purposes of analysis, several additional subscores were defined: percentage of original responses; absolute number of original responses; absolute number of responses (admissible plus original).

Here are some examples:

1. Stimulus image:
   A candle burning low
   Admissible responses:
   Life ebbing away   (scored 1)

A basin of water emptying down a drain   (scored 2)
The last drops of coffee going through a filter   (scored 3)
The last pages of a faded book   (scored 4)
The last hand in a gambler's last card game   (scored 5)

2. Stimulus image:
   Empty bookcase
   Admissible responses:
   A hollow log   (scored 1)
   An empty sack   (scored 2)
   An abandoned beehive   (scored 3)
   An arsenal without weapons   (scored 4)
   A haunted house   (scored 5)

3. Stimulus image:
   Sitting alone in a dark room
   Admissible responses:
   Lying awake at night   (scored 1)
   An unborn child   (scored 2)
   A stone under water   (scored 3)
   A king lying in a coffin   (scored 4 or 5)
   Milton   (scored 5)

Even the lowest ranking of admissible responses moves some distance from the literal correspondence, as these examples show. To be admissible at all, the response must reproduce the main features of the stimulus image, which included formal properties as well as functional relationships among them. A candle burning low, for example, includes prominently (1) a source of light and perhaps heat, (2) a process that uses up a supply of something, and (3) visible evidence that the process is coming to a close. An empty bookcase has the characteristics that (1) it is a container, (2) its earlier or usual contents are many and can be numbered, and (3) the contents were valuable or useful. Sitting alone in a dark room (1) implies a personal presence, (2) combines solitariness with darkness, and (3) specifies an enclosure.

Original responses are, first of all, unusual. Once a catalogue of responses has been assembled from many subjects, an unusual response is easily recognized. To be highly original, or to get the highest rating, the response should have additional dimensions: It grabs you, it surprises you, it gives you a chill as a great line of poetry can do. And even here there are degrees of elegance. A king in a coffin is unusual and gripping as an image; a king in his grave might perhaps be better (or perhaps not); Milton (after his blindness, we are left to understand) is the greatest of kings in the darkest of rooms.

Needless to say, there are problems in scoring, in this as in all imaginal productions. Literal (concrete, physical) complexity must be distinguished from conceptual complexity; the preferences of the raters for complex versus simple phenomenal fields must be taken into account; the ability of the rater to recognize transformations and to differentiate them as to quality must be reckoned with.

The Symbol Equivalence Test as a measure of individual differences in symbolic scope

Eventually the Symbol Equivalence Test was administered to several hundred very creative people in the IPAR studies of artists, architects, writers, mathematicians, scientists, and mountain climbers (these mountain climbers, by the way, were the first American team to ascend Mount Everest, and the first team ever to do it by the West Ridge – a strenuous way to challenge assumptions, take advantage of chance and the weather, see things in a new way, take risks, and so forth). The climbers were "assessed" just before they left San Francisco for Nepal in 1963, accompanied, to be sure, by an IPAR staff member, Dr. James T. Lester, Jr., who made the climb with them and assiduously got them to tell him their dreams en route.

The validity of the Symbol Equivalence Test as an ability measure proved quite substantial. First of all, it provided a clear rank ordering by creativity of samples studied, highly correlated with group rank when they were rated independently for overall verbal creativity. Famous writers topped all groups, followed by famous architects, and then in turn by (1) mathematicians at the Institute for Advanced Study in Princeton, (2) women mathematicians who had been rated as the most creative in their field in the United States, (3) successful entrepreneurs in Ireland, (4) the Mount Everest team, (5) research scientists, (6) student artists at the San Francisco Art Institute, and finally a mélange of "opportunity samples" who were assessed by test only and for a variety of reasons during the 1950s and early 1960s at IPAR. An important point here is that the test responses were scored by an elaborate, laborious, and expensive procedure in which every response image was rated independently by three skilled raters without knowledge of other responses given by the same subject, and also, of course, without knowledge of the individual's name or group membership. (Later, by the way, I used the norms thus established to develop a mechanically scored multiple-choice form of the test, Symbol Equivalence II.)

The Symbol Equivalence Test scores were then correlated with external criterion ratings of creativity of each subject in relation to all others in the relevant professional group. Substantial positive, statistically significant correlations were found for writers, architects, artists, and entrepreneurs. Details of these studies are available elsewhere (Barron, 1969).

In brief, a relatively short and simple test, taking half an hour of administration time and another half hour for a trained scorer to evaluate, has demonstrated substantial validity for measurement of a key component of creativity: the ability to make original and apt transformations of a given image, received in words and expressed in words.

Originality in producing symbol equivalences has been correlated with other measures as well in several of the samples. Research with student artists provides a good example (Barron, 1972b). In that study, the subjects were 92 art students in studio classes at the San Francisco Art Institute. They took a battery of psychological tests at the beginning of their first year of studio work. The test battery included a scale for rating oneself on creativity, an adjective self-description questionnaire scored on an "artistic self-concept" key, the Barron Independence of Judgment and the Barron Complexity of Outlook scales, and the following set of performance measures: the McGurk Perceptual Acuity Test, the Barron M-Threshold Inkblot series, the Gottschaldt Embedded Figures, the Franck Drawing Completion Test (Barron, 1958), and two forms of Symbol Equivalence: Form I, free response (scored for originality) and Form II, multiple choice (scored for "recognition of originality").

The two forms of the Symbol Equivalence Test used were SE-I, scored for overall quality, and SE-II, scored for recognition of originality, a multiple-choice format presenting two alternative responses to each stimulus image, one of which had been rated "commonplace" and the other "original" in the earlier normative study. The instruction to the test respondent on SE-II was to "pick the more original response." The overall free-response quality score showed a high positive correlation with other variables in the test battery and in studio performance were quite similar: significant positive r's with perceptual acuity (accuracy of perceptual judgment and resistance to illusion), ability to recognize a previously seen pattern embedded in a more complex pattern, quality of drawing on a standardized drawing completion test, and independence of judgment and complexity of outlook on two inventory scales, and finally, and most important to the Admissions Office, substantial correlations (.60) with studio grades. Grades, in turn, by the middle of the third year at the Art Institute, were correlated positively in the neighborhood of .50 to .60 with initial self-ratings, complexity of outlook, consequences, and a strong tendency to perceive human movement in the Barron M-Threshold Inkblot series (as well as with the scores on SE-I and SE-II).

These findings reflect what is generally considered the core of the metaphoric or analogical process. They add up to a picture of substantial construct validity as well as predictive validity for the Symbol Equivalence procedure. But what of transformations more dependent on rational imagination, logical processes, contingent thinking? These, too, are decisively important in creativity, particularly in the disciplines and professions that make things happen in the great world – science, technology, law, politics, business, the military.

Transformations in the service of prediction and control

Poets are supposed to be impractical. Planners are not. Contingent thinking, or discursive reason applied to problems of prediction, is the mark of the practical individual. These are stereotypes, of course, but like most stereotypes, there is some truth to them.

Stereotypes become most misleading when they are personified. John Doe is a poet – ergo, impractical. Jane Roe is in business – ergo, bound to dollars and cents, the bottom line.

There are indeed archetypal poets and archetypal merchants, but we avoid the danger of stereotypes if we think in terms not of persons but of modes. In creativity, the analogical mode often is at war with the logical, but the creative act issues from the tension between the two. One without the other is lost.

Creative people are equally capable of the logical and the analogical, are open alike to the rational and the nonrational, are at home to image and to abstraction. This hypothesis argues for another sort of test, a measure of rational thinking in the domain of action, or at least of anticipation of the consequences of an action or event.

Several such tests had already been developed elsewhere by 1950, and IPAR put two of them to use in its assessment program. One was the Bennett Test of Productive Thinking. For an example of its use, see the chapter "An Odd Fellow" in *Creativity and Psychological Health* (Barron, 1963b). It asks questions such as "What would happen if the mean level of the oceans were to drop 5 feet?" Another test, developed by J. P. Guilford and his colleagues, was the Consequences test cited earlier, similar in format to the Bennett test. For example: "What would be the result of . . . if everyone could read everyone else's mind?" The tests were scored in slightly different ways, but basically they were made to measure the ability to produce ideas about the future given certain contingencies.

I developed a scoring scheme for the Bennett test based on the dichotomies of banality–originality and practicality–cosmicality. It was evident from the outset that the content of the test (i.e., the specified contingencies) was highly modifiable, and I soon began using the test with items composed for specific purposes. In our study of Irish entrepreneurs, for example, I made up a "Consequences for Ireland" form of the Consequences Test. Working with State of California heads of divisions in a workshop sponsored by the California Management Institute, I proposed contingencies relevant to planning for the future in California (water, population, immigration, the master plan for education, etc.). For a meeting of the Society of Gynecological Laparoscopists, I gathered data on "what would happen if *in vitro* methods for fertilization of human ova became medically safe and inexpensive?" This latter question is part of my own form of the test, now known as the "What-If Test," to elicit people's thinking about what would happen given certain contingencies in the "nuclear–space–computer" age, especially concerning nuclear arms and nuclear energy situations.

The point of all this is that tests like Symbol Equivalences and What-Ifs can be adapted to virtually any set of problems and can be coordinated with one another. They are extremely effective as points of departure for workshops and can be used not only to activate imaginal processes but also to focus practical discussions. By choosing stimulus images from the contingencies themselves, the analogical mode can be used to enrich the analytic and predictive mode. I am sufficiently encouraged by results I have obtained in workshops to believe that rigorous experimentation along this line would pay off. In effect, the construction of symbolic equivalences for practical terms in a contingent thinking problem is a way of "looking aside" and of energizing abstract reason by metaphor and nonliteral images.

One example may suffice. In a group workshop setting, I divided the participants into two working committees. The task of Committee A was to bring in recommendations on how to spend a given amount of civic funding for a Senior Citizens Center. The task of Committee B was set by reading to them the opening lines of Coleridge's poem "Kubla Khan," known in the creativity literature because of the alleged interruption of Coleridge's reverie by the infamous "traveler from Porlock."

> In Xanadu did Kubla Khan
>   A stately pleasure dome decree
> Where Alph the sacred river ran
>   Through caverns measureless to man
>   Down to a sunless sea.

The question for Committee B was, "What sort of stately pleasure dome would *you* decree?" (The symbolic equivalence is here quite complex, of course, because the poem hints of last pleasures before descent to the eternal shade.)

This was an unpublished study, but I did count the ideas and evaluate their originality under two conditions for each subject: serving on Committee A first versus Committee B first. The prior "thinking-aside" condition employing the Coleridge poem as a symbolic equivalent led to much greater originality when the "real contingency" was presented.

Personal philosophy and creativity

Recall that symbolic scope as measured by the Symbol Equivalence Test proved to be highly correlated in art students with two of the measures I had developed in the early 1950s as part of the "tooling-up" process for the IPAR studies: (1) independence of judgment and (2) complexity of outlook. These two variables, measured by inventory scales, are now part of the "Inventory of Personal Philosophy" (an unpublished values inventory developed for research by the present author and available from him on request). Both measures were found in early studies to be substantially predictive of a wide range of characteristics associated with creativity, including cognitive measures of flexibility as well as social traits indicative of acceptance of racial group differences (low ethnocentrism), changing mores sexually, ecumenical attitudes in matters of religious belief, and internationalism.

The scale for measuring independence of judgment was developed in collaboration with Solomon Asch and was based on significant item correlations with independent (nonyielding to conformity pressures) behavior in the Asch experiments (Barron, 1953b). The Complexity of Outlook scale was developed (Barron, 1953a) by successive item analyses in several samples against preference for complex-asymmetrical versus simple-symmetrical visual displays (the Barron-Welsh Art Scale). Extensive use of the verbal scale in succeeding samples provided the basis for naming it Complexity of Outlook.

The two scales rest on a powerful theoretical base with ramifications in scientific and artistic creativity. To see things as they are, not as the conforming masses would have one see them, is the hallmark of realistic unconventionality. It requires accuracy of perception, persistence in seeking the truth, and personal force and courage in resisting the inevitable pressures to conform. The famous Asch experiments condensed these requirements into the experimental social situation he devised.

To prefer a complex phenomenal display is not in itself a mark of creativity, unless it is coupled with an unrelenting drive to find a simple order. Simplicity in complexity, unity in variety – these are the criteria for beauty and elegance, in art, mathematics, science, and personal consciousness in general.

A coupling of these two characteristics, independence of judgment and complexity of outlook, is potentiated by symbolic scope and by contingent thinking that is both realistic and searching.

Strong support for this idea is provided by recent results. In a 1983 lecture (Barron, 1983) I reported correlations between scales of the Inventory of Personal Philosophy and originality as measured by What-If Test responses to nuclear contingency items. (Examples: What would happen if the ozone layer were destroyed? What if terrorists were to obtain possession of a dozen thermonuclear weapons? What if one country and no others were to develop an impenetrable defense against ICBMs? What if a limited nuclear war were to begin in the Middle East? Originality in responding to these questions was correlated positively in the neighborhood of .50 with both Independence of Judgment and Complexity of Outlook, and negatively with Ethnocentrism (.35).

An item analysis of the entire inventory in its 1983 revision showed that many items specific to attitudes about nuclear arms control, scored so as to reflect a belief that an immediate freeze on nuclear testing and substantial reductions in nuclear weapons worldwide would be highly desirable, were also correlated highly with both Independence of Judgment and Complexity of Outlook. The Inventory of Personal Philosophy (IPP) had been expanded in 1983 to include 45 items related not only to arms control but also to ecological concerns, space exploration, belief in the likelihood of extraterrestrial intelligence, and internationalism or "global consciousness" in general. Twenty-nine of these new items were found to constitute independent factors in the IPP, and further work established the scale as an important differentiator of attitudes in samples in West Germany as well as in Arizona and California (Bradley, 1984). A subset of 10 of these 29 items, scored as the Nuclear Arms Reduction Scale, was later correlated in those and in additional U.S. and European samples with Independence of Judgment and Complexity of Outlook, yielding *r*'s once again ranging around a mean of .50. Because there was no item overlap, the finding is strongly indicative of a possibility that has been largely overlooked in U.S.–Soviet negotiations: that the true attitudes of negotiators and the actual determinants of outcomes at the negotiating table are personality variables. Political scientists, and even social psychologists, have resisted such interpretations, but these findings deserve further exploration. It is quite possible that creativity is not being put to work on this most critical problem simply because personal traits and tangential philosophical preferences are blocks to creative thinking.

Symbols for self and career

It is easy to lose sight of the self when one is thinking in terms of test factors, even when they refer to such dynamically important variables as personal philosophy, symbolic scope, and contingent thinking. But only the self creates in a sustained manner. To achieve unity of being requires a self to integrate the schemata, the part-selves. And the more original, complexly inclusive, and deeply experienced the self, the greater its power of creativeness.

Note here that I speak of the self, not of "personality." Creative people come in all shapes and sizes, all colors and ages, and all sorts of personality types. There are introverts and extroverts, manics and depressives and manic-depressives, schizothymes and hysterics, sociopaths and good citizens – in brief, a wide variety of temperaments among people who are especially creative. It is not, in my judgment, the personality type that makes the difference, but the self. To the self I ascribe motivation and style, the choice of meaning, and *the making of meaning,* in work, career, life course. It is in the self that opposites are in strife, calling for choice.

"A career is a general course of action through life." This dictionary definition does ask us to think further about "the life course." For psychology, a conceptualization of the life course is very important. The course of life is by no means a straight line, or a series of unbroken circles on the face of the clock. It is not just a progress through time. Lives and careers are spatiotemporal processes that spill over in all directions, hodologically, topologically, hologrammatically. They exist as structures and as ensembles – of other people, of documents, of buildings, of compositions, of the trees we plant and all the other living things we shelter and help to grow; offspring and creations of all sorts, including ruins, alas! These ensembles endure through time and ramify in space; they undergo changes as the world changes and time passes; and some of their effects may be very distant indeed from their point of origin. Start a style, write a poem, provide a method, enjoin others to action – who plants a tree plants a hope – these are creative works not only in themselves but also in their capacity to create new conditions in which the creativity of others may find expression. I like the poem Seamus Heaney wrote for Harvard's 350th birthday, and because we have been hearing from poets in this essay, I yield to the temptation to quote:

> A spirit moved. John Harvard walked the Yard.
> The atom lay unsplit, the West unwon.
> The books stood open, and the gates unbarred.

These words and images celebrate an idea, a place, a space, time and events unforeseen, a moral and intellectual career; they give us a hint of the sometimes brooding quality of creative thought. It is not John Harvard's personality that would interest me, but his self.

Self and creative career

A creative career is the sustaining of creativity in a coherent enterprise, such as a profession or vocation or institution, over a fairly lengthy period of time, from months to years to a virtual lifetime.

To choose a career that is merciless in its demand for creativity is to make a life-staking, often lifelong, commitment. Even to consider such a choice is to engage the deepest resources of the self. This sort of career is intrinsically moral and intellectual in nature. It is not to be chosen idly. It requires an exacting discipline, toil without stint, and sacrifices, and it yields an uncertain reward. And in the eyes of the world, there are losers as well as winners in such careers.

Of course, not all careers need engage the individual in such intense self-development, either as a requirement or as an opportunity. There is a middle ground between that archetypal artist and the archetypal burgher that is being claimed increasingly today. People do want their occupations to be self-expressive. And with increasing mobility and leisure there is more opportunity for us to use our creative potential ad lib. Further, as work itself changes, part of it may call for creativity at times, but not all the time. Creativity in work is a potential whose vitality may endure through long stretches of inactivity and then come into action when called on. There is no *need* to be creative as a life work.

One's life itself is there to create. Family, friends, and associates, personal style, inner experience, general behavior, dress, character – these are creations in the opportunity available to us all as human beings.

It is in personal style, as aspect of selfhood, that I find the ingredients of creativity. Openness to new ways of seeing, intuition, alertness to opportunity, a liking for complexity as a challenge to find simplicity, independence of judgment that questions assumptions, willingness to take risks, unconventionality of thought that allows odd connections to be made, keen attention, and a drive to find pattern and meaning – these, coupled with the motive and the courage to create, give us a picture of the creative self.

Practical steps toward applied creativity

The term "brain drain" is not fully appreciated. The drain is not from one country to another – the emigration of talent from less rewarding places of employment to more rewarding is a small and not very important adjustment. The real drain is the loss of the creativity that stays at home but is not employed properly. And *that* is a worldwide waste: brains down the drain (if one likes that metaphor; I prefer Thomas

Grey's "Elegy in a Country Churchyard," where a "mute inglorious Milton" lies interred). The word is *waste* – a waste of talents.

There are numerous ways in which our resources of creative intelligence are wasted:

1. Creative potential is not identified systematically and nurtured responsibly.

This failure begins in the school system in the elementary grades, and it continues right through the undergraduate years at most colleges. Not until graduate school is there any explicit crediting of creativity as an important qualification for admission to training in independent intellectual work and social leadership.

There are effective means now available for identifying creative potential. In this essay I have focused on three measures of what I consider significant characteristics of creativity: symbolic scope (analogical power), rational imagination (applied to contingent thinking), and two personality traits: (1) independence of judgment and (2) a dynamic tension between the striving for simplicity and the entertaining of complexity. Add to these the *motivation to be creative,* which is open to education and responsive to incentives, and we have the means for identifying and nurturing creativity.

The nurturing of creativity in schools requires, it seems to me, direct instruction aimed at increasing creative thinking abilities: new curricula, new incentives, new teacher training.

2. Established organizations in government, industry, and education do not take creativity as a value and consequently do not make provision for creative use of the creative individuals they employ.

Consider the creativity of university faculties, as an example close at hand for the most likely readers of this essay. Routine committee assignments and routine clerical tasks are uniformly accepted as part of most faculty jobs, and to some extent this is unavoidable and perhaps as it should be. But surely some other institutional means can be found, short of sending people on leave to "think tanks" (small in number), for allowing highly trained academic talent to get together with the explicit goal of considering society's needs for innovation. Interdisciplinary programs may founder when their purpose is defined solely as interdisciplinary, but if the purpose is socially transcendent, rather than merely accommodative of interdisciplinary viewpoints, surely something more creative is possible. I would like to see this tried, not just on university campuses but in other organizations of already highly trained people whose innovative talents are being wasted simply for lack of an organizational structure that would facilitate creative thinking. Explicit use of techniques of rational imagination and the search for symbolic equivalences, as well as other procedures known from research and development in the area of creativity, should be given a chance.

3. There is at present no national or international recognition that creativity is itself a product. We are accustomed to indices such as Gross National Product, the Consumer Price Index, and so on; but where is there the faintest hint that the important reality, a nation's creativity, can be measured, studied, and influenced?

The components of such a National Creativity Index would have to be identified, and the means of measurement established, but the problem surely can be solved. There are countable evidences of artistic, musical, and literary creativity, of technological innovation, of influential changes in government through court decisions, legislation, and executive initiatives. Medicine is already highly organized for appraisal of outcomes from new diagnoses and treatments, delivery of health care, and so on. With effort, we should be able to appraise our level of creativity, nationally and internationally, and pay heed to the cultivation of this human resource. (Nor should we forget creativity's other face: "destructivity.")

4. There are virtually no "centers for research on creativity" in existence, certainly none at the national level. Perhaps we should be wary of a recommendation that there should be. Institutionalization can easily become the burial vault of creativity, and one would want to watch such centers closely. But certainly there is a place for concerted new research efforts in creativity as a discipline. There are untapped resources crying out for research: the creativity of women; use of new technologies (computers, audiovisual educational methods, new environments for creativity); the genetics as well as social psychology of creativity; the role of memory in creation (about which virtually nothing is known); psychotropic drugs and creativity (a topic on which the books should not be closed); emergent social forms in the developing nations; creativity in relation to religion and philosophy.

These are merely hints at the topics needing research. Considering the vastness of this human resource and its crucial importance at this juncture in human development, shamefully little is being done. Where should we begin?

We must first recognize that creativity *is* a human resource, the gift of life to the human species. It is a unique force in the universe.

The main ingredients of creativity have by now been identified. What shall we do with all these ingredients? Put them together properly, and put them to work. There are rivers to be washed, air to be cleaned, mouths to be fed, guns to get rid of, diseases old and new to be conquered, justice to be ensured to all, new opportunities to be created, communication and empathy to be increased, secrets of the cosmos and of the mind to be understood, a changed reality to be comprehended and adapted to.

Applied creativity is not a barbarism, so far as I am concerned. The more we know about creativity, the more use we can make of it for the good of all. It is a gift, a talent to be exercised in the measure to which we have it – one talent or ten, we should put it to work.

The transformative power of imagination, coupled with the will to apply it, and given the means for its cultivation in education, government, and the world economy, is the main source of hope to counter what may otherwise become a pessimism about the human future as the millennium comes to an end. The dark side of the millennium is the possibility that earth, too, may die, even in this generation. Creativity in the face of this darkness is above all a reason for hope, a symbol of the renewal of earth, when new growth begins.

References

Barron, F. (1953a). Complexity–simplicity as a personality dimension. *Journal of Abnormal and Social Psychology, 48*, 163–172.

Barron, F. (1953b). Some personality correlates of independence of judgment. *Journal of Personality, 21*, 287–297.

Barron, F. (1955). Threshold for the perception of human movement in inkblots. *Journal of Consulting Psychology, 19*, 33–38.

Barron, F. (1958). The psychology of imagination. *Scientific American, 199*, 150–166.

Barron, F. (1963a). Creativity (psychology of). *Encyclopaedia Britannica, 6*, 711–712. University of Chicago Press.

Barron, F. (1963b). *Creativity and psychological health.* New York: D. Van Nostrand.

Barron, F. (1969). *Creative person and creative process.* New York: Holt, Rinehart & Winston.

Barron, F. (1971). Genius. *Encyclopedia Americana, 12*, 420. New York: Americana Corp.

Barron, F. (1972a). Towards an ecology of consciousness. *Inquiry, 15*, 95–113.

Barron, F. (1972b). *Artists in the making.* New York: Seminar Press.

Barron, F. (1979). *The shaping of personality.* New York: Harper & Row.

Barron, F. (1983). *The influence of personal philosophy on creative thinking in the nuclear gun-pointing situation.* Faculty research lecture, University of California, Santa Cruz (available from Laboratory for the Study of Lives, UC Santa Cruz).

Barron, F., & Harrington, D. (1981). Creativity, intelligence, and personality. In Rosenzweig, M. R., & Porter, L. W. (Eds.), *Annual Review of Psychology* (Vol. 32, pp. 439–476). Palo Alto, CA: Annual Reviews.

Barron, F., & Harrington, D. (1985). Creativity. *Social Sciences Encyclopedia* (pp. 167–169). London: Routledge & Kegan Paul.

Bartlett, F. C. (1932). *Remembering.* Cambridge University Press.

Bradley, P. (1984). Dimensions of personality and attitudes towards the nuclear situation: A study of West German values. *Master's Abstracts* (University Microfilms No. 39791/1984/361).

Chambers, J. A., Sprecher, J. W., & Barron, F. (1980). Identifying gifted Mexican-American students. *Gifted Child Quarterly, 24*, 123–129.

Lewis, C. D. (1946). *The poetic image.* London: Jonathan Cape.

Williams, W. C. (1949). *Pictures from Breughel.* New York: New Directions.

4   Various approaches to and definitions of creativity

Calvin W. Taylor

Creativity is "a many splendored thing," as Guilford has pointed out repeatedly. To us, as displayed in our own studies, creativity is a very complex human performance and occurrence, one of the highest-level performances and accomplishments to which humankind can aspire. To many in the arts, including poets and creative writers, the highest degree of the creative process is almost a combined total-human-being response, involving all aspects of such a person's response repertoire. Many subcomponents of creativity are combined simultaneously and/or successively to approach this almost total-human-being response.

Our initial focus and opportunity to undertake major studies on creativity was among scientists and engineers in large research centers. These studies measured products, performances, and other accomplishments in their careers, plus their needs to have better organizational climates for creative scientific work. As we studied the processes scientists used in their work, we contemplated what is meant by "the scientific method." To us, the colorful and best description is that creative scientists use the approach of "no holds barred" to tackle the challenges in an existing field or to open a new field for scientific investigation. The best scientists seem to get extremely involved in a problem. They become so immersed that they stick to the problem, and the problem sticks to them. One fellow scientist described his colleague by saying that the only way one could stop him from working on his problem would be to shoot him. All this led to the book that summarized our first three creativity research conferences: *Scientific Creativity: Its Recognition and Development* (Taylor & Barron, 1963).

A few years after completing a dissertation on fluency in ideas (ideational fluency) and on expressional versatility (or fluency), I was invited by the National Science Foundation (NSF) to take a 2-year leave of absence to work on NSF's challenge of selecting the best scientists both for the future of science and for the good of the nation. By then, fellowship support was provided for predoctoral and postdoctoral work through the NSF's new Fellowship Program. My base was the Office of Scientific Personnel's first director of research in the National Academy of Science–National Research Council (NAS-NRC). Through its past fellowship awardees, the NRC Fellowship Program had already attained a distinguished reputation.

As I left to return to Utah, the leaders and advisors of both NSF and NAS-NRC gave me the *time-unlimited challenge* of studying and learning how to identify highly creative scientists, a few of whom can make such a tremendous difference in a field, as had occurred, for example, in the splitting of the atom and the opening of the Atomic Age. This challenge also included stimulation of others to work in this realm by holding periodic and timely research conferences among researchers who had done the best studies on creative scientists. Eventually this led to *Widening Horizons in Creativity* (Taylor, 1964), the volume from our Fifth Creativity Research Conference, with its coverage being expanded to include all areas of human endeavor in which creativity can function and flourish.

A few comparisons of a highly general nature will be made between the early Intelligence movement (including its current outcomes) and the early Creativity research-and-implementation movement, as well as its recent and possible future outcomes. A concern here is that the Creativity research-based movement definitely should *not* follow all the same paths and outcomes of the Intelligence movement efforts. It appears, in hindsight, that the potentially vast concept of Intelligence converged and comparatively rapidly was reduced to a much smaller concept, as measured by group-tested IQ scores (already obtained for probably over a hundred million persons).

The much earlier Intelligence movement rushed prematurely and noncreatively to considerably simplified, functional solutions. It materialized in objective, tangible, reachable concepts. It definitely oversimplified, so that even four decades ago, basic research on the dimensions (factors) of the mind had expanded far beyond the IQ, and the number of dimensions discovered is now way, way beyond the IQ. IQ measures only small fish and has failed to catch and hold onto the truly big fish that the word "intelligence" signifies to most people. The general public has been misled and still readily believes that IQ is the "total intelligence" that encompasses all of the dimensions (factors) of the mind, including all creative factors (and possibly all other dimensions not yet discovered and measured in the total mind-power).

This measured concept of intelligence is much narrower than Dr. Machado's recent concept of the "development of intelligence," which was included in his minister's title in the Venezuelan cabinet. Along with the program he initiated in his country, he energetically sought teammates for his concept in many nations around the world. Far more than being concerned just with increasing IQ scores of students, he was essentially talking about developing the total potential mindpower of each and every person. He emphasized the real powers of the mind, especially the creative and other thinking and producing powers, not merely the less powerful processes of learning from the library of knowledge of the past.

Four major approaches to creativity

According to Ross Mooney (1963), there are "four significantly different approaches to the problem of creativity, depending on which of four aspects of the problem a person uses to gain his initial hold.'' Mooney's phrasing about a person gaining his initial hold suggests that each person may have his own explicit or implicit definition or subdefinition of creativity or even definitions of one or more subcomponents of creativity going along with his approach in order to get an initial start on the problem of creativity. Mooney's four approaches are

1. the *environment* in which the creation comes about, that is, the *creative environment* (or climate or situation or *place*),
2. the *product* of creating, that is, the *creative product,* or
3. the *process* of creating, that is, the *creative process,* or
4. the *person* who is creative, that is, the *creative person.*

In all the creativity research conferences, and also in the work of our own Utah team, all of these four approaches have been found to some degree as an approach or set of approaches used by investigators in their projects and/or programs of research. As research findings have started to accumulate in each of these four areas, some predictive equations have been set up and validated. The creative process and the creative product have typically been seen as the criteria of creativity; the creative person has been the main basis of the predictors in the equation; and the environment has been used variously as a modifier in the equation as well as the stimulus situation through which the inner creative processes are activated.

Both the conferences and our work have been strong in the criterion area, especially in multiple measures of the creativity of products, including performances, behaviors, publications, ideas, and other types of accomplishments. We are possibly as well prepared as anyone to write a full article on the complexity of the criterion problem. In one conference, possibly the only one on the general problem of the criterion, we definitely had the most data and the widest variety of experiences in working on criterion problems (Henry, 1967). In our own projects we have worked on the creative processes as belonging in the criterion area in some cases and in the person-predictor area in other cases, such as in our development of a Creative Process Check List.

In covering these four approaches in greater detail, we are focusing not only on basic research studies but also on implementation efforts. These include research on implementation in schoolrooms and in other settings in education, business, industry, and government organizations.

The creative environment

Typically this includes the total complex situation in which the creative processes are initially stimulated and sometimes sustained through to completion. The environmental situation can be a natural or a typical environment. It can even be one in which very deliberate attempts have been made to design a *total environment,* such as specially designed instructional media used to spark and sustain creative processes in one or more individuals.

Our first in-the-world Architectural Psychology Program could be used to design total collective environments for this purpose. One of the program's slogans is "Peace of Mind from the Well-Designed." This could alternatively be stated as "Activating a Creative Mind from the Well-Designed." For example, the large Salk Institute building in La Jolla was described by a San Diego newspaper as "An Architectural Experiment in Creativity."

In our Sixth Creativity Research Conference report, *Instructional Media and Creativity* (Taylor & Williams, 1966), the first two chapters were entitled "creativity through Instructional Media: A Universe of Challenges (Parts I and II)." This report was drawn from notes about the impact of instructional materials on the creativity of students. A total of 36 of the 42 pages in my first chapter contained discussions (with each person named when sparked to comment from the challenges in the think piece). It provided a marvelous kick-off session for the conference, because all 14 persons around the table entered into the discussion multiple times. A shortened and further edited example of this discussion from pages 16–19 in *Instructional Media and Creativity* (Taylor & Williams, 1966) follows, with the discussants being identified by name:

Rogers: The "mind set" of the person doing the teaching is so important. A leading physicist at the California Institute of Technology has been very much involved in trying to free up their teaching of physics. In addition to the rather standard material, he purposely put in his new text lots of little peripheral issues – puzzles that no one knows the answer to – to get the students thinking about them. Now there is a strong tendency for the graduate assistants who teach the quiz sections to include quiz questions on these peripheral things just to stimulate students and let them feel that there are a lot of unanswered questions.

Taylor: There are both knowns and unknowns in a field. We must learn somehow to give attention in the classroom to the unknowns as well as to the knowns, even though this has hardly ever been done to date.

Hughes: I am convinced that teachers will have to acquire new concepts of their jobs and new concepts of their relationship to students in order to eventually do any of these new things. One of the things research shows is that, in general, teachers behave very much the same in all American classrooms. Current concepts of what a teacher does are much more similar than dissimilar. The personality factors of teachers that have been investigated do *not* show a relationship to teaching pattern – they just show that teachers work under a cultural, societally defined set of expectations. In some way the basic concepts of the role of the teacher will have to be reevaluated or restated.

Beck: Does this suggest that we train teachers according to a pat formula, and then we put them into cells where they operate for the rest of their lives with practically no feedback?

Hughes: Yes, there is very little feedback as long as they keep control of the classroom – as long as the classroom doesn't go to pot.

Beck: Then they have no opportunity to watch others teach. Each one is in his or her little cell working alone and working according to the ways that he or she has been taught.

Hughes: I would even go further than that. Our training of student teachers has practically no effect later on what they do later as teachers in the classroom. How they teach in the classroom emerges from the concept they have gotten as a teacher, through the years in school under teachers plus the cultural stereotypes and clichés and so on, rather than through the training that as student teachers they obtained in colleges and universities.

MacKinnon: Are you suggesting that as they later teach, they do something quite different from what they have been taught to do as student teachers in training?

Hughes: Yes. Indeed they do something quite different from what they have been taught about teaching. But instructors in education, in educational psychology and so on, teach as they have been taught, too, but they tell their student teachers to teach in a different way than they themselves teach.

Guilford: The student teachers use their own teachers as models of how to teach.

Hughes: Yes, and they are responding to the models.

Rogers: At Wisconsin we tried an experimental program where we really taught the student teachers quite differently, where they gained quite a different kind of experience than occurs in typical teaching. The data still are very tentative on this thing. Many of them found that the kind of teacher they had been taught to be couldn't live in the educational subculture; so they dropped the way they were taught to teach and simply became conventional teachers because there was no place for them.

Taylor: That's the same as for supervisory development programs. You deliberately take supervisors out of their work situation and train them. But when you put them back into the old situation, the old system generally overpowers them and their training.

Edling: What I think is unique about new media is that we are introducing something new into the system, and it makes this new kind of a role for a teacher more possible, provided that the new media come in sufficient quantities for every teacher to use in the entire system.

Parnes: A situation at our institute relates to this idea that new media might provide a new opportunity for teachers who might not otherwise be willing to change. One man in particular came through our 3-day program where we taught our methodologies of creative problem solving, and then he participated in a follow-up 2-day program where we have them teach novice students the same concepts. At the end of the first 3 days he didn't think that the whole business was worth a darn. He didn't see anything in it. But he said that when he taught this to students and when he observed what happened to them, it opened up his eyes completely to this approach. I think the new media might tend to help the teacher do this.

Williams: We have been experiencing in film learning for a number of years. It is not the passiveness of the observer when he observes someone else teach by new approaches, but the activeness of the person himself when he takes over to do this new type of teaching.

Parnes: Yes, but it wasn't so much this man's active participation in teaching as it was his observation of what was happening to the students when they were learning it. Initially he didn't think there was anything to the methods, but the final 2 days he reevaluated his opinions when he saw that something different was happening to the students.

Williams: In designing new media devices, then, the point may be how to get the classroom student and even the teacher himself active in observing what happens to students rather than passively showing a film.

Hughes: What experience did this man have that made him sensitive or allowed him to be sensitive to the reaction of students? Because this is one of the things to which our teachers are generally not sensitive. And so I am interested in how he became aware of the consequences of his teaching in terms of what was happening in the students.

Torrance: That gives me another idea about our experience. Maybe what we have put into our own experiment of having the teachers write their own reactions and observations of the pupils' reactions might have been more powerful than anything else we did, including having the teachers write their own reactions to their new teaching experiences.

Hughes: This is a sensitizing process that is sorely needed.

Three of the 10 articles in *Clues to Creative Teaching* (Taylor, 1963–1964) contribute to the environmental approach. One article points out that existing library knowledge may be an asset or a deterrent to creativity. Furthermore, accumulation of past knowledge by a person certainly provides no assurance that such a person will be a producer of new knowledge beyond that which is known.

These discussions and my research show that past knowledge can be learned and retained with such great force that a person might be unlikely to stretch out beyond that knowledge into the unknown or even to break away from that knowledge to revise it or to produce future knowledge that has not yet been produced. Conversely, other persons may use past knowledge as stepping-stones – standing on the shoulders of past knowledge. One can thereby rise above the past level to create new knowledge at a higher level. A step toward creating an atmosphere conducive to new knowledge could be to have a unit of existing knowledge be presented in a provocative way so that students would process that knowledge creatively. The stimulus nature of the input knowledge and the method used in its presentation can be important in whether such knowledge is an asset or a liability in activating creative processes in a person.

Along with this issue of the nature of stimulus and form of presentation is the issue whether the person's mode and channel of reception are favorable or unfavorable toward creative use of environmental stimuli. The first input stage can help determine whether or not the inner processes will start to be creative. These are dealt with, to some degree, in two of the *Clues to Creative Thinking* articles, "Learning and Reading Creatively" and "Listening Creatively" (Taylor, 1963–1964).

In these two articles we talk about marginal reading, which can produce marginal thinking – a play on the ambiguous word "marginal." In reading a printed page creatively, a person can write notes in the margin of the printed page either about the message on the printed page or about ideas of one's own that are sparked from reading the page. In the latter case, the person considers the printed page to be "what has [already] been written," and the marginal notes can later be expanded into another column of "what is now being written by oneself that has not been written before."

The creative product

The products of creativity can include behaviors, performances, ideas, things, and all other kinds of outputs, with any of all channels and types of expressions. The criteria of creativity define the targets against which a predictor or batteries of predictors are validated through correlation and multiple regression methods.

Our first major criterion study entailed 52 different measures of career contributions of U.S. Air Force scientists, including eight different sources from which data on each scientist were collected. These included 10 ratings and 1 ranking by immediate supervisors; 4 ratings by laboratory chiefs; 6 ratings, rankings, and nominations by peers; 12 quantity (from vitae) and quality (judged by senior scientists) scores on publications and research reports from the researchers who worked on the project; 1 score on membership in professional societies; and 5 "control" variables (to determine if they influenced any of the preceding criterion scores).

These 52 scores were factor-analyzed to yield 14 criterion factors (plus one control factor in a 15th separate dimension). The rotated factor analysis matrix is presented in *Scientific Creativity* (Taylor, Smith, & Ghiselin, 1963, pp. 60–61).

In further analyses of these U.S. Air Force project data in *Widening Horizons in Creativity* and in the Seventh Creativity Research Conference report on *Climate for Creativity* by Taylor and Ellison (1964, 1972), 130 predictor scores derived from 14 different tests were validated against each of 14 criteria. The predictabilities for these 14 criterion factors mentioned earlier are listed in rank order below. The percentage of the battery test scores found to be valid against each criterion, in turn, is listed in parentheses. In addition to the results below, the predictabilities of three of the initial (unfactored) criterion scores were 35% for Peer Rankings on Productivity, 29% for Supervisor Ratings on Creativity, and 25% for Supervisor Ratings of Drive-Resourcefulness.

> Likableness as a research team member (44%)
> Scientific and professional society membership (43%)
> Current organizational status (38%)
> Judged work output (35%)
> Supervisory ratings of overall performance (35%)
> Productivity in written work (32%)
> Creativity rating by laboratory chiefs (29%)
> Originality of written work (20%)
> Visibility (20%)
> Recognition for organizational contributions (17%)
> Recent publications (14%)
> Contract monitoring load (11%)
> Status-seeking, "organization-man" tendencies (8%)
> Quality (without originality) of research reports (2%)

Six of the foregoing criterion factors were selected as separate targets using multiple regression equations. Appropriate indices were also computed to analyze the percentage of criterion variance overlapped by each of the 52 scores in the predictor test battery, as reported in a later section. A somewhat different set of six criterion factors was also used to derive subscore predictors and total score predictors from a specially constructed lengthy biographical inventory, as also described later.

Process versus product in creativity: a spontaneous discussion

Consider the following edited discussion of process versus product in creative thinking (Taylor, 1964):

Barron: It has been assumed in most of our discussion that we can determine whether or not a person is creative by observing his or her behavior or discovering what his or her products are. This kind of definition is probably basic to the kinds of prejudices that psychologists have. One could just as well construe creativity as an internal process continually in action but not always observable – or perhaps in some cases fundamentally unobservable.

Fiedler: Yes, but creativity surely must be identified eventually by its product – no?

Barron: No.

Hyman: You mean that a person can go through life being creative and nobody will be able to identify him or her?

Barron: Yes, by this type of definition.

Fiedler: But not by mine.

Hyman: But how are we going to be able to try to identify creativity, then?

McPherson: There are at least 28 definitions, expanding almost toward or beyond 50 or more. Take you choice. [See the appendix to this chapter.]

Westcott: What do you mean by an internal process, as opposed to products or the results of processes?

Barron: I think of it as something that is happening in the central nervous system. My own basic interest in research on creativity stems from the hope it offers that one may find in psychic creation the same formal variables that can be used to describe creative process in all of nature.

Hyman: There are several different gradations between "process" and "product." A lot of good work has been done toward measuring cognitive structure operationally. The product, then, could emerge from different cognitive structures. You could see this if you had effective ways to index changes in the meaning and structure of the individual's experience. I think these changes can be indexed with present techniques. In this way we may be getting very close, actually, to what Barron is talking about.

Westcott: One place where this might be very "studyable" would be in the development of children, who, as they grow up, have to discover for themselves and invent for themselves the millions of things that all adults know anyhow. It is my feeling that children are doing this constantly. The processes whereby they reach the new views of the world are very much, I would think, like the same processes whereby a scientist reaches a new view of his field.

Mullins: You say that no product is necessary for creativity. How do you define product? Is it some useful product, or is there no sign of a product?

Barron: It would be unusual to find no evidence of creativity in behavior even though creative process was occurring, but I would argue that this sometimes happens – that is, that no sign of it appears.

McPherson: Even to the person himself or herself?

Barron: He or she might not be able to compare himself or herself sufficiently with others to see the signs.

McPherson: Do you think that he or she might be creative but not know that he or she is creative?

Barron: Yes.

Fiedler: But how do you operationally define this?

Barron: I cannot, without considerable further thought, offer an operational definition of creative process occurring in the central nervous system without evidence in behavior and without the fact of its occurrence being known subjectively. Yet from analogy to other internal processes of which we are unaware, I shouldn't think this to be impossible in principle.

Parnes: But wouldn't the person know that something is happening, whether he or she would call it creativity or not?

Leary: I can't understand how there can be any question about what Barron is saying. I can't understand how anybody would disagree with him.

Guilford: It is not very clear what he means.

Levine: Sprecher reports that somebody asked an engineer about his creativity, but he didn't consider himself as being creative. Everybody else said that he was. His approach was novel. He was solving problems. But the engineer didn't think that he was creative – he was just doing his job.

Sprecher: He said, "I'm doing things which are routine to a scientist or a knowledgeable person with my background. These other people think I'm wonderful in producing novel ideas." He had a good opinion of himself, but he said, "The things that they praise about me are developed."

Westcott: I think that the only thing we can say is that if a person does put out productive creative materials, then it seems possible that he's indulging in creativity. But if he doesn't do this, or you don't see any of these products, if he doesn't manifest any of this outwardly, then you really don't know what to say about him.

Barron: Yes, there are virtually no false positives in identifying "creatives," but there may be a great many false negatives (true creatives not identified).

Sprecher: People can produce creative acts or novel acts without having creative thinking. I would expand my definition of creativity (I've seen lots of shaking of heads around here, but you're all wrong) to say that a person can be creative in the sense that he produces a novel product by a very routine, plodding, technical way, with perhaps little thought.

Mednick: What I mean to say is that recognizing the usefulness of a product is an important part of the creative act. The question that no one asked me when I discussed my notions relating to creativity was, "How is it that a person who is creative can pick the appropriate combination of associations from the many, many he has presented to him?" It seems to me that this is a crucial question.

Hyman: If you read Edison's story, you'll see that it's not trial and error.

Sprecher: Yes, it is. It's a very deliberate research of many substances. Well, it's not trial and error in that sense, but it's a technician's search.

Hyman: Edison's criterion was a complete system of what he needed to find. He had a very clear-cut, planned strategy.

Sprecher: No. I've read Josephson's biography of Edison, too, if that's what you're talking about. I'm not referring to the fact that he had a grand conceptual scheme which would encompass more than the light bulb. I'm talking about the fact that in one specific sense he had a problem to solve: "I want this darn filament to last."

Hyman: He had all the specifications of exactly what he wanted in that filament, too.

Sprecher: Then he produced this novel, valuable product in a routine way by just collecting all possible materials in encyclopedic fashion.

Hyman: But first he formulated the complete problem of exactly what he wanted and how he would recognize the product even before he saw it. It is this formulation of a context for searching and for evaluation of his trials that I want to emphasize.

Leary: I venture to predict that creative performance or the production of creative expressions will increasingly be seen as a systematic combining of elements which have not been combined before. Many people who are seen as creative writers, artists, and so forth are technicians who have wanted to be creative, wanted to play the creative game, and fiddled around rearranging symbols. Henry Miller's chapter in Ghiselin's book (1955) is a very nice account of how this author went at the technical problems of being a creative writer. He experimented extensively with imitations of other authors. Finally, he quit imitating, plunged deeply into the "ocean of reality" on his own, and went on to what I would call a creative experience. [A few short exchanges about machines and creativity next occurred.]

Holland: We have a place in Chicago where you buy your own paints and drop them down on a spinning wheel. You can get some very nice pictures.

Hyman: Leary, the point that you're making is that if you can explain the process a man uses and duplicate it with a machine in some way, then that's not creativity. You feel that creativity is some kind of – well, whatever it is I don't know – but something that man can't simulate on a machine, is that it?

Leary: I'm distinguishing between the (inner) creative experience (or the inner creative process) and the outcome of a so-called creative product.

Harmon: Couldn't you perhaps duplicate these same processes on a machine and, if you did a good simulation, have a creative process – when there's a human being involved?

Barron: That's a critical point. If you can get a proper, full description of the creative process, can it be entirely mechanical?

Westcott: Isn't it true that a machine which produces some of these kinds of things uses almost infinitely more work than a person does in accomplishing a comparable end? From what we know about the machines, they can whir . . . and in fifteen seconds do five years' work.

Barron: But only on what's fed into them. We do more work than anything else in the universe – we are the biggest workers.

Leary: We have experimented by using cut-up recombinations with convicts who've had mystical experiences and who can't report them verbally because they don't have adequate vocabulary. We can sometimes come out with very striking images which reduce this tremendous gap between experience and the expressive communication of it which has bothered all of us for a long time.

Mednick: I think that the role of random behavior in the construction of this "cut-up" poetry is a bit exaggerated. The creative act in cut-up poetry occurs once after the fiftieth or so rearrangement of the cut-up words. The constructor has an "Aha!" experience and selects this order of words as meeting some requirements. Incidentally, this is a way of assessing the degree of creativity; that is, *the more requirements a product meets, the more creative the product is.* Let me expand on the questions of requirements a bit more. I believe that we can judge how creative a product is by the number of requirements it meets. This sounds very simple-minded, perhaps, but it meets a minimum requirement itself in that *it begins to be a researchable definition.* In terms of the definition, except under special circumstances, it is difficult to specify what reliable requirements such products meet.

Sprecher: You are saying that *this is creativity for Mednick.* This is legitimate, so long as you recognize it as yours, *but allow other people to define creativity however they wish.*

Beittel: Yes, that's a good point. I was going to mention it. I can see why we perhaps study architects and painters, because painters have set themselves a problem of constant innovation at present. I want to throw in one more thing. Our culture in the arts is heavy in this expressionistic ego-centered feedback with the problem. I like the point that Murray made in the essay in the Michigan symposium about what he called *biotic creativity.* He thought that there was a way to transfer this into the social realm where you don't have the ego-centered relationship to the product. I think that type of transfer presents some hope as an image, for the feedback would concern an almost pure process, and the product would be a little bit sharable, in a sense.

Westcott: Certainly, in the realm of haikai poetry, a requirement of usefulness is not directly met, so *such poetry falls outside of this requirement of usefulness.* I wonder whether this criterion of usefulness does not fit in this case in the sense of the particular task that the artist or the poet is trying to accomplish.

Mednick: If you can reliably specify this task, then you have a researchable problem. It seems likely to me that often the aim of a particular artistic work was to communicate a given emotional state to a given group of people. In this case we can ask, Does the painting do this? Yes. It does? It does it beautifully? Then it is wonderful.

McPherson: What about time? It might do it at one time and not at another.

Westcott: Yes, this is true.

Taylor: I'm sure that we can't solve many things here, but there is merit in getting these issues out on the table, as all of you have just done. I suggest you note our studies wherein we obtained at least crude measures, separately, for processes and for products and found the relationships between these different measures of processes and products. (Ghiselin, Rompel, & Taylor, 1964; Taylor & Ellison, 1964)

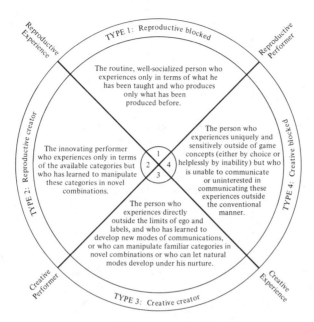

Figure 4.1. Categories for diagnosing creativity in terms of performance and experience. The diagnostic grid is defined by two axes: experience and performance. Each axis runs a continuum from creative to reproductive. (From Leary, 1964, with permission.)

This is the end of the discussion. The next few paragraphs and graphs are from Leary's chapter (1964).

Because there is creative experience (i.e., creative awareness) and there is creative performance, a multidimensional Diagnosis of Creativity is possible. *Awareness can be creative –* our experience can be direct and fresh; *or it can be reproductive,* i.e., within the interpretative framework of the already learned, in which case we see only what we have been taught to see.

Performance can be creative – we can produce new combinations; *or it can be reproductive –* a repeating of old combinations.

When we oppose these two dichotomous continua of experience and performance in orthogonal axes, a diagnostic circle is obtained. Four "types" of creativity are defined by the four quadrants of the diagnostic circle shown below in Figure 4.1.

Type 1. *The reproductive blocked* (no novel combinations, no direct experience), which I estimate to comprise about 75% of our American population.

Type 2. *The reproductive creator* (no direct experience, but crafty skill in producing new combinations of old symbols), comprising, let us say, the most visible, successful 12% of our population.

Type 3. *The creative creator* (new experience presented in novel performances), of which we can hope for 1% in any Golden Age.

Type 4. *The creative blocked* (new direct experience expressed in conventional modes), a somewhat cryptic 12%.

These four "types" of creativity are obvious by definition and seem to require no elaboration. What does deserve amplification is the social perception of these four types. A person in

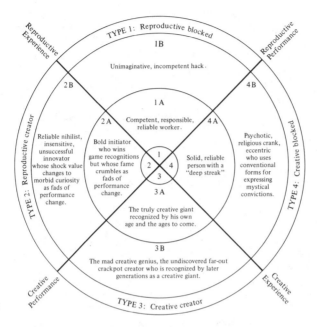

Figure 4.2. Schematic diagrams of social labels used to describe types of creativity. Inner circle illustrates positive social labels, and outer circle negative labels. (From Leary, 1964, with permission.)

any of these four quadrants can be seen as effective or as incompetent by his culture – and, for that matter, by cultural subgroups.

If we divide each type into those labeled by their contemporaries as (a) effective and (b) ineffective, we obtain the eight categories presented in Figure 4.2. These two-dimensional circular grids can be used to plot test scores or content-analysis indices along the two coordinates in order to diagnose the individual. Thus we can work not just in terms of eight types but in terms of two continua which define a wide expanse of diagnostic space. The same mathematical and psychometric methods apply. We can plot the location of scores on check lists of creative experience and creative behavior executed by the subject or by appraisers of this performance. Multilevel discrepancy indices can thus be calculated which provide opportunities for differential approaches in the development of creative behavior.

The creative process

In all our approaches we have always been interested in what a supervisor or teacher and other medium can do for workers and students. Also, we try to discover what the surrounding environment can do and what kinds of persons it takes to have their inner processes functioning creatively. My teaching style is to use provocative methods and rewards, so that students are treated as thinkers in class, after which they keep thinking, intermittently, between classes about the subject matter and about the stretching of their own minds and mind powers. One student volunteered that in my class he learned "not only what education is doing *for us* but also what education is doing *to us*." This concurs with what Sam Proctor (1978) has emphasized: *A mind is a terrible thing to waste.* A high percentage of students' minds are not being developed and utilized in typical schoolwork; to challenge education to improve, students could write a book titled "Don't dwarf our minds!" It is also true that *a large part of anyone's mind is a terrible thing to waste.*

Brewster Ghiselin worked with R. Rompel (a graduate student) and me on constructing and developing a Creative Process Check List with 225 adjectives as items (Ghiselin, Rompel, & Taylor, 1964). There were different types of responses to these items. The first was on "States of Attention" before, during, and after the moment of a person's shaping a new insight. The second measured "States of Feeling" before, during, and after the moment of insight. We divided our scientists by their criterion measures into those high in creativity but not in material recognition and success and those high in material recognition and success but not in creativity. The Creative Process Check List appeared to be a promising research instrument for investigation of the psychological processes of scientists. It also appeared likely to prove useful as a predictor of scientific accomplishment. The check list could be improved if we would now use phrases as well as adjectives in expanding and revising the check list items.

One of our most successful studies in the classroom was accomplished in Project Implode in the Bella Vista School in Utah's Jordan School District. "Implode" appropriately means an internal explosion – in this case, in students. Consequently, it called for a lot of internal action in the brain processes in the students. The teachers and even the principal became effective in activating these inner processes; so the students produced tangible products, first in quantity, and then with some traditional quality and occasionally even some creative quality features. Practically all of the students became quite effective in at least one or more of the high-level brain-power talents being activated and developed.

The creative person

Intellectual, personality, motivation, and group indicators provided the predictor scores against the previously cited criterion measures in our validation equations. Generally, creative thinking has been developed much more than have creative characteristics. The latter is an area as yet remarkably untried in schooling.

In this section it is appropriate to talk about research by Taylor and Ellison (1964), in which we found that the product of beta weights and validity coefficients for each of 52 predictor scores showed the percentage of the variance of the criterion target overlapping with each predictor score. The four most creative criterion targets and two other criteria with some creative features were selected for further validation work.

All of the 52 scores in the battery, in combination, overlapped approximately half or more of what each criterion measured (i.e., the criterion variance). These percentages were 50.0%, 46.8%, 70.7%, 71.0%, 66.0%, and 65.4%. The overlapping of each criterion was accumulated mainly from a large number of small contributions from the 52 predictor scores. In fact, for a single score, the contribution of 6%

is quite infrequent, and a contribution of 10% is definitely rare for any criterion. Therefore, no single test score usually adds much to the total contribution. In other words, the large total overlap is obtained through many small, separate, low contributions. Through these analyses, we have also learned to have considerable respect for low validities, even in the range of .20, especially if we have enough of them. If high validities are not being found and if low validities are all that are available, then we would like to have as many of these low validities as we can get.

Our well-developed and continually improved "dynamic" biographical inventories yield scores that have proved to be the best predictors by far and to cover the most relevant number of dimensions of intellectual and nonintellectual attributes in our test batteries. Our factor analyses of items in biographical inventories discover great complexity in the number of separate dimensions that such inventories measure. In our Form U inventory (Taylor & Ellison, 1983) the creativity score measures from 7 to 10 different subcomponents or subdimensions of the total creativity score. The research on biographical inventories suggests that it takes what we call "a lot of little oars, each pulling its share in the general direction of the target, to build up high validity coefficients." Collectively these little oars bring about a strong total pull in the right direction. However, no one of these oars usually produces much validity by itself; so we advise persons not to lean too much on any single oar.

The most sound approach and the one recommended here is to use first and foremost the predictive efficiency of a complex, well-developed, valid, biographical inventory. Then, afterward see how much other types of tests (or measures) of intellectual talents, special abilities, grades, achievement test scores, and personality scores may add to the predictive efficiency of the biographical inventory scores. Any early measurement of creative potentials should also involve a complex battery of scores in order to account for a very high percentage of all that is involved. In other words, one may need to measure 10, 15, 20, or more dimensions in any predictor battery if one wants to account for very much of any performances, products, and processes that are highly creative.

These analyses argue that creative performances are very complex and that no single-variable test, no single-variable training program, no single-variable change in working conditions, and no single-variable theory of creativity will account for much of the total phenomenon unless the single variable happens to be a mighty complex one in itself. In other words, our evidence from multiple studies argues strongly that creative performance is a very complex multivariable phenomenon.

In addition to the definitions in this chapter's Appendix (Repucci, 1960), we want to report our own uses and experiences with definitions of creativity, with help from Arnold Toynbee of Great Britain, Brewster Ghiselin of our university, and Robert Lacklen of NASA. Fortunately we received permission by correspondence to publish in *Widening Horizons in Creativity* (Taylor, 1964) a challenging question by Arnold Toynbee (1964): Is America neglecting her creative minority?

Toynbee declares that

to give a fair chance to potential creativity is a matter of life and death for any society. This is all-important, because the outstanding creative ability of a fairly small percentage of the population is mankind's ultimate capital asset. . . .

Creation is a disturbing force in society because it is a constructive one. It upsets the old order in the acts of building a new one. This activity is salutary for society. It is, indeed, essential for the maintenance of society's health; for the one thing that is certain about human affairs is that they are perpetually on the move, and the work of creative spirits is what gives society a chance of directing its inevitable movement along constructive instead of destructive lines.

A creative spirit works like yeast dough. But this valuable social service is condemned as high treason in a society where the powers-that-be have set themselves to stop life's tide from flowing. This enterprise is foredoomed to failure. . . .

In present-day America [or so it looks to Toynbee] the affluent majority is striving desperately to arrest the irresistible tide of change. It is attempting this impossible task because it is bent on conserving the social and economic system under which this comfortable affluence has been acquired. With this unattainable aim in view, American public opinion today is putting an enormously high premium on social conformity; and this attempt to standardize people's behaviour in adult life is as discouraging to creative ability and initiative as the educational policy of egalitarianism in childhood.

Egalitarianism and conservatism work together against creativity, and, in combination, they mount up to a formidable repressive force. . . . America rose to greatness as a revolutionary community, following the lead of creative leaders who welcomed and initiated timely and constructive changes, instead of wincing at the prospect of them. . . . It is ironic and tragic that, in an age in which the whole world has come to be inspired by the original and authentic spirit of Americanism, America herself should have turned her back on this, and should have become the arch-conservative power in the world after having made history as the arch-revolutionary one.

What America surely needs now is a return to those original ideals that have been the sources of her greatness. . . . America's need, and the world's need, today, is a new burst of American [creative] pioneering, and this time not just within the confines of a single continent but all round the globe.

America's [needed spirit and her] manifest destiny in the next chapter of her history is to help the indigent majority of mankind to struggle upward towards a better life than it has ever dreamed of in the past. . . . If this spirit is to prevail, America must treasure and foster all the creative abilities that she has in her.

Later, after Toynbee spoke at my 1967 summer creativity workshop on our campus, he wrote us on April 18, 1968, a letter from London that

my impression – and indeed my conviction – is that, if America is to treasure and foster all the creative ability that she has in her, a new and right spirit of change has to be injected into her educational philosophy. The rather rigid egalitarian models of educational selection and treatment will, I should press, have to be refashioned to include the creative talents of the coming generations.

It would follow from this, if I am right in my diagnosis, that new educational philosophies and new institutions of learning need to be constructed to provide an opportunity for creative individuals to enhance their talents in schools. If the American people, or any other people, are unwilling to change their minds and hearts to remold their educational establishment in ways that foster creative talents, they cannot expect to be able to persist in this negative attitude with impunity. This is surely true, particularly of the American people, conceived, nurtured, and guided, as it has been, for almost two hundred years by its creative leadership. "Where there is no vision, the people perish."

Our first major study on creativity of scientists involved U.S. Air Force scientists. One member of our team was Brewster Ghiselin, who suggested that the measure of the creativeness of a product should be "the extent to which it restructures our universe of understanding" (Taylor and Ellison, 1964, p. 228). His formulation, which is applicable across disciplines, was also suitable for our measurement of the performance and contributions of Air Force scientists. That is, the more creative the contribution, the more it restructures one's universe of understanding. Conversely, the less creative the contribution, the less it affects and requires any restructuring of our total universe of understanding.

In our studies of NASA scientists (Taylor & Ellison, 1964, p. 229) we used the breadth-of-applicability definition, which Robert Lacklen, NASA's first personnel director, produced and which was widely accepted by NASA. The degree to which a NASA scientist's contribution is creative is found by determining the extent of the area of science that each contribution underlies. The more basic a contribution, the wider its effects. In the NASA creativity scale, the highest degree is as follows:

The impact of his work has been quite exceptional. His creative solutions to complex problems have broad generality and have even opened up important areas of investigation with wide implications.

NASA's lowest degree of creativity is described as follows:

His work has demonstrated very little creativity or originality. It usually has provided no more than a rather simple solution to the immediate problem.

To deal with the inner processes of individuals majoring in liberal arts on campus, a pertinent restatement of Ghiselin's definition would be as follows: "The creative process is the process of change, of development, of evolution, in the organization of subjective life." This implies an internal restructuring of a student's own universe of understandings and insights – even a reorganization of one's inner established order, especially if it is too entrenched. Students who are most adept at their own individual creativity are the ones who most easily break out of their established order and restructure it as needed.

At our Third Creativity Research Conference (Taylor, 1959), Golovin and Kuhn engaged in an unrecorded debate about whether definitions are prerequisites to progress or outcomes of progress. Both had doctorates in physics, Golovin as the space expert in the Advanced Research Projects Agency of the Department of Defense, and Kuhn was becoming eminent as a philosopher of science from his writings on the structure of scientific revolutions. The relation of definition to progress is an important one, with Golovin taking the first position (definition as a prerequisite) and Kuhn the second (definition as an outcome).

Recently, Joe McPherson, another major creativity researcher, remarked that "closure is not a way of life to recommend to anyone." Nor is it particularly wise to recommend to any growing movement, such as the creativity research and implementation movement. Increasing openness is more in tune with creativity and longevity.

Once I thought I heard a person say "hopenendedness," a word I liked because it

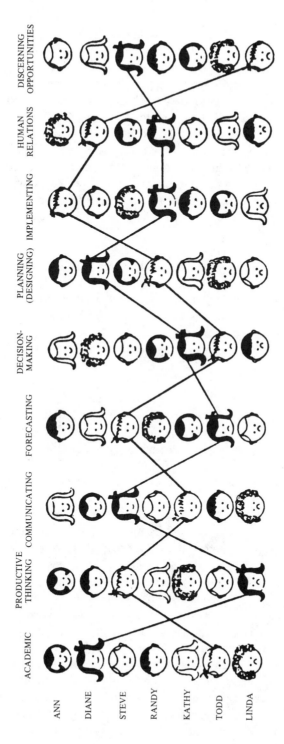

Figure 4.3. Taylor's talent totem poles, 1984 extended version. (Copyright 1984, Calvin W. Taylor.)

was full of hope. However, I checked with him and found that he had said "openendedness" instead, which also provides opportunities for hope. Controls and restrictions that limit the meaning and scope of creativity are contrary to the spirit of creativity. They are also contrary to the characteristics found in creative persons, such as flexibility, discernment of opportunities, tolerance of ambiguity, and avoidance of premature closure, especially rigid closure. The expanding field of creativity could be stifled by curtailing divergence and diversity, by maximizing convergence, and by crystallizing too solidly. It would be an injustice to the current lively movement and could result in failure to reach the highest level of creativity that is now being sought after and being approached gradually and asymptotically. At this time, any person interested in creativity can find a subcomponent or combination of subcomponents of creativity to get hold of and move ahead to make whatever contribution possible.

Another relevant area of our work has been in teaching for multiple creative talents beyond the academic talent, which essentially covers traditional teaching and testing for knowledge. Initially, while still at the theoretical stage, we had two talents in mind, namely, academic and creative talents, with the latter being the breakthrough and breakaway talent. As we moved into classroom practices, we retained the academic talent and replaced the second talent with the five talents of productive thinking, planning, communicating, forecasting, and decision making, which were shown in a set of theoretical totem poles as first sketched by Darrel Allington.

In 1969, Beverly Lloyd first put 28 live second grade students, four sets of seven at a time, on the six totem poles listed earlier. Later, she followed them through high school as her dissertation research at our university (Lloyd, 1983). Figure 4.3 shows nine talent totem-pole illustrations, the first six described earlier plus three new ones added in the last 4 years, namely, implementing, human relations, and discerning opportunities. The last eight talents are all thinking, producing, and creating types of talents.

After these analyses, we recently decided to do a synthesis, because all these eight totem poles can be used to function creatively. A group of experienced creativity researchers assigned weights to yield a Creativity Composite Score to return to a two-totem-pole illustration of Academic versus Creativity, as seen in Figure 4.4. The point here is that this is another way to use the last eight subcomponents (totem-pole scores) in combination to define and yield a Creativity Composite Score for each student on the total set of talent totem poles. This classroom implementation and research evaluation work has now been going on for nearly 25 years in some schools all around the nation.

In summary, in our work on the *creative environment* (or *place*) we used from 7 to over 15 different dimensions or subcomponents in studying the "total" environment in classrooms and large organizations. In our studies of the *creative product* we covered up to 14 factored dimensions from a vast number of criterion scores. In our *creative process* study we used over 200 items in two different ways to probe initially into this complex, vital area. Finally, in our numerous studies of the

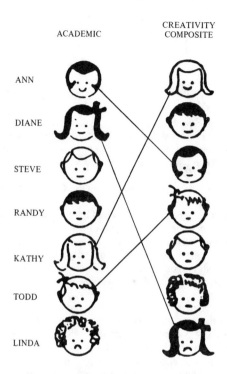

Figure 4.4. Totem poles for two broad talents. (Copyright 1984, Calvin W. Taylor.)

creative person we used seven or more dimensions in our biographical inventory scores and tested the validity of up to 52 predictor scores in our large study of predictors and criteria of U.S. Air Force scientists.

Each different approach involved somewhat different problems of what description and measures to use. Great complexity was found in terms of the numbers of dimensions in these different types of studies of creativity. Consequently, it provides a great unmet challenge for anyone who seeks to produce one definition that fits well and satisfies all these different approaches.

In conclusion, we hope to encourage the diversity of approaches necessary to keep the creativity movement growing and thriving. We believe that the importance and complexity of the highest level of creativity are worthy of a continually diversifying movement with increasing support. The movement should not miss the "big creativity fish" and settle prematurely for a "little fish," as the group-IQ movement seems in hindsight to have done.

We move toward Creative and not just Traditional Excellence, because the latter focuses on perpetuating the past and defaults the future creative-history-making to others elsewhere. We therefore insist on improvements through cultivating both *Creative Excellence* and *Traditional Excellence*, not either one without the other.

Appendix

Definitions of creativity

L. C. Repucci
Dow Chemical Company

A review of the literature on thinking and problem-solving reveals a variety of theoretical orientations and a whole host of experimental investigations. To sift through this mass of data is a separate task in and of itself. Consequently, we shall focus on one specific aspect of the thinking-problem-solving dimension. This is the area referred to as creativity or creative problem-solving.

In order to orient ourselves, we must briefly consider the semantics of the word itself. That is, what is creativity? What does the word mean?

A great deal of effort has been spent to reach some understanding of the word. At present, our investigation reveals the existence of some 50 or 60 definitions and list is expanding every day. If we examine the many definitions which have been offered, we can classify them into six major groups or classes. These groupings are not mutually exclusive since each definition may contain elements which fall into different classes. To overcome this difficulty, the class into which a definition was placed was determined by the main theme of the definition.

The first class of definitions will be labeled *"Gestalt"* or *"Perception"* type definitions wherein the major emphasis is upon the recombination of ideas or the restructuring of a "Gestalt." Certainly, Wertheimer's (1945) definition that creativity is the "process of destroying one gestalt in favor of a better one" belongs in this category. So also the definition of Keep (1957) that it is "the intersection of two ideas for the first time" and Duhrssen's (1957) notion that it is the "translation of knowledge and ideas into a new form" belong in this category. Mooney (1955), Von Fange (1954) and others utilize this approach.

The second class of definitions may be called *"end product"* or *"innovation"* oriented definitions. A representative member of this class is Stein's definition (1953) that "Creativity is that process which results in a novel work that is accepted as tenable or useful or satisfying by a group at some point in tie." Even Webster's dictionary (1953) is oriented in this direction for "to create" is defined as "To bring into being," "To produce as a work of thought or imagination." Harmon (1955) prefers to speak of it as "any process by which something new is produced – an idea or an object, including a new form or arrangement of old elements."

A third class of definitions can be characterized as *"Aesthetic"* or *"Expressive."* The major emphasis here is upon self-expression. The basic idea seems to be that one has a need to express himself in a manner which is unique to him. Any such expression is deemed to be creative. Hence we have Lee's definition (1957) that "the creative process can be defined as ability to think in uncharted waters without influence from conventions set up by past practices." In this vein, Lange (1957) offers that "The creative process is God, the creator, working through his creation, man." Northrop (1952) speaks of it in terms of stimulating our sensibility to dissatisfaction and Compton (1952) sees the essence of creativity as being the decision to do something when you are irritated. Thurstone (1954) thinks of it in terms of problem sensitization and Ghiselin (1955) defines it as "the process of change, of development, of evolution, in the organization of subjective life."

A fourth class of definitions can be characterized as *"psychoanalytic"* or *"dynamic."* In this group, we find creativity defined in terms of certain interactional strength ratios of the id, ego and superego. In this respect, Bellak (1958) assumes that all forms of creativity are

First section of an unpublished 1960 report to Dow Chemical Company titled *Definitions and Criteria of Creativity.*

permanent operant variables of personality and he subscribes to the notion that to be creative the ego must regress in order for preconscious or unconscious material to emerge. Leading proponents of this type of definition are Anderson (1959), Kris (1951) and Kubie (1958).

A fifth class of definitions can be grouped under the classification of *"Solution Thinking."* Here the emphasis is upon the thinking process itself rather than upon the actual solution of the problem. Spearman (1931), for instance, defines creativity in terms of correlates. That is, creativity is present or occurs whenever the mind can see the relationship between two items in such a way as to generate a third item. Guilford (1959) on the other hand, defines creativity in terms of a very large number of intellectual factors. The most important of these factors are the discovery factors and the divergent-thinking factors. The discovery factors are defined as the "ability to develop information out of what is given by stimulation." The divergent-thinking factors relate to one's ability to go off in different directions when faced with a problem. This is similar to Dunker's notion (1945) that in order to solve a problem one often must move tangentially from common types of solutions. Other proponents of this class of definitions are Poincaré (1913) and Wallas (1926).

The sixth and last class of definitions is labeled *"Varia"* simply because there is no easy way of characterizing them. There is, for instance, Rand's (1952) definition that creativity is the "addition to the existing stored knowledge of mankind." Lowenfeld (1957) speaks of it as the result of our subjective relationship with man and environment. Porsche (1955) sees it as the integration of facts, impressions, or feelings into a new form. Read (1955) feels that it is that quality of the mind which allows an individual to juggle scraps of knowledge until they fall into new and more useful patterns and Shepard (1957) speaks of it as a destructive process much like Wertheimer when he spoke of creativity in terms of destroying one Gestalt in favor of another.

References

Anderson, H. H. (1959, May). *External and internal criteria of creativity.* Paper presented at a symposium on creativity, Midwestern Psychological Association, Chicago, IL.

Bellak, L. (1958). Creativity: Some random notes to a systematic consideration. *Journal of Projective Techniques, 4,* 363–380.

Compton, A. H. (1952). Case histories: Creativity in science. In F. Olsen (Ed.), *The nature of creative thinking* (pp. 23–31). New York: Industrial Research Institute, Inc.

Duhrssen, A. (1957). Discussant in *The Arden House conference on motivating the creative process.* Harriman, NY.

Dunker, D. (1945). On problem solving. *Psychological Monographs, 58,* No. 270.

Ghiselin, B. (1955). *The creative process.* New York: Mentor.

Ghiselin, B., Rompel, R., & Taylor, C. W. (1964). A creative process check list: its development and validation. In C. W. Taylor (Ed.), *Widening horizons in creativity* (pp. 19–33). New York: Wiley.

Guilford, J. P. (1959). Intellectual resources and their value as seen by creative scientists. In C. W. Taylor (Ed.), *The third (1959) University of Utah research conference on the identification of creative scientific talent* (pp. 128–149). Salt Lake City: University of Utah Press.

Harmon, L. R. (1956). Social and technological determiners of creativity. In C. W. Taylor (Ed.), *The 1955 University of Utah research conference on the identification of creative scientific talent* (pp. 42–52). Salt Lake City: University of Utah Press.

Henry, E. R. (Ed.). (1967). *Conference on criteria for research and application of research in management, leadership and creativity.* Greensboro, NC: Smith Richardson Foundation.

Keep, O. A. (1957). Discussant in *The Arden House conference on motivating the creative process.* Harriman, NY.

Kris, E. (1951). On preconscious mental processes. In D. Rapport (Ed.), *Organization and pathology of thought* (pp. 474–496). New York: Columbia University Press.

Kubie, L. S. (1958). *Neurotic distortion of the creative process.* Lawrence: University of Kansas Press.

Lange, G. C. (1957). Discussant in *The Arden House conference on motivating the creative process*. Harriman, NY.

Leary, T. (1964). The effects of test score feedback on creative performance and of drugs on creative experience. In C. W. Taylor (Ed.), *Widening horizons in creativity* (pp. 94–96). New York: Wiley.

Lee, W. J. (1957). Discussant in *The Arden House conference on motivating the creative process*. Harriman, NY.

Lloyd, B. (1983). *Longitudinal effects of multiple talent training on 28 second grade students – the totem pole kids*. Unpublished dissertation, University of Utah, Salt Lake City.

Lowenfeld, V. (1957). *Creative and mental growth*. New York: Macmillan.

Mooney, R. L. (1955). Cultural blocks to creative activity. In J. E. Arnold (Ed.), *Creative engineering seminars*. Cambridge: Massachusetts Institute of Technology.

Mooney, R. L. (1963). A conceptual model for integrating four approaches to the identification of creative talent. In C. W. Taylor & F. Barron (Eds.), *Scientific creativity: its recognition and development* (pp. 331–340). New York: Wiley.

Northrop, R. S. C. (1952). Philosophy's statement of the problems of creativity. In F. Olsen (Ed.), *The nature of creative thinking* (pp. 16–22). New York: Industrial Research Institute, Inc.

Poincaré, H. (1913). Mathematical creation. In G. H. Halsted (Trans.), *The foundations of science* (pp. 383–394). New York: Science Press.

Porsche, J. D. (1955, October). *Creative ability – its role in the search for new products*. Paper presented at special conference on managing product research and development, American Management Association, New York.

Proctor, S. D. (1978). A mind is a terrible thing to waste. *Phi Delta Kappan*, pp. 201–203.

Rand, H. J. (1952). Creativity – its social, economic and political significance. In F. Olsen (Ed.), *The nature of creative thinking* (pp. 12–15). New York: Industrial Research Institute, Inc.

Read, G. M. (1955). *Profile of human materials*. Paper presented at a centennial symposium on modern engineering, University of Pennsylvania, Philadelphia.

Shepard, H. A. (1957, August). The destructive side of creativity. *The Chemist*, pp. 303–307.

Spearman, C. (1931). *Creative mind*. New York: Appleton.

Stein, M. I. (1953). Creativity and culture. *Journal of Psychology, 36*, 311–322.

Taylor, C. W. (1959). *The third (1959) research conference on the identification of creative scientific talent*. Salt Lake City: University of Utah Press.

Taylor, C. W. (1963–1964). Clues to creative teaching (featured 10-year series usually starting on p. 5). *The Instructor*.

Taylor, C. W. (Ed.). (1964). *Widening horizons in creativity*. New York: Wiley.

Taylor, C. W. (Ed.). (1972). *Climate for creativity*. New York: Pergamon Press.

Taylor, C. W., & Barron, F. (Eds.). (1963). *Scientific creativity: its recognition and development*. New York: Wiley.

Taylor, C. W., & Ellison, R. L. (1964). Predicting creative performances from multiple measures. In C. W. Taylor (Ed.), *Widening horizons in creativity* (pp. 242–253). New York: Wiley.

Taylor, C. W., & Ellison, R. L. (1972). *Predictors and criteria of creativity – a Utah progress report*. In C. W. Taylor (Ed.), *Climate for creativity* (pp. 149–165). New York: Pergamon Press.

Taylor, C. W., & Ellison, R. L. (1983). Searching for student talent resources relevant to all USDE types of giftedness. *Gifted Child Quarterly*, pp. 99–106.

Taylor, C. W., Smith, W. R., & Ghiselin, B. (1963). The creative and other contributions of one sample of research scientists. In C. W. Taylor & F. Barron (Eds.), *Scientific creativity: its recognition and development* (pp. 60–61). New York: Wiley.

Taylor, C. W., & Williams, F. E. (Eds.). (1966). *Instructional media and creativity*. New York: Wiley.

Thurstone, L. L. (1954, April). Criteria of scientific success and the selection of scientific talent. In W. J. Brogden et al. (Eds.), *Criteria of success in science* (pp. 29–34) (Technical Report 4, Office of Scientific Personnel). Washington, DC: National Academy of Sciences–National Research Council.

Toynbee, A. (1964). Is America neglecting her creative minority? In C. W. Taylor (Ed.), *Widening horizons in creativity* (pp. 3–9). New York: Wiley.

Von Fange, E. K. (1954). *The creative process in engineering.* General Electric Co., Creative Engineering Program.

Wallas, G. (1926). *The art of thought.* New York: Harcourt, Brace.

Webster's New Collegiate Dictionary. (1953). Springfield, MA: G. & C. Merriam Co.

Wertheimer, M. (1945). *Productive thinking.* New York: Harper.

Cognitive approaches

5   A three-facet model of creativity

Robert J. Sternberg

Alice should have been the ideal graduate student: She entered Yale's graduate program with 800-level scores on the Graduate Record Examination, close to a 4.0 undergraduate academic average, excellent letters of recommendation, and all of the apparent undergraduate socialization that should have taught her what counts in academe. During her first year, when course work, multiple-choice tests, and writing brief critical papers were stressed, Alice was everything her record promised she would be. But by the time she left the graduate program, her record did not look promising at all. Alice continued to show excellent memory and critical-thinking skills. But once having creative ideas started to matter, Alice proved not to be competitive with even the typical students in the program. She was a good critical thinker, but not a good creative thinker. Nothing in her undergraduate record prepared the faculty – or Alice – for this unwelcome surprise. In contrast, Barbara, who entered the program with relatively low test scores and only typical undergraduate grades, as admitted students go, fared much better. Her critical ability was good, but it was not critical abilities that propelled her to great success. Rather, she proved to be among the most creative researchers we had. Only her letters of recommendation praised her creativity. There was nothing in the hard data – test scores and grades – to indicate that Barbara would be an exceptional student.

In her book *Whatever Happened to the Quiz Kids?* Ruth Feldman (1982) describes the childhood feats of the television quiz kids. These children dramatically impressed the world with their extraordinary demonstrations of learning and recall. It was hard to believe that young children could be so smart. Indeed, Feldman reported that all of them had very high IQs. Yet, in reading their biographies, one cannot help but be struck by how much less creative they were than they were intelligent. Certainly, their creative performances in their later lives have nowhere near matched their intelligent performances in their earlier lives.

In the film *Amadeus,* both Mozart and his rival, Salieri, are portrayed as highly intelligent as well as professionally ambitious. Had one given each of them a standard intelligence test suitable for the times, it is unlikely that the test scores would much have distinguished their relative levels of musical expertise. But Mozart was far more creative than Salieri, as Salieri and Mozart both recognized. In the long run, Mozart was remembered, and Salieri all but forgotten.

These three vignettes are only a small sample of the vignettes, as well as the data, that indicate that for whatever overlap there may be between intelligence and creativity, it is not complete. Reviews of the empirical literature (Perkins, 1981; Vernon, 1970) reveal that creativity is unlikely to be understood merely as an

Preparation of this research was supported by Contract N00014-85-K-0589 from the Office of Naval Research. Requests for reprints should be sent to Robert J. Sternberg, Department of Psychology, Yale University, Box 11A, Yale Station, New Haven, CT 06520.

adjunct of some other cognitive or personality phenomenon. Creativity overlaps with other psychological phenomena, such as intelligence, cognitive style, and personality, but it is not identical with any of them. The goal of this chapter is to attempt to understand what creativity is and how it can be understood at a peculiar intersection between three psychological attributes: intelligence, cognitive style, and personality/motivation. Taken together, these three facets of the mind help us understand what lies behind the creative individual.

The chapter will be divided into five basic parts. In the first, I review some research that helps delineate the boundaries of creativity – what the phenomenon is that needs to be understood. In the next three parts, I discuss those aspects of intelligence, cognitive style, and personality/motivation that seem most to contribute to the phenomenon that we label creativity. In the last part, I attempt to integrate these various aspects of creativity into a tentative, unified account of this elusive psychological attribute.

The nature of creativity

What is creativity? Few psychological constructs have proved more elusive to define. Sometimes creativity is defined in terms of products, such as products that are statistically unusual and also adjudged to be of high quality (Perkins, 1981). But such a definition tells us little about the psychology of the creative person. In studying phenomena that are not well understood, it is sometimes helpful to start with a study of people's implicit theories – or conceptions – of a given phenomenon. This is a course we took in the study of intelligence (Sternberg, Conway, Ketron, & Bernstein, 1981) and have more recently applied to the study of intelligence, wisdom, and creativity and the interrelations among them (Sternberg, 1985b). Through such a study it is possible to understand what people perceive creativity to be and how they see it as distinguished from intelligence and wisdom. Such a study does not tell us what creativity "really is." But it serves as a start toward defining the core as well as the boundaries of the phenomenon.

Intercorrelational relations among creativity, intelligence, and wisdom

I began (Sternberg, 1985b) by sending questionnaires to professors of art, business, philosophy, and physics. The questionnaires asked these individuals to list behaviors that were characteristic of people who were highly intelligent, wise, or creative in their respective fields of endeavor. A comparable questionnaire was given to laypersons – people from the New Haven area who answered an advertisement in a local newspaper. The number of individuals responding averaged 25 per group. The number of behaviors listed averaged 131 for each of the three attributes of intelligence, wisdom, and creativity, so that the listing procedure generated quite a large number as well as variety of behaviors for each attribute.

A new questionnaire was then sent out to different people within the same subject population. These "new" people were asked to rate how characteristic each of the set of behaviors was of an ideally intelligent, wise, or creative individual in their respective groups. The rating scale ranged from extremely uncharacteristic (1) to extremely characteristic (9). The average number of subjects per group was 65, and all subjects provided all three ratings (for intelligence, wisdom, and creativity), although in different orders. For example, some of the people would provide ratings for creativity first, others would provide creativity ratings second, and still others would provide creativity ratings last. The ratings obtained in each of the groups proved to be highly reliable, meaning that there was substantial agreement among the members of the various groups as to what constituted intelligent, wise, or creative behavior.

The various ratings were intercorrelated in order to determine how closely related the people in each of the groups thought intelligence, wisdom, and creativity to be. Three findings of particular interest emerged from these intercorrelations.

First, I found that, in general, intelligence and wisdom are perceived as most closely related (median $r = .68$), intelligence and creativity as next most closely related (median $r = .55$), and wisdom and creativity as least related (median $r = .27$). The only departure from this pattern was for philosophers, for whom intelligence and creativity were considered to be more highly related ($r = .56$) than were intelligence and wisdom ($r = .42$).

Second, all of the interrelationships were positive, meaning that greater amounts of a given attribute were associated with greater amounts of each other attribute. However, there was one exception to this trend: The business professors saw greater amounts of wisdom as being associated with lesser amounts of creativity ($r = -.24$). In other words, in business, the wiser people are seen as less creative, and vice versa.

Third, there were some interesting differences in magnitudes of interrelations across groups. For example, the art, philosophy, and physics professors all saw intelligence and creativity as being highly related (r's $= .55, .56, .64$, respectively), but the business professors and laypersons saw them as only weakly related (r's $= .29$ and $.33$, respectively). Moreover, the relation between creativity and wisdom reached moderate levels in the opinion of the art professors and philosophy professors (r's $= .48$ and $.37$, respectively), but was low for the other groups and, as mentioned earlier, was actually negative for the business group.

To conclude, the first study was critical in showing that whereas intelligence, wisdom, and creativity are all viewed as being positively related, on the average, the relations among them differ. Creativity is less closely related to the other two constructs than these two constructs are to each other. Moreover, the positive relation between wisdom and creativity actually becomes negative in the opinion of the business group. Finally, the strength of the relation between intelligence and creativity, although always positive, varied among groups. Business professors and laypersons saw them as being less closely related than did the others.

The structure of implicit theories of creativity

In a second study, 40 college students were asked to sort three sets of 40 behaviors into as many or as few piles as they wished on the basis of which behaviors are "likely to be found together" in a person. These behaviors were from the listings for intelligence, wisdom, and creativity from the first study. Only the top 40 behaviors (i.e., behaviors rated by laypersons as highly characteristic of ideally intelligent, wise, or creative individuals) were used in each sorting task. Different subjects did the sortings for intelligence, wisdom, and creativity in different orders.

A method of data analysis called nonmetric multidimensional scaling was used to analyze the sortings. This method enables one to determine the latent structure in a set of sorting or rating data. A latent structure was determined for each of the three attributes. The scalings provided an excellent fit, statistically, to the data.

The multidimensional scaling for creativity yielded six major elements (Stress, Formula $1 = .14$. $R^2 = .87$):

1. *Lack of conventionality* (e.g., one makes up rules as one goes along; has a free spirit; is unorthodox).
2. *Integration and intellectuality* (e.g., makes connections and distinctions between ideas and things; has the ability to recognize similarities and differences; is able to put old information, theories, etc., together in a new way).
3. *Aesthetic taste and imagination* (e.g., has an appreciation of art, music, etc.; can write, draw, compose music; has good taste).
4. *Decisional skill and flexibility* (e.g., follows gut feelings in making decisions after weighing the pros and cons; has the ability to change directions and use another procedure).
5. *Perspicacity* (e.g., questions societal norms, truisms, assumptions; is willing to take a stand).
6. *Drive for accomplishment and recognition* (e.g., is motivated by goals; likes to be complimented on work; is energetic).

For comparative purposes, it is useful to say something of the dimensions that emerged for the constructs of intelligence and wisdom. For intelligence, six basic elements also emerged: practical problem-solving ability, verbal ability, intellectual balance and integration, goal orientation and attainment, contextual intelligence, and fluent thought. For wisdom, six basic elements were found: reasoning ability, sagacity, learning from ideas and environment, judgment, expeditious use of information, and perspicacity.

To summarize, there is some overlap, though it is far from total, in the perceived dimensions of intelligence, wisdom, and creativity. The amounts of overlap reflect the findings of the previously described correlational study: Intelligence and wisdom show the most overlap, and creativity and wisdom the least. Most important, from the present perspective, the emerging view of creativity shows aspects of intelligence, intellectual style, and personality/motivation. Lack of conventionality will be viewed here as a matter of style – a way of approaching problems and situations. The aspect of integration and intellectuality is defined as primarily an aspect of intelligence, similar to the intellectual-balance-and-integration dimension that emerges for intelligence. The aspect of aesthetic taste and imagination contains elements of intelligence, style, and personality/motivation. The aspect encompassing decisional skill and flexibility is a matter of intelligence and intellectual style, as is perspicacity. Drive for accomplishment and recognition would seem to be primarily in the personality/motivational domain. Thus, it probably makes some sense to attempt to understand the psychological antecedents of these aspects of perceived creativity in terms of something like the three-facet approach used in this chapter.

Use of implicit theories of creativity in evaluating the creativity of others

In the last of the series of studies, 40 individuals, all of whom were adults in the New Haven area, were presented with 54 simulated letters of recommendation. Two typical letters were as follows:

> *Gerald*
> He possesses ability for high achievement.
> He has the ability to grasp complex situations.
> He has good problem-solving ability.
> He attaches importance to well-presented ideas.
>
> *Doris*
> She is motivated by goals.
> She questions societal norms, truisms, and assumptions.
> She thinks quickly.
> She is not materialistic.
> She is totally absorbed in study.

Descriptions were generated to vary predicted levels of intelligence, wisdom, and creativity. Each description was either four, five, or six sentences in length and was paired equally often with names of males and with names of females. A given subject, however, saw a given description only once – either with a male name or with a female name. The subject's task was to rate the intelligence, wisdom, and creativity of each of the described individuals. Ratings of the individuals were made on a 9-point scale ranging from not at all intelligent, wise, or creative (1) to extremely intelligent, wise, or creative (9). The order of ratings was varied across subjects in the study.

It was possible to obtain predicted ratings of intelligence, wisdom, and creativity by summing up the ratings of laypersons from the first study on each attribute for each subject, and then dividing by the number of attributes given for the hypothetical individual. Averages rather than sums of ratings were used because the number of behaviors was not the same for each of the descriptions.

Suppose, for example, that five behaviors were given for Susan. The predicted intelligence ratings would be the average of the characteristicness ratings for intelligence in the first study (plus an additive constant). The predicted wisdom rating would be the mean of the ratings for wisdom in the first study (plus an additive constant), and the same held true for predicted creativity. Thus, the closer the description of the hypothetical individual represents the ideal of the first study on each of the three attributes of intelligence, wisdom, and creativity, the higher the rating that the hypothetical individual receives in the present study.

Average ratings of the hypothetical individuals were highest for intelligence (5.8), intermediate for wisdom (5.3), and lowest for creativity (5.0). The ratings were highly reliable (median reliability = .98), meaning that there was agreement among subjects as to who was relatively more or less intelligent, wise, or creative. Intercorrelations (degree of relationship) of ratings were extremely high between intelligence and wisdom (r = .94), high between intelligence and creativity (r = .69), and moderately high between wisdom and creativity (r = .62). Thus, the rank order of the correlational relations was the same as that in the past studies, although in this study, intelligence and wisdom were almost indistinguishable. Use of male versus female names had no effect either on level or on correlational pattern of ratings.

The relations between observed and predicted ratings (with predictions deriving from the first study) each showed an excellent fit of the predictions to the data. In each case, the correlation between the predicted and observed values for a given attribute was extremely high (median r = .89). Moreover, this correlation of predicted with observed values for a given attribute (e.g., predicted values for creativity with observed values for creativity) was always higher than the correlation of predicted with observed values across attributes (median r = .51) (e.g., predicted values for creativity with observed values for wisdom). Thus, people seem not only to have implicit theories of intelligence, wisdom, and creativity but also to use these implicit theories in predictable and somewhat distinguishable ways to judge others.

To summarize, people have implicit theories, and they use these theories to evaluate others. It is possible to predict people's evaluations of others on the basis of knowledge about their implicit theories. The results of their judgments closely mirror the results of their mental structures as revealed by the previous correlational and multidimensional scaling analyses.

Differences among laypersons and various experts in their conceptions of creativity

To this point, implicit theories have been discussed primarily as though they are the same from one group of people to another. Indeed, the studies described here show a high degree of overlap between implicit theories across different groups. However, there are some interesting differences as well as commonalities. Consider these differences for the analyses of creativity.

For laypersons, conceptions of creativity overlap with those of intelligence, but there is much less emphasis in implicit theories of creativity on analytical abilities, whether they be directed toward abstract problems or toward verbal materials. For example, the very first dimension shows a greater emphasis on nonentrenchment, or the ability and willingness to go beyond ordinary limitations of self and environment and to think and act in unconventional and even dreamlike ways. The creative individual has a certain freedom of spirit and unwillingness to be bound by the unwritten canons of society, characteristics not necessarily found in the highly intelligent individual. Implicit theories of creativity encompass a dimension of aesthetic taste and imagination that is absent in implicit theories of intelligence, and they also encompass aspects of inquisitiveness and intuitiveness that do not seem to enter into the implicit theories of intelligence. Implicit theories of creativity go far beyond conventional psychometric creativity tests. A person's abilities to think of unusual uses for a brick, or to form a picture based on a geometric outline, scarcely do justice to the kind of freedom of spirit and intellect captured in people's implicit theories of creativity.

For specialists, implicit theories of creativity in the specialized fields are highly overlapping across fields and also highly overlapping with the implicit theories of laypersons; nevertheless, there are some differences worthy of note. Professors of art place heavy emphasis on imagination and originality, as well as on an abundance of and willingness to try out new ideas. The creative artist is a risk-taker and persists in following through on the consequences of risks. Such a person thinks metaphorically and prefers forms of communication other than strictly verbal forms. Business professors also emphasize the ability to come up with new ideas and to explore these ideas, especially as they relate to novel business services and products. The creative individual escapes traps of conventional thinking and can imagine possible states that are quite different from what exists. Philosophy professors emphasize the ability to toy imaginatively with notions and combinations of ideas and to create classifications and systematizations of knowledge that differ from the conventional constructs. Creative individuals never automatically accept the "accepted," and when they have novel hunches, these hunches often pay off. The creative person is particularly adept at generating insights regarding connections between seemingly unrelated issues and forming useful analogies and explanations. Physics professors share many of these same ideas about the creative individual, but show a particular concern with inventiveness, the ability to find order in chaos, and the ability to question basic principles. The physicists emphasize creative aspects of problem solving, such as the ability to approximate solutions, the ability to find shortcuts in problem solving, and the ability to go beyond standard methods of problem solving. Finally, the physicist thinks a creative person has the ability to make discoveries by looking for reasons why things happen the way they do. Such discoveries may result from the perception of physical and other patterns that most others simply overlook.

Conclusions

What are the main conclusions to be drawn from this work on implicit theories? First, people have implicit theories of creativity, as well as of intelligence and wisdom, and they use these theories both in conceptualizing these attributes and in evaluating themselves and others. Second, the three constructs are distinct, although interrelated. A complete theory of creativity would have to account for both the overlap and the distinctness. Third, assessments of creativity are in need of serious reconsideration and especially broadening. The measures of creativity presently available to us measure creativity in a less meaningful (some might say more trivial) way than would correspond to people's implicit theories of creativity. Thinking of unusual uses for a paper clip, for example, and similar tasks, would seem to draw relatively little on the lack of conventionality, integration and intellectuality, aesthetic taste and imagination, decisional skill and flexibility, perspicacity, and drive for accomplishment and recognition that are seen as essential aspects of creativity. But then, how can we understand creativity so that we might better measure it? The remainder of this chapter is devoted to developing a psychological account of creativity that is consistent with, but in at least some respects goes beyond, people's implicit theories.

The intellectual facet of creativity

The intellectual facet of creativity refers to those aspects of creativity that can be accounted for in terms of the theory of intelligence. The particular theory on which I shall draw here is my own triarchic theory (Sternberg, 1985a). According to this theory, intelligence can be understood as comprising three aspects: its relation to the internal world of the individual, its relation to experience, and its relation to the external world of the individual. It is through experience that the individual mediates the relation between the internal and external worlds.

The relation of intelligence to the internal world

In order to understand creativity, we need to understand the mental processes of the intellect that underlie it. The triarchic theory of intelligence, through its componential subtheory, specifies some, although almost certainly not all, of these processes. These processes can be executed in more or less creative ways. The creativity of the way in which they are executed depends on the originality and quality of the component execution. The relevant processes are of three kinds.

Metacomponents. Metacomponents are higher-order executive processes used in planning, monitoring, and evaluating one's problem solving. The metacomponents most relevant to creativity per se are the planning metacomponents, or what I sometimes call the "legislative" ones, in that they legislate what one is going to do.

   1. *Recognizing the existence of a problem.* An important aspect of creativity is the recognition of problems – not just any old problems, but problems that are (a) large in scope, (b) important in their potential consequences, and (c) potentially soluble, at least to some meaningful degree. Creative individuals are not just good problem solvers but also good problem finders (Getzels & Csikszentmihalyi, 1976).

They know a good problem when they see one, and indeed, they might best be characterized as having "good taste" in problems (Zuckerman, 1983). In my own experience of editing large numbers of manuscripts for a prestigious journal in the field of child development, I found that what distinguished the more eminent from the less eminent scientists was not always how well they designed or executed their experiments but rather what experiments they deemed worthy of performing in the first place. The greatest experiments are not always the most well-designed experiments. In psychology, for example, the seminal experiment on semantic memory, that of Collins and Quillian (1969) on semantic networks, had a number of methodological holes and proved to be subject to a variety of alternative interpretations. Similarly, the classic Shepard and Metzler (1971) experiment on mental rotation, which was intended to show the analogue nature of mental representations, actually yielded results that could be interpreted as consistent with a propositional representation (Palmer, 1975); again, Tulving's classic experiment (1966) on negative transfer in part-whole free recall, deemed to show the importance of organizational effects in episodic memory, could be interpreted entirely in terms of list-discrimination effects (Sternberg & Bower, 1974). What made these experiments great was not the flawlessness of their designs but the vision that went into selecting important problems, and then approaching them in what at the time seemed like a compelling way. Problem selection was far more important than problem solution in determining the classic role of these experiments in the history of psychology.

2. *Problem definition.* Once we have recognized an important problem, we still have to define it. Sometimes we know we have problems facing us in life, but we cannot quite figure out what the problems are, or what their structure looks like. Problem definition requires the structuring of the problem in a way that makes the problem both meaningful and soluble. In my own primary field of intelligence, for example, what has changed over the past decade is only secondarily the way the problems in the field have been approached. Rather, what has changed primarily is the way the problems are structured. The goal of research is no longer seen as understanding what conventional intelligence tests are measuring, but rather as understanding what they should measure and how this differs from what they actually do measure.

A classic problem showing the importance of problem definition – or redefinition – can be found in the so-called nine-dot problem. In this problem, subjects are presented with three rows of three dots and are asked to connect the dots with a pencil, using no more than four straight lines and never lifting the pencil from the paper. People unfamiliar with the problem usually define it in terms of connecting the dots with lines that remain within the confines of the implicit border of the nine dots. In fact, the problem can be solved only if one extends one's pencil beyond the nine dots. There was nothing in the statement of the problem to suggest that one must stay within the implicit border of the nine dots. People tend to define the nine-dot problem narrowly rather than broadly and hence miss out on the opportunity to solve it at all.

Consider a second problem of a slightly different ilk:

A monk wishes to pursue study and contemplation in a retreat at the top of a mountain. The monk starts climbing the mountain at 7:00 a.m. and arrives at the top of the mountain at 5:00 p.m. of the same day. During the course of his ascent, he travels at variable speeds and takes a break for lunch. He spends the evening in study and contemplation. The next day, the monk starts his descent at 7:00 a.m. again, along the same route. Normally, his descent would be faster than his ascent, but because he is tired and afraid of tripping and hurting himself, he descends the mountain slowly, not arriving at the bottom until 5:00 p.m. of the day after he started his ascent. Must there be a point on the mountain that the monk passes at exactly the same time of day on the two successive days of his ascent and descent? Why or why not?

The answer is affirmative, but it is extremely difficult to figure out if the problem is defined in the way it is originally presented. The problem becomes much easier to conceptualize if, rather than imagining the same monk climbing the mountain one day and going down the mountain the next, the reader imagines two different monks, one ascending and the other descending the mountain on the same day. In this redefinition of the problem, the monk's descent on the second day is reconceptualized isomorphically as a different monk's descent on the same day as the first monk's ascent. If there were two monks, their paths of ascent and descent would necessarily cross each other at the same time of day. Obviously, their meeting must be at a given place and point in time, although one cannot specify in advance exactly when or where the meeting will take place. Note that the problem becomes easily soluble only when it is creatively redefined.

Creative redefinition of problems is not limited in its applicability or importance to academic problems such as those cited. One instance relevant to many people's lives is what to do when one is involved in an intimate relationship and one is more involved with the other person than the other person is with oneself. Most people define the problem as one of equalizing levels of involvement by trying to get the other person to be more involved – to reach one's own level of involvement. Our research suggests that such a strategy usually is nonoptimal (Sternberg & Barnes, 1985). A better strategy is to redefine the problem as one of more nearly equalizing the levels of involvement by reducing one's own level of involvement. Although this reduction of one's own level of involvement may be difficult to achieve, it is more likely to lead to continuation and, ultimately, success of the relationship.

3. *Formulation of a strategy and mental representation for problem solution.* I am not a great spatial visualizer. When I was younger, I would take tests of spatial visualization ability and turn in some truly marginal performances. Somewhere along the line, I realized that I did not have to perform at a marginal level on many of these problems, because many of them could be solved verbally rather than spatially. Once I had this realization, I no longer tried to solve the problems in the way the test constructors intended. Rather, I would first try to determine if there was a nonspatial means of solution and use this means of solution if I was able to find one; I would use spatial processing only if no verbal strategy seemed to be available. My scores on these tests improved substantially.

Many problems can be solved in multiple ways. Often, some of these ways are more creative than others.

Performance components. The performance components of intelligence execute the instructions of the metacomponents. In most cases, the execution of these components is straightforward. However, in some instances, performance components can be executed more or less creatively. For example, inferences can be more or less creative, depending on how far beyond a given set of data one is able to go. A creative inference is one that is unusual and high in quality or veridicality. Similarly, mappings – recognition of second-order relations (relations between relations) – can be more or less creative, depending on their nontriviality.

Tourangeau and Sternberg (1981) have proposed a theory of metaphorical thinking that is relevant to determining the level of creativity of an analogy. One can imagine concepts as occurring in sets of local subspaces, with each subspace containing a set of related concepts (i.e., a semantic field). Thus, one can conceive of the mind as comprising a large set of such local subspaces, which may overlap with respect to certain concepts. In this conceptualization, it is possible not only to compute the distance between points within a given local subspace (using Euclidean distance) but also to compute the distance between subspaces. Some semantic fields are rather closely related (e.g., sets of fruits and sets of vegetables), whereas other fields are more distantly related (e.g., sets of animals and vehicles of conveyance).

In an analogy or metaphor, one relates two sets of two terms (which may be stated either explicitly or implicitly). A good analogy is one in which the two sets of terms are at correspondent points within their respective local subspaces. For example, "the Rolls-Royce is the lion of automobiles" will be a good metaphor to the extent that one perceives the Rolls-Royce as the "king" of cars, as the lion is often viewed as the "king" of the animals. A creative analogy is one in which the between-subspace distance is large, but the corresponding within-subspace distances are small. In other words, the two sets of two terms are at roughly correspondent points in their respective local subspaces, but the two sets of terms are in relatively distant local subspaces. Thus, the correspondence between the two sets of terms is good, but the two sets of terms are not trivially related. For example, "the Rolls-Royce is the lion of automobiles" is a creative metaphor to the extent that "Rolls-Royce" and "lion" are at correspondent points in their local subspaces, but also to the extent that "automobiles" and "animals" are in relatively distant local subspaces. The unusualness of the analogy or metaphor will be largely a function of between-subspace distance. The accuracy of the analogy or metaphor will be largely a function of alignment of corresponding points in their respective local subspaces.

Knowledge-acquisition components. Knowledge-acquisition components are involved particularly in a specialized form of creativity: insight. Janet Davidson and I (Davidson & Sternberg, 1984; Sternberg & Davidson, 1982) have suggested that three knowledge-acquisition components form the bases for three different kinds of potentially creative insights.

1. *Selective encoding.* An insight of selective encoding involves sifting out relevant from irrelevant information. Significant problems generally present large

amounts of information, only some of which is relevant to problem solution. Insights are involved in many fields of endeavor. For example, an insightful detective needs to sift out relevant clues, and an insightful doctor needs to sift out relevant symptoms in making a diagnosis. Davidson and I have found that a major distinguisher between better and lesser scientists is the ability of the better scientists to recognize what is important in their data. The better scientists seem to know what findings to emphasize and what findings to deemphasize or ignore. The lesser scientists are less able to distinguish what matters more in their data and what matters less. A famous example of a selective encoding insight in science can be found in Sir Alexander Fleming's discovery of penicillin. Fleming had been attempting to grow bacteria in a petri dish, but his culture was spoiled by a mold that had killed the bacteria. A typical scientist might have despaired, his experiment having been spoiled. Fleming noticed that what had started off as a mundane experiment had become a monumental one: He had discovered a way of killing bacteria via a mold, which later came to be called penicillin.

2. *Selective combination.* An insight of selective combination involves synthesizing what might originally seem to be isolated pieces of information into a unified whole that may or may not resemble its parts. Whereas selective encoding involves knowing which pieces of information are relevant, selective combination involves knowing how to blend together the pieces of relevant information.

There are many examples in real-world performance of how the insight of selective combination operates. For example, once a detective has decided what clues are relevant to the solution of a particular case, a way must be found to put them together in order to pinpoint the perpetrator of the crime. A doctor must figure out how the observed symptoms fit together in order to provide a basis for a diagnosis. Also, we have found that the more competent scientists seem better able to fit their findings together into a coherent package, or story. Less competent scientists are less able to comprehend the interrelationships. They tend to present facts as isolated, rather than as part of a finely woven story relating to the phenomenon under investigation. A famous instance of selective combination can be found in Darwin's formulation of the theory of evolution. The facts that compose the basis for this theory had been available for a long time; what Darwin realized was how to put these facts together to serve as the basis for a new theory of how life evolves.

3. *Selective comparison.* An insight of selective comparison involves relating newly acquired information to information acquired in the past. Problem solving by analogy, for example, is an instance of selective comparison: One realizes that new information is similar to old information in certain ways (and dissimilar in other ways) and uses this old information in better understanding the new information.

One could cite many instances of how selective comparison insights operate in real-world activities. For example, a detective draws on experience in order to solve a crime. The detective may recall a previous case in which the clues fit into a similar pattern and use the earlier case as a basis for solving the newly committed crime. A doctor may recollect a previous patient whose symptoms resembled those of a current patient. The diagnosis relevant in the earlier case might be relevant in the current case. We have found that better scientists seem better able to relate their new work to past endeavors in the field. They have a sense of where their work fits into the current scientific picture, and they may carry on their work without a clear understanding of why it is, or is not, really worth doing. A famous example of the application of selective comparison is in Kekulé's discovery of the structure of the benzene molecule. Kekulé had been trying for some time to decipher the structure of this molecule; one night he had a dream in which a snake danced around and bit its tail. The next morning, Kekulé made the association between the dream and his quest: The snake biting its tail was a visual image for the structure of the ring.

The relation of intelligence to experience

The components of intelligence can be applied to problems at various levels of experience, ranging from tasks and situations that are wholly unfamiliar to problems and situations that are highly familiar, and possibly overlearned. Creativity can come into play in both kinds of tasks and situations, either when an old and familiar problem is seen in a new way or when a new and unfamiliar problem is seen in an old way, that is, when one realizes how to apply what one already knows to a new kind of task or situation.

Coping with novelty provides one of the best opportunities for display of creativity. When one confronts something that is quite different from what is already known, one has the opportunity to approach the problem in a particularly creative way. In some of our research, for example, we present subjects with novel kinds of tasks or situations, then ask the subjects to imagine what would follow if some of these novelties were true. In one experiment, for example, subjects were told to imagine themselves on the planet Kyron, where there are four kinds of people: plins, who are born young and die young; kwefs, who are born old and die old; balts, who are born young and die old; and prosses, who are born old and die young (Sternberg, 1982; Tetewsky & Sternberg, 1986). In another experiment, subjects were asked to solve analogies as though a counterfactual statement were true, for example, that villains are lovable. We were interested in how well subjects would reason in a world in which it is assumed that this statement is true (Marr & Sternberg, 1986). Although almost everyone can solve problems of these kinds, we have observed that some people can easily adjust to the demands of these non-entrenched problems, whereas others have trouble imagining the world to be any different from the way it is.

In recent times, cognitive scientists have more and more emphasized the role of knowledge in intelligence (Chi, Glaser, & Rees, 1982), and knowledge would seem to play a role in creativity as well. In particular, it is impossible to have novel ideas about something if one knows nothing about it. One needs knowledge to extend from in order to see how to apply or extend it creatively. At the same time, too much knowledge can be (although need not be) a dangerous thing. One can become so entrenched in set ways of seeing issues and problems that one is unable to go beyond the existing paradigms and points of view. Thus, often the most creative work in a given area is done by people who are relatively new to the field and who know a fair amount about that field, but not too much about it.

The relation of intelligence to the external world

Intelligence has a contextual element, and so does creativity. According to the triarchic theory, intelligence in the everyday environment can serve any one of three contextual functions: adaptation to an existing environment, shaping of an existing environment into a new environment, or selection of a new environment.

Creativity is probably most associated with environmental shaping. The great creative thinkers in almost any field are those who shape the field to their own conception of what that field should be. For example, a writer such as Hemingway, an artist such as Picasso, an educator such as Dewey, and a scientist such as Herbert Simon have all been viewed as creative in part because of their enormous impact in shaping their respective fields. Sometimes, the shapers actually create new fields. For example, Newton and Leibniz independently invented the field of calculus, thereby shaping much mathematical thinking for centuries to come. Shaping an environment so as to take a new form allows many possibilities for creativity, although environments differ in the extent to which they can be shaped, and hence in the extent to which one is able to exercise one's creativity through shaping.

Environmental selection also enables one to exercise one's creativity if one moves into an unusual but nevertheless appropriate environment vis-à-vis one's abilities, propensities, and possibilities. This creativity can be exercised in even as routine a decision as to where to go on a vacation. Some choices of vacations (environmental selections) will turn out to be fairly routine, whereas others may be much more exciting and creative.

Adaptation probably allows the fewest opportunities for true creativity, although some adaptations to an existing environment can certainly be more creative than others. For example, one may be able to stay within a given system because one finds a way to work around that system, without actually changing the system. Students in school often are able to adapt to the school environment precisely because they find ways of working around it.

To summarize, a first facet of creativity is in the application of intelligence in a creative – statistically unusual and highly appropriate – way. But there is more to creativity than intelligence. A second facet of creativity derives from intellectual style – the way in which intelligence is utilized in one's thought and action.

Intellectual styles

A second aspect of creativity derives from the manner, or style, with which one directs one's intelligence. Some level of intelligence probably is a necessary condition for creativity, but not a sufficient condition, in part because the style with which one uses one's intelligence is as important as the level of intelligence in determining whether or not one is creative.

My comments regarding intellectual styles are drawn from my theory of mental self-government as a basis for intellectual styles (Sternberg, 1986). The styles serve to bridge between intelligence, on the one hand, and personality, on the other.

If one views intellectual functioning as mental self-government, then one can view certain kinds of mental self-government as more potentially creative than others. According to the theory, mental self-government can be characterized in terms of five major aspects: (a) functions, which can be legislative, executive, or judicial; (b) forms, which can be monarchic, hierarchic, oligarchic, or anarchic; (c) levels, which can be global or local; (d) scope, which can be internal or external; and (e) leaning, which can be conservative or progressive. Each of these aspects of mental self-government has at least some relevance for understanding creativity.

Functions of government

Mental self-government, like societal government, serves three basic political functions: legislative, executive, and judicial. Consider each of these three styles in turn.

The legislative style is found in people who (a) like to create their own rules, (b) like to do things their own way, (c) prefer problems that are not prestructured or prefabricated, (d) like to build structure as well as content, (e) prefer kinds of activities that involve legislation, such as writing papers, designing projects, and creating new business or educational systems, and (f) gravitate toward legislative occupations such as creative writer, scientist, artist, sculptor, investment banker, policymaker, or architect.

People with an executive style (a) like to follow rules, (b) like to figure out which of existing ways to do things, (c) prefer problems that are prestructured or prefabricated, (d) like to fill in content within existing structure, (e) prefer activities that are executive in nature, such as solving math problems, applying rules to problems, giving talks or lessons based on others' ideas, and enforcing rules, and (f) gravitate toward executive kinds of occupations, such as lawyer, policeman, engineer, builder (of others' designs), surgeon, soldier, and proselytizer (of others' systems).

Individuals with a judicial style (a) like to evaluate rules and procedures, (b) like to evaluate existing structures, (c) prefer problems in which one analyzes and evaluates existing things and ideas, (d) like to judge structure and content, (e) prefer judicial kinds of activities such as writing critiques, giving opinions on things, judging people and their work, and evaluating programs, and (f) prefer judicial kinds of occupations such as judge, critic, program evaluator, admissions officer, grant or contract monitor, systems analyst, or consultant.

I would argue that creative individuals tend to be those with a primarily legislative style, or at least those who combine a legislative style with one of the two other styles. Legislation is an activity that is creative by its nature. However, it is possible to perform executive or judicial tasks in a way that emphasizes their legislative functions. Note that a proclivity toward legislation does not guarantee an ability for it. Whereas the preceding section of this chapter concerns the level of ability needed for creative performance, this section deals with proclivity in the utilization of abilities. And if one looks at creative performances in the world, these performances tend to be legislative, whether they are in creating art, literature, governmental legislation, scientific theories, or whatever. A creative administrator is one who brings a legislative style to bear, at least in part, on administrative work, whereas a "creative critic" is one who goes beyond just evaluative comments and perhaps creates a new and exciting framework in which these comments are made.

Forms of mental self-government

Mental self-governments, like societal governments, come in multiple forms. Some of these forms are more likely than others to lead to creative performance. The monarchic style is shown by people who (a) tend to be motivated by a single goal or need at a time, (b) are single-minded, (c) are driven, (d) believe that ends justify means, (e) believe in going full speed ahead, and damn the obstacles, (f) are oversimplifiers, (g) are un-self-aware, (h) tend toward intolerance, (i) are inflexible, and (j) have little sense of priorities. People with the hierarchic style (a) tend to be motivated by a hierarchy of goals, with the recognition that not all goals can be fulfilled equally well and that some goals are more important than others, (b) tend toward a balanced approach to problems, (c) believe that the ends do not justify the means, (d) can deal with competing goals, (e) are complexifiers, (f) are self-aware, (g) are tolerant, (h) are flexible, and (i) have a good sense of priorities. People with the oligarchic style (a) tend to be motivated by multiple, often competing goals of equal preceived importance, (b) follow multiple, possibly competing approaches to problems, (c) are driven by goal conflict and tension, (d) believe that ends do not justify means, (e) believe that competing goals and needs tend to interfere with task completion, (f) are complexifiers, sometimes to the frustration point, (g) are self-aware, (h) are tolerant, (i) are very flexible, and (j) have trouble setting priorities. People with an anarchic style (a) are motivated by a potpourri of needs and goals that are often difficult to sort out, (b) exhibit what seems like a random approach to problems, (c) are driven by "muddle," and sometimes seemingly inexplicable forces, (d) believe that ends justify means, (e) are often unclear as to their goals, (f) tend to be simplifiers, (g) are un-self-aware, (h) tend toward intolerance, and (i) cannot set priorities because they have no basis for them.

Creativity probably is not as strongly linked to form of mental self-government as it is to function. Nevertheless, one of the forms lends itself particularly to creative potentialities, namely, the anarchic form. Anarchics have the ability to remove themselves from existing constraints, ways of seeing things, and ways of doing things. They are particularly drawn to problems that require a departure from existing rules and principles. Insight problems, for example, are often best solved by people who can escape from existing mental sets and perceive problems in new ways. But not all anarchics demonstrate creativity. Some of them lack the intellectual ability to be creative. Others lack the legislative style that needs to be combined with the anarchic style in order to generate creative performance. Still others are punished so strongly for their anarchic style that their creative ability is channeled into antisocial pursuits. Anarchics generally are not to the tastes of either teachers or parents, because the anarchics go against the existing grain. As a result, it is likely that they will come into conflict with existing authority structures, and unless this conflict is canalized in a constructive way, it may be defeating both to the anarchics and for the society that ultimately could stand to benefit from the anarchics' creative performance.

True monarchics probably are the least likely to exhibit creative performance. They are so susceptible to fixation on a single goal or means to a goal that they are blinded to the alternatives. They simply do not seek or even envision alternative ways of doing things. Creativity is possible within a hierarchical pursuit of a single goal. But if both the means and the ends are monarchic, creativity is unlikely to display itself.

Levels of mental self-government

Globalists are individuals who (a) prefer big issues, (b) ignore or eschew details, (c) tend to be conceptualizers and idea-oriented, (d) enjoy abstract thinking, (e) show an occasional or possibly frequent tendency to get lost on cloud 9, and (f) may see the forest but overlook the trees. In contrast, localists (a) prefer details, (b) deal well with details, (c) are oriented toward pragmatics, (d) tend toward concrete thinking, (e) are down-to-earth, and (f) may miss the forest for the trees.

Most people are some combination of the global and local styles, and indeed the two styles represent a continuum rather than a discrete bifurcation. Nevertheless, at least some global inclination is needed for creative performance. Individuals who get lost in details and who eschew the ''big picture'' are unlikely to put themselves in a position where they can even imagine the creative possibilities of a problem situation. They are too concrete and too detail-oriented. Global tendencies are certainly not sufficient for creativity, but at least some sense for and desire to achieve a big picture is necessary in order to approach a problem creatively.

Scope of mental self-government

Individuals with an internal style tend to be (a) introverted, (b) task-oriented, (c) aloof, (d) socially less sensitive, (e) interpersonally less aware, and (f) alone when they work. In contrast, those who emphasize the external scope of mental self-government tend to be (a) extroverted, (b) people-oriented, (c) outgoing, (d) socially sensitive, (e) interpersonally aware, and (f) with others when they work.

Creativity is certainly possible within either internal or external scope of mental self-government. However, at least some internal scope is needed, even in one's dealings with people, in order fully to display creativity. Creativity requires working with the world of ideas, and this work is almost always, at least in part, a solitary process. Some people gain from interactions with others, and they benefit if they work well with others, but at some point along the way some solitary endeavor is needed. To be creative, one needs to be able to be by and with oneself and also needs to engage with ideas as well as things and others. People who are too external in their orientation can be so busy seeking and enjoying the company of others that they do not allow themselves the time and mental investment needed in order to pursue creative endeavors.

Leaning of mental self-government

People with a conservative style (a) like to adhere to existing rules and procedures, (b) like to minimize change, (c) prefer familiarity in life and work, and (d) avoid ambiguous situations. In contrast, people with a more progressive style (a) like to go beyond existing rules and procedures, (b) like to maximize change, (c) prefer unfamiliarity in life and work, and (d) seek ambiguous situations.

Clearly, at least some progressivism is needed in order to display creative behavior. An individual who is conservative with respect to existing ways of seeing and doing things is unlikely to look beyond them and hence is unlikely to find either creative solutions or creative means toward problem solutions. The creative individual is one who expresses at least some dissatisfaction with existing principles and procedures and directs this dissatisfaction in the constructive direction of seeking new principles and procedures rather than merely criticizing or destroying old ones. (Note that anarchics need not be progressives. Some anarchics may not care in what directions things move so long as there is change, whereas true progressives wish change in a forward direction and no other.)

To conclude, I have argued in this part of the chapter that the creative individual not only needs certain intellectual abilities in order to be creative but also needs an intellectual style that directs these abilities in a creative way. I have used my theory of intellectual styles as mental self-government in order to argue this point. Certain styles are more conducive than others to creative behavior. The most important aspects of creative intellectual style is in a legislative bent toward problems. The legislator is a person who enjoys looking for new things to do and for new ways of doing old things. At least some progressivism in one's approach to these legislative problems facilitates the creative process, as does at least some internal orientation. A creative person may approach problems from the standpoint of any of the various forms of mental self-government, but true monarchics are unlikely to allow themselves the mental and emotional freedom to be creative. In conclusion, creativity is as much a function of the direction of one's intelligence as it is of the level of one's intelligence. Both must be taken into account.

Personality

It has been argued that two important facets of creativity are to be found in aspects of intelligence and in aspects of the ways in which intelligence is utilized through intellectual styles. A third and equally important ingredient of creativity is to be found in personality. In particular, certain personality attributes are more conducive to creative performance than are others.

Tolerance of ambiguity

As has been noted before (Vernon, 1970), tolerance of ambiguity is almost a sine qua non of creative performance. Creative ideas rarely hatch in mature form. Rather, as Gruber (1986) has pointed out, they evolve as systems. Although there may be a few individuals who hatch their creative ideas whole, they are the exception rather than the rule. The majority of creative people must learn to tolerate ambiguity and incompleteness in the development of their creative products. The development of this chapter, for whatever level of creativity it may involve, was an example of this point. The idea for how to combine intelligence, intellectual styles, and personality into a unified account of creativity evolved slowly, after many false leads regarding how the chapter might be written. I found myself having to tolerate ambiguity as I struggled for a synthesis that would make at least some contribution to the literature on creativity. Had I not been willing to tolerate some ambiguity, the chapter would never have been written. Similarly, in their work, scientists pursuing a problem rarely solve it immediately, or with their first-pass attempt. Rather, their solutions tend to be arrived at through a series of successive approximations, and these successive approximations require them to know when they are closing in on a solution but not quite there. Scientists who cannot tolerate this ambiguity may declare themselves at a solution before they actually arrive. As a result, their solution may be incomplete or simply wrong. Indeed, a constant struggle for many scientists is the fear that their next idea or even their present idea will be their last. They have to tolerate the ambiguity of not knowing if their creativity will continue to manifest itself in future endeavors. The general point, then, is that to be creative, one must be willing and able to tolerate at least some ambiguity in order fully to manifest one's creativity.

Willingness to surmount obstacles

Creative people inevitably encounter obstacles. So does everyone else. Such an obstacle can be either an impediment to future creative performance or a spur toward it. I have seen many a fine graduate student "go under" because of an unwillingness or inability to persevere beyond the obstacles that always crop up in graduate careers. Scientists have some articles rejected and grant proposals turned down. Writers have manuscripts rejected or unfavorable reviews of some of their work. Similarly, artists of various kinds also almost inevitably receive at least some unfavorable reviews in the news media. Their ability to sustain their creativity requires an ability to overcome these hurdles and not be dragged down by them. The question is not whether or not an individual will encounter obstacles but rather how one will handle them. A creative individual perseveres.

Willingness to grow

There exists a category of creative individuals in which one has one's last and also one's major creative idea when one has one's first major idea. These individuals are unable or, more likely, unwilling to grow in their ideation. They come up with creative ideas early in their careers, and then are afraid to move beyond those ideas. Sometimes, perhaps, one of these individuals is overly reinforced for this first idea, and continues to thrive on this reinforcement, all the more so when the reinforcement becomes intermittent, as it often does when one stays with a given idea for too long a period of time. It is important to note that in Gruber's theory, the systems of creative people are evolving, not static. Those individuals whose systems are static or show only minor evolution never achieve the true heights possible for creative performance.

Intrinsic motivation

Amabile (1983) has pointed out the critical importance of intrinsic motivation for creative performance. Ultimately, creative people receive much of their push from their own internal desire to be creative. They motivate themselves. Individuals who are largely extrinsically motivated are less likely to be creative, if only because they are so dependent on reinforcement from others in the assessment of their work. Hence, they are likely to be less willing to take the risks needed for creative performance.

Moderate risk-taking

Creative people have a sense of acceptable levels of risk. In order to be creative, they need to take some risk. At the same time, they need to recognize that there are some projects, whatever the field, that are simply too risky to justify the investment of their effort. Scientists, for example, often are aware of problems they would like to study, but they do not tackle those problems because they are too difficult or too unlikely to be susceptible to solution within a reasonable period of time. The successful scientists choose the most difficult problems that they have a reasonable expectation of being able to handle, not problems that are easier, and not ones that are impossible for them.

Desire for recognition

Creative individuals often balance high levels of intrinsic motivation with a desire for recognition. Creativity does not exist in a vacuum; it is in part an ascription by others. Hence, the creative individual will be identified as creative by virtue of being so labeled by others. To achieve such a label, the person must seek it to at least some extent and do what is necessary in order to achieve it.

Willingness to work for recognition

Some people wish to achieve recognition but are not willing to do what they need to do in order to attain it. Ultimately, the individual recognized as creative not only wishes to attain recognition but also actively seeks it in ways that are rewarded by the groups making the relevant ascription.

To summarize, certain personality attributes tend to be associated with creative performance. In this section of the chapter, I have described what some of these personality attributes are. The list is not exhaustive, nor need a creative person exhibit all these attributes. But at least some of them are likely to be present in individuals recognized as creative.

Integration

People are creative by virtue of a combination of intellectual, stylistic, and personality attributes. This chapter has listed a subset of the attributes in each of these three categories that contribute toward the generation and display of creative behavior. Moreover, it has outlined the scope of creativity as revealed by implicit theories. In some domains, implicit theories probably are of little use: Fire, for example, is what it is, regardless of what people think it is. The same cannot be said of creativity: Because creativity is largely an attributional phenomenon, it is important to know what people believe creativity is in order to know how they attribute creativity to people.

Creativity can take many forms and come in many blends, in part because its intellectual, stylistic, and personality facets can combine in essentially an infinite number of ways. Some people will have more of the intellectual attributes, others more of the stylistic attributes, and still others more of the personality attributes. As a professor, for example, I am aware of students with creative intellectual abilities who simply do not have the stylistic or personality attributes for their creativity to come through; other students have the right personality attributes, but frustrate others and usually themselves by not having the intellectual wherewithal to produce creative products. The general point is that creativity will manifest itself in different forms depending on the blend of characteristics one brings to one's attempts at creative performance.

Different blends result not only from individual differences across the three facets of the model of creativity but also from different blends within each facet. Some individuals, for example, may have something of the anarchic style that would free them from past constraints, but may be so local in their anarchistic tendencies, or so executive rather than legislative (e.g., the individual who carries out the revolution that others plan) in their functioning, that their tendency toward anarchism does not manifest itself at all in creative behavior. In order fully to understand the mental bases of creativity, we need to understand both the interrelations and the intrarelations within each of its facets.

Even this is not enough, though. It seems likely that certain blends are more likely to be synergistic (and other blends antagonistic) with respect to generating creative behavior. It does not seem likely that the parts are merely additive, so that the whole represents a simple sum of its parts. For example, a legislative style would seem to be particularly synergistic with excellence in the execution of the legislative metacomponents: problem recognition, problem definition, component selection, strategy selection. and representation selection. In contrast, an executive style combined with excellence in these metacomponents might be antagonistic to the display of creativity: The legislative metacomponents might well end up being used in the service of executive functions.

The notion of "service" of one aspect of mental functioning to another is one that I believe is particularly important in the display of creativity. All styles represent a continuum rather than a discrete partition, and no one is completely dedicated to one style or another: In order to function in the world, they could not be. As a result, people will display different styles as a function of their predispositions, as well as of the tasks and situations in which these predispositions function. Someone who is primarily executive may use legislative activities in the service of the executive, or vice versa. Someone who has a great desire for recognition may seek to turn even executive tasks into legislative ones that are likely to lead to increased recognition. In seeking to understand creativity, therefore, we need to understand the interactivity among its parts as well as their independent functioning.

The emphasis in this chapter has been on the internal attributes that are likely to lead to creative functioning. But a complete model of creativity would have to take into account the environmental as well as the personal variables that facilitate as well as impede the manifestation of creativity. A potentially creative individual may wither in an environment that does not foster, or that actively inhibits, a display of creative behavior. Such environments, unfortunately, are not rare. I have argued elsewhere (Sternberg, 1986) that certain types of schooling, for example, can inhibit creativity, and there are certainly job settings in which creative displays are punished rather than rewarded. A complete theory of creativity, therefore, will ultimately be as much a theory of environments as of persons, and some of the other chapters in this volume deal with the environmental variables that tend either to foster or to impede a display of creativity.

In conclusion, creativity is a multifaceted phenomenon, of which three critical facets would seem to be aspects of intelligence, style, and personality. This chapter has described what some of these aspects might be and how they might be utilized in ways that render people more or less creative in their thought and action.

References

Amabile, T. M. (1983). *The social psychology of creativity*. New York: Springer-Verlag.

Chi, M. T. H., Glaser, R., & Rees, E. (1982). Expertise in problem solving. In R. J. Sternberg (Ed.), *Advances in the psychology of human intelligence* (Vol. 1, pp. 7–75). Hillsdale, NJ: Lawrence Erlbaum.

Collins, A. M., & Quillian. M. R. (1969). Retrieval time from semantic memory. *Journal of Verbal Learning and Verbal Behavior, 8,* 240–248.

Davidson, J. E., & Sternberg, R. J. (1984). The role of insight in intellectual giftedness. *Gifted Child Quarterly, 28,* 58–64.

Feldman, R. D. (1982). *Whatever happened to the quiz kids?* Chicago: Chicago Review Press.

Getzels, J., & Csikszentmihalyi, M. (1976). *The creative vision: A longitudinal study of problem-finding in art*. New York: Wiley-Interscience.

Gruber, H. E. (1986). The self-construction of the extraordinary. In R. J. Sternberg & J. E. Davidson (Eds.), *Conceptions of giftedness*. Cambridge University Press.

Marr, D. B., & Sternberg, R. J. (1986). Analogical reasoning with novel concepts: Differential attention of intellectually gifted and nongifted children to relevant and irrelevant novel stimuli. *Cognitive Development, 1,* 53–72.

Palmer, S. E. (1975). Visual perception and world knowledge: Notes on a model of sensory-cognitive interaction. In D. A. Norman & D. E. Rumelhart (Eds.), *Explorations in cognition*. San Francisco: Freeman.

Perkins, D. (1981). *The mind's best work*. Cambridge, MA: Harvard University Press.

Shepard, R. N., & Metzler, J. (1971). Mental rotation of three-dimensional objects. *Science, 171,* 701–703.

Sternberg, R. J. (1982). Natural, unnatural, and supernatural concepts. *Cognitive Psychology, 14,* 451–458.

Sternberg, R. J. (1985a). *Beyond IQ: A triarchic theory of human intelligence*. Cambridge University Press.

Sternberg, R. J. (1985b). Implicit theories of intelligence, creativity, and wisdom. *Journal of Personality and Social Psychology, 49,* 607–627.

Sternberg, R. J. (in press). Mental self-government: A theory of intellectual styles and their development. *Human Development*.

Sternberg, R. J., & Barnes, M. (1985). Real and ideal others in romantic relationships: Is four a crowd? *Journal of Personality and Social Psychology, 49,* 1589–1596.

Sternberg, R. J., & Bower, G. H. (1974). Transfer in part-whole and whole-part free recall: A comparative evaluation of theories. *Journal of Verbal Learning and Verbal Behavior, 13,* 1–26.

Sternberg, R. J., Conway, B. E., Ketron, J. L., & Bernstein, M. (1981). People's conceptions of intelligence. *Journal of Personality and Social Psychology, 41,* 37–55.

Sternberg, R. J., & Davidson, J. E. (1982, June). The mind of the puzzler. *Psychology Today, 16,* 37–44.

Tetewsky, S. J., & Sternberg, R. J. (1986). Conceptual and lexical determinants of nonentrenched thinking. *Journal of Memory and Language, 25,* 202–225.

Tourangeau, R., & Sternberg, R. J. (1981). Aptness in metaphor. *Cognitive Psychology, 13,* 27–55.

Tulving, E. (1966). Subjective organization and effects of repetition in multi-trial free-recall learning. *Journal of Verbal Learning and Behavior, 5,* 193–197.

Vernon, P. E. (1970). *Creativity*. Harmondsworth, UK: Methuen.

Zuckerman, H. (1983). The scientific elite: Nobel laureates' mutual influences. In R. S. Albert (Ed.), *Genius and eminence: The social psychology of creativity and exceptional achievement* (Vol. 5, pp. 241–252). New York: Pergamon Press.

6   Problem solving and creativity

Robert W. Weisberg

It has long been believed by psychologists that research in problem solving will illuminate broad issues in the study of creative thinking, defined as the thought processes involved in producing work of acknowledged greatness in art or in science. The gestalt psychologists, for example, explicitly equated the productive thinking involved in true problem solving with the thought processes occurring in more esoteric situations, such as the work of great scientists (Wertheimer, 1959). However, the direct connection between research on problem solving and study of creative thinking has been slow in coming. Modern cognitive psychologists have only very recently begun to extend conclusions drawn from laboratory research in problem solving to the thought processes used by scientists and artists (Greeno, 1980; Perkins, 1981; Weisberg, 1986). As one example of this separation of the problem-solving literature from that on creativity, Newell and Simon's (1972) influential analysis of problem solving does not even have entries for creativity or creative thinking in the index. Thus, even though Newell and Simon had proposed an analysis of creative thinking in earlier publications (Simon, 1979), the relevance of the work on problem solving to an understanding of creativity was at most implicit in their magnum opus. As a further example of this conceptual bifurcation, examination of several modern texts on cognitive processes (Bransford, 1979; Gilhooly, 1982; Martindale, 1981) indicates a lack of connection between discussions of problem solving and creative thinking, if both are even mentioned in the same work. For the most part, then, cognitive psychologists have devoted their efforts to the study of laboratory problems of various sorts and seem to have assumed that creative thinking would ultimately be illuminated by this work, without explicitly dealing with creative thinking per se.

Perhaps in part because of this lack of direct involvement by experimental psychologists, the literature on creativity was until recently dominated by what one could call the ''genius'' view of creativity, which also pervades our society. This view, which has many sources, ranging from Plato to Koestler (1964) to Osborn (1953) to psychometric theorists such as Guilford (1950), assumes that truly creative acts involve extraordinary individuals carrying out extraordinary thought processes. These individuals are called geniuses, and the psychological characteristics they possess – cognitive and personality characteristics – make up what is called genius.

Some support for the genius view came from self-reports by acknowledged creative geniuses, such as the following from Samuel Taylor Coleridge, which describes the circumstances leading to his writing "Kubla Khan." At the time, Coleridge had been ill and was living in the country. One afternoon, because of "a slight indisposition," he took "an anodyne" (opium) and fell asleep while reading a book describing Kubla Khan's capital city. According to Coleridge (Ghiselin, 1952, pp. 84–85), the following events then occurred:

The Author continued for about three hours in a profound sleep, at least of the external senses, during which time he had the most vivid confidence that he could not have composed less than from two to three hundred lines; if that indeed can be called composition in which all the images rose up before him as *things,* with a parallel production of the concurrent expressions, without any sensation or consciousness of effort. On awakening he appeared to himself to have a distinct recollection of the whole, and taking his pen, ink, and paper, instantly and eagerly wrote down the lines that are here preserved. At this moment he was unfortunately called out by a person on business from Porlock, and detained by him above an hour, and on his return to his room, found, to his no small surprise and mortification, that though he still retained some vague and dim recollection of the general purport of the vision, yet, with the exception of some eight or ten lines and images, all the rest had passed away like the images on the surface of a stream into which a stone has been cast, but alas! without the after restoration of the latter!

Thus, an entire poem appeared full-blown, with no conscious work on Coleridge's part. This example has been taken as evidence for the importance of unconscious processes in creativity. A similar report was made by Mozart in an often-quoted letter (Ghiselin, 1952, pp. 44–45):

When I feel well and in a good humor, or when I am taking a drive or walking after a good meal, or in the night when I cannot sleep, thoughts crowd into my mind as easily as you could wish. Whence and how do they come? I do not know and I have nothing to do with it. Those which please me, I keep in my head and hum them; at least others have told me that I do so. Once I have my theme, another melody comes, linking itself to the first one, in accordance to the needs of the composition as a whole.

Mozart's report may be even more remarkable than that of Coleridge, because Mozart seems to have needed no help from stimulants or other external sources in order to have creative products come to him. Again, unconscious thought is assumed to have been crucial here.

A final famous example of the extraordinary nature of creative thinking is Friedrich August von Kekulé's report of his discovery of the ring structure of benzene. According to Kekulé, he had the following dream during days of thinking about the problem (Rothenberg, 1979, pp. 395–396):

I turned my chair to the fire and dozed. Again the atoms were gamboling before my eyes. This time the smaller groups kept modestly to the background. My mental eye, rendered more acute by repeated vision of this kind, could now distinguish larger structures, of manifold conformation; long rows, sometimes more closely fitted together; all twining and twisting in snakelike motion. But look! What was that? One of the snakes had seized hold of its own tail, and the form whirled mockingly before my eyes. As if by a flash of lightning I awoke. . . . Let us learn to dream, gentlemen.

In discussions of this incident (Koestler, 1964), two points are emphasized. First, Kekulé was dreaming, which points again to the difference between creative thinking and ordinary conscious thinking. Second, Kekulé used a visual analogy in order to solve his problem. He represented the strings of atoms as snakes, and then one of them bit its tail. Thus, the use of a remote analogy (snakes are far removed from atoms) points to still another difference between creative thinking and ordinary conscious thinking. Many theorists have emphasized the role of analogy in creative thought (Perkins, 1981). Another often-cited example is Bohr's use of the solar system as a model for the structure of the atom. The genius view emphasizes the fact that these two cases involved remote analogies (i.e., the domains involved in each example are not ordinarily considered to be closely related). Strings of atoms do not seem to be closely related to snakes, and neither do atoms and solar systems seem closely related, but creative thinkers found these remote analogies useful. Thus, according to the genius view, the creative thinker finds connections where ordinary individuals do not (Koestler, 1964).

In sum, these examples make clear the purportedly extraordinary aspects of great creative acts and the individuals who produce them. Mozart reported that melodies came to him unbidden, and by themselves expanded into complete works, without his conscious participation. Coleridge reported a similar experience, helped along by a dose of opium. Finally, Kekulé used a visual analogy in a dream to solve the problem of the structure of benzene. In these examples we see unconscious thought processes, as well as modes of conscious thought (e.g., use of a remote analogy), that are beyond the reach of ordinary individuals.

The genius view of creativity has motivated students of creativity to examine those characteristics that lead to the production of great artistic and scientific works (Weisberg, 1986). One stream of research has focused on isolating those personality characteristics that supposedly separate the creative genius from ordinary individuals. There have also been examinations of the brains of geniuses, such as Einstein, in order to determine the areas of the brain that might underlie the capacity to be creative. Finally, much research has been concerned with the mode of thinking involved in creativity. The genius view assumes that creative thinking involves some kind of thought processes (and related personality characteristics) that allow one to break away from the habitual, away from one's past experience, and thereby produce something truly novel, in a leap of insight. As was seen in the foregoing quotations, unconscious processes, altered states of conscious, and use of remote analogies are three characteristics that have been attributed to creative thinkers.

My purpose in this chapter is to explore the implications of laboratory research in problem solving for an understanding of significant creative acts, and thereby to raise questions about the genius view of creativity. The analysis will begin with a consideration of several potentially significant findings from laboratory study of undergraduates' performances on a problem-solving task. These findings will then be supported by results from other laboratory investigations of problem solving. This will lead to a discussion of several case studies from the literature on creativity in science, technology, and the arts. Although the data from such case studies are not as rigorous as those from laboratory experiments, it is my belief that one must directly address the literature concerning individuals of acknowledged greatness. If not, the question always remains whether or not one can generalize from undergraduates solving problems in an experiment to, say, Darwin, Watson and Crick, Edison, Picasso, Mozart, and so on. In making any such generalization, the burden is on the one who would make the generalization from undergraduates to creative geniuses, and so I shall make clear what I see as the connection between laboratory work in problem solving and specific events in the careers of great artists and scientists. The conclusions to be drawn may not at first glance appear to be relevant to true creative thinking, given the genius view. I shall take those conclusions seriously, however, in order to show that the thought processes underlying problem solving by ordinary undergraduates may be similar to those involved in much more esoteric activities, such as developing a scientific theory or painting a mural.

Solution of the candle problem

Duncker's (1945) candle problem asks that the problem solver attach a candle to the wall, with the available materials being a book of matches and a box of tacks or nails. This problem was originally of interest to gestalt psychologists because it was assumed to be an example of a situation in which past experience interfered with productive thinking, in a manner supposedly comparable to that seen in the Luchins water-jar experiments (Luchins & Luchins, 1959). It was argued by Duncker and others that one very effective but infrequent solution to this problem (using the tack box as a platform or holder for the candle) was infrequent because subjects were "fixated" on the use of the box as a container for the fasteners and therefore were not able to conceive of the box as a platform for the candle.

Research by Weisberg and Suls (1973) pointed to a more straightforward explanation of why subjects produced or failed to produce the box solution. First, comparisons of thinking-aloud verbal protocols produced by box-solvers with those of non-box-solvers indicated that all individuals began to work by attempting to apply their knowledge relatively directly to the problem, in response to the instructions (Weisberg & Suls, 1973, Exp. 3). Thus, all individuals started by trying to follow the problem instructions as straightforwardly as they could – by attempting to attach the candle to the wall using the fasteners or melted wax as glue. If these initial attempts were found to be inadequate in some way (e.g., the candle started to split when the fastener was pushed into it; the candle was too thick for the fastener to pass through; or the wax-glue was not strong enough), then attempts would be made to correct this inadequacy. Other solutions, including the box solution, evolved out of these attempts to correct inadequacies in seemingly straightforward solutions.

This research indicated that creative solutions to problems were based on interaction between the subject's knowledge and the problem itself. The subject sets the criteria for solution, based on the instructions and knowledge, and then uses these criteria as the basis for judging the adequacy of any attempted solution. Inadequacies in any solution then become further problems to solve, and so on, recursively, until all criteria are met.

This solution process could be conceptualized as multiple searches of memory, in the sense that each step in the solution, if judged to be inadequate, serves as the cue for further retrieval of information. One could say that the problem becomes reformulated, or changed into a new problem, as the problem solver works through it. New information constantly becomes available as the subject realizes that what was conceived of as an adequate solution is inadequate in some way. This recursive search is similar to Newell and Simon's (1972) discussion of means–ends analysis as a problem-solving heuristic. In contrast to the genius view, which postulates leaps of insight based on remote analogies, this recursive memory search is "local" in nature, because it depends at any time only on the inadequacy the individual is attempting to deal with.

It must be emphasized, however, that this process is more than simply retrieval and use of some old knowledge, because the problem situation is new to our subjects. Therefore, by definition, they cannot be simply retrieving something previously done in this situation. Any retrieval that occurs must be brought about through only a partial match between the present situation and past experience. In this sense, then, all solutions to the candle problem (and perhaps all solutions to any problem) should be considered creative, so long as they are novel as far as the problem solver is concerned, and they solve the problem at hand. I shall therefore assume that the various solutions to the candle problem are equivalent psychologically; production of one solution rather than another depends on the particular tack taken by a given problem solver, which in turn depends on those specific factors in the problem that the problem solver considers important. One subject might respond to the weakness of the wax-glue by trying to increase the area of contact between the candle and the wall, whereas another might try to provide additional support for the glue. The former subject might try to flatten the candle, whereas the latter might try to use the box as a shelf under the candle. Although earlier investigators emphasized lack of production of the box solution, from the present perspective all the various solutions are equivalent, because they are responses to a novel situation, they meet the criteria, and, I believe, they are the results of the same thought processes.

Implications

This work has several implications for understanding problem solving in particular and creative thinking in general. The first implication is that all attempts to solve problems are firmly based on past experience. Individuals initiate work on a problem based on a match between that problem and their knowledge. Furthermore, any inadequacies discovered in an initial solution are also dealt with on the basis of past experience (Greeno, 1980). Second, novel solutions to problems come about in an evolution, as one gradually moves away from the conception with which one began, through local memory searches. No great leaps of insight occur in the production of any solution, whether or not that solution is judged by the experimenter to be particularly creative. However, in order to see the incremental nature of problem solving, one must have available more than simply the initial problem and the final solution. That is, if one knew only that a subject had produced the box solution to the candle problem, one might be tempted to assume that that solution had come about in a modest leap of creativity. With a detailed problem-solving protocol available, on the other hand, one might see that the subject began with an attempt to glue the candle to the wall with melted wax. The box was then used in an attempt to shore up the wax. Thus, the incremental nature of creative problem solving is revealed by a fine-grained analysis of the situation. Third, as just mentioned, this incremental process based on local memory search is set in motion by feedback concerning the inadequacy of some proposed solution. This new information transforms the problem situation and thereby makes possible new solution types. To continue with the same example, a subject who finds that the wax-glue is not strong enough to keep the candle affixed to the wall is now faced with a new problem: How does one hold up a falling candle if glue does not work? This new problem can result in an evolution of the initial solution into something new. Fourth, if it is true, as mentioned earlier, that all solutions to problems are "creative," so long as they are novel and they meet the demands of the problem, then the capacity to think creatively must be a basic human capacity, and not the exotic trait or skill envisioned by the "genius" view. This has potentially important implications for teaching creative thinking.

Research with other problems

These implications, though evolving out of work on a single laboratory problem, have support from other laboratory research in problem solving.

Dependence of creative problem solving on past experience

There has been a small but steady stream of research concerning what are called "insight problems." This is a heterogeneous class of problems that are assumed to be difficult to solve because subjects are inhibited by past experience. Supposedly, the only way to solve such problems is to break away from past experience, which allows one to approach the problem in a novel way (Adams, 1979; Scheerer, 1963). An example of such a problem is the nine-dot problem, shown in Figure 6.1. According to the traditional analysis, the nine-dot problem would be very easy if subjects could simply break away from their tendency to keep their lines within the square formed by the dots. Once subjects break out of this fixation on the square

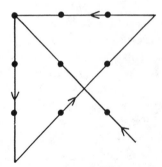

Figure 6.1. Nine-dot problem.

shape, and thereby approach the problem on its own terms, solution should be effortless.

Two studies (Burnham & Davis, 1969; Weisberg & Alba, 1981) tested this view by instructing subjects that in order to solve the nine-dot problem, they had to draw their lines outside the square formed by the dots. Contrary to the traditional view, in both studies only a small percentage of subjects solved the problem, and those subjects took a relatively long time to do so. In addition, both studies found that subjects needed relatively specific information in order to solve the problem. Weisberg and Alba were also able to facilitate or inhibit solution of the nine-dot problem by giving subjects experience solving dot problems of different sorts.

These results were extended by Lung and Dominowski (1985), who facilitated solution of the nine-dot problem by giving subjects practice with six simple dot problems that required that the lines be drawn outside the dots, as well as by giving subjects more detailed instructions concerning what they had to do once they drew lines outside the square formed by the dots. This study supports the earlier ones in showing that the nine-dot problem demands relatively extensive knowledge concerning dot problems on the part of the problem solver.

Similar conclusions can be derived from recent research on expert problem solving in a variety of domains. This work, which began with DeGroot's (1966) analysis of problem-solving skills of master chess players, has resulted in the conclusion that master-level problem solving in any domain depends on the acquisition of deep knowledge about the domain in question (Greeno, 1980). Studies that have compared problem-solving performances of experts and novices in such domains as computer programming, mechanics, and geometry have all indicated that experts are able, because of their knowledge, to "home in" on the important aspect of any novel problem. The expert is able to relate a novel problem to something already known and to use this knowledge as the basis for dealing with the new problem. As Greeno (1980) notes, there has been a blurring of the distinction between "real" problem solving and behavior based on "mere knowledge," as it has been realized that all problem solving is based on knowledge. Any differences between doing something by rote versus as a result of creative thinking may be matters of degree rather than of kind.

Thus, research indicates that rather than being independent of past experience, truly efficient problem solving comes about only when an individual has acquired a deep knowledge of the domain in question. As mentioned earlier, it may be reasonable to assume that all problem solving, if the problem is novel, is creative. This in turn leads to the speculation that creative thinking in other domains, such as science and the arts, may also depend on extensive knowledge in those domains. Evidence relevant to this speculation will be considered in a later section.

Stimuli to novelty

It was mentioned earlier that evidence indicates that the candle problem can become changed as the individual works through it. More specifically, as the problem solver realizes that an initial solution will not work, this information serves as the basis for a new search of memory, in an attempt to overcome the difficulty. Novel solutions to a given problem thus come about because the new information moves the individual away from the original conception. It should therefore be possible to isolate the information that pushes the problem solver in a given direction and use it to induce naive problem solvers to approach the problem in that way. That is, it ought to be possible to short-circuit the incremental processes that lead to innovation in problem solving by presenting the critical information at the very beginning. This hypothesis was tested by Weisberg and DiCamillo (1986) in a series of experiments using what we call the Charlie problem:

Dan came home and found Charlie dead on the floor and Tom in the same room. On the floor Dan saw some broken glass and water. How did Charlie die?

This problem was studied by having subjects ask yes/no questions of the experimenter, which enabled us to keep track of the information they acquired as they worked. (The solution: Tom [a cat] knocked over a fishbowl. Charlie [a fish] died from lack of oxygen.)

When subjects are presented with this problem, all initially assume that the characters are human and that the pieces of glass and the water came from a broken drinking glass. These initial assumptions follow directly from the way the problem is presented. The characters have human names, and no information is given that would cause the subject to question whether or not they are in fact human. In order to solve the problem, however, the subject must come to the realization that the characters are not human, and so on. The research indicated that the solution to the problem only gradually developed, as subjects acquired information in response to their yes/no questions.

As in the candle problem, all subjects begin the Charlie problem in the same way: They ask questions about human deaths. Eventually subjects acquire the information that Charlie died from lack of oxygen. This information alone is not enough to push them to the realization that Charlie is a fish. For about half our subjects, once they found out that Charlie died from lack of oxygen and that the glass and water came from a broken fishbowl, they then inferred rather directly that Charlie was a fish. Thus, subjects' novel analysis of the situation seemed to be the result of their acquisition of two critical pieces of information that changed the situation they were dealing with.

The other subjects did not go directly from "Charlie is human" to "Charlie is a fish." These individuals first made an intermediate deduction, that Charlie was not human, which then led them to "Charlie is a fish." The switch to "Charlie is not human" was stimulated by new information that was inconsistent with the initial assumption that Charlie was human. As an example, one subject asked about Charlie's age and found that though he might be a year old, he was not an infant. That information led rather directly to the conclusion that Charlie was not human.

Thus, two modes of solution were found, one going directly from "Charlie is human" to "Charlie is a fish," and one going indirectly, through "Charlie is not human." Furthermore, different sorts of information seemed to trigger the two modes. This was verified in later experiments in which naive subjects who were given the supposedly relevant information not only solved the problem more quickly but also solved it using the expected mode of solution.

In sum, research using the Charlie problem has demonstrated that novel solutions evolve out of the relatively prosaic solutions with which all subjects begin, in this case proposals concerning human deaths. Furthermore, it has been possible to isolate the crucial pieces of information that result in formulation of the novel solution. Thus, in this case at least, novelty in problem solving comes about through ordinary thought processes in interaction with the information available in the problem. As this information changes, so does the solution produced by the subject, but the thought processes remain the same.

Problem solving, predictability, and insight

Metcalfe (1986) has recently presented evidence to support the view that there is a mode of problem solving that does not depend on past experience and that should be characterized as resulting from leaps of insight. Metcalfe has asked subjects to predict how well they will perform on a task, before they begin to work on it. When the task involves answering trivia questions, the subjects are able to predict which questions they will be able to answer. However, when the task involves problem solving, there are cases in which subjects cannot predict how they will perform. Thus, in tasks involving retrieval of information from memory, subjects are able to predict their performance, whereas they are not always able to do so in tasks involving problem solving.

Metcalfe takes this discrepancy as evidence for the view that in some cases problem solving does not depend on retrieval of information from memory, contrary to the view presented here. According to Metcalfe, because subjects can predict how well they will be able to retrieve information from memory, then if problem solving were based on retrieval of information from memory, they should also be able to predict how well they will solve problems.

However, Metcalfe's analysis is based on an oversimplification of the processes involved in problem solving. Whereas the present view argues that problem solving always depends on the use of past experience, and there is no need to postulate a special process called insight, this does not mean that subjects must be able to predict their problem-solving performance. Indeed, most of the "insight" problems studied by psychologists are so designed that prediction of performance is essentially impossible (Weisberg, 1980, chaps. 10 and 12), which was what made such problems interesting in the first place. Problems like the Charlie problem are so designed that the initial direction taken by the subject is incorrect, which means that any initial predictions by naive subjects are certain to be unrelated to final performance. Solution of such problems depends on feedback from the environment, which informs the problem solver that the initial attempt is incorrect. Therefore, Metcalfe's finding that subjects cannot predict their performance is not surprising. From my perspective, even though problem solving is firmly rooted in past experience, this does not mean that problem solving will be predictable on the part of the subject.

"Local" memory search

A number of studies support the claim that individuals do not widely search memory when attempting to solve problems. The general theme of this research is to provide problem solvers with information demonstrably relevant to the problem at hand, and then to determine the factors that influence the utilization of that information. Over the years there have been studies of the effectiveness of hints of various sorts during problem solving; see Bourne, Ekstrand, and Dominowski (1971) for a review. I shall concentrate on more recent research.

In one study (Weisberg, DiCamillo, & Phillips, 1978), subjects received paired-associate training before trying to solve the candle problem. For the experimental subjects, the critical pair was "candle-box," which was presumably relevant to the candle problem. Control subjects learned "candle-paper" in place of the critical pair. It was found that without an explicit hint that the previously learned pairs might help them solve the problem, experimental subjects produced box solutions no more frequently than did control subjects. This was true even when actual objects, identical with those in the candle problem, were used in the paired-associated training. In this condition, learning the candle-box pair involved the subjects actually putting the candle into the box, but facilitation in using the box to solve the candle problem still was not achieved. On the other hand, all subjects given a hint that one of the pairs might help them solve the problem did produce box solutions, indicating that the candle-box association was potentially useful. In explaining these results, it seems that any memory search stimulated by the candle problem was very limited in nature and was restricted to previous situations involving attaching things to walls. If so, then without an explicit hint to refer to the paired associates, one would not expect them to help, even though the experimenter, from outside the situation, knows that one pair is potentially relevant.

This conclusion is further strengthened by results of studies using verbal problems of the following sort (Perfetto, Bransford, & Franks, 1983):

A man in a certain town has married 20 women in the town. The women are all still alive. The man is neither a Mormon nor a bigamist, he is not divorced, and he has not broken any law. How is that possible?

A police officer watched an individual go against a red light, ignore a stop sign, and go the wrong way down a one-way street, and yet the officer did nothing. Why not?

The solution to the first problem is that the man in question is the clergyman who performed the service marrying each of the 20 women to her husband. In the second problem, the police officer did nothing because the individual in question was a pedestrian.

In their research, Perfetto and associates first presented subjects with sentences to study, ostensibly as part of a memory task. Several of the sentences were potentially relevant to the word problems presented in the second part of the experiment. An example: A minister may marry several people in a single week. Although such a sentence seems of obvious relevance to the problem presented earlier, Perfetto and associates, like Weisberg and associates (1978), found no effect of previous exposure to the critical sentences, unless subjects were explicitly told that some of the earlier-studied sentences might be relevant to the problems.

The local nature of memory search during problem solving has also been shown in recent studies investigating the role of analogy in problem solving. As mentioned earlier, one component of the genius view is that creative products sometimes result from leaps of insight based on remote analogies. In one set of studies on the role of analogy in problem solving, Gick and Holyoak (1983) used Duncker's (1945) radiation or tumor problem as the target problem. In this problem, a doctor is faced with a patient with an inoperable stomach tumor and has available a source of rays that at sufficient intensity will destroy it. However, the rays at that intensity will also destroy healthy tissue, which is unacceptable. How can the doctor use the rays to destroy the tumor while not destroying any healthy tissue? The solution is to use two or more weak bundles of rays, which are so positioned that they cross just at the tumor. The intensity of the rays at the tumor will then be sufficient to destroy it, while the lower-intensity individual bundles will not destroy healthy tissue.

Gick and Holyoak gave subjects prior experience with stories analogous to the radiation problem and then compared their performance to that of control subjects who had preexposure to nonanalogous stories. An example of an analogous story used by Gick and Holyoak involves a general who wishes to attack a fortress, which has roads radiating out from it like the spokes of a wheel. The general has his army massed, ready to attack the fortress, but the roads leading to it have been mined, so that if the whole army is sent down any one road, the weight of soldiers and machines will set off land mines, causing destruction of the army as well as widespread damage to houses of citizens who live along the road. The general therefore divides his army into small groups and positions each group at the head of one of the roads leading to the fortress. At a signal from the general, the small groups move together toward the fortress, and because each group is too small to set off the mines, they are all able to reach the fortress at the same time, and so the general can have his entire army attacking the fortress at once.

Gick and Holyoak (1983) found that preexposure to two stories like the general story facilitated performance on the radiation problem. Most important in the present context, this facilitation was found even among subjects who were not informed of the relationship between the stories and the radiation problem. These results support the view that creative problem solving can use remote analogous relations as the basis for memory search.

However, there is one potential contaminating factor in Gick and Holyoak's studies that raises questions about how wide a search of memory was actually made by their subjects. In addition to the analogous structural relations that existed between the stories and radiation problem, they were also linked by context: They were presented closely in time in one session by a single experimenter. Although Gick and Holyoak told their subjects that the stories and problems were parts of different experiments, there is still the possibility that the context served as a cue whereby the stories were brought to bear on the radiation problem. That is, on receiving the radiation problem, the subjects may have thought back to the stories only because they had just been presented in the same session, not because they were structurally analogous to the radiation problem. The subjects may have been trying to figure out why they were given two tasks to do in the same session, which may have led to the conclusion that the two tasks were related. This, in turn, could lead them to try to relate the stories to the radiation problem. According to this view, analogical thinking is not the cause of the facilitation of the tumor problem brought about by prior exposure to the stories.

In a test of this hypothesis, Spencer and Weisberg (1986) replicated Gick and Holyoak's study, except that the context was changed from the stories to the tumor problem. This was done by having the stories presented as part of an experiment at the beginning of a class, conducted by a visitor unknown to the students. After the experimenter left, the instructor presented the radiation problem as part of a class discussion of problem solving, without making any mention of a relation between the stories and the radiation problem. Spencer and Weisberg found that no transfer occurred from the analogous stories to the radiation problem if subjects were not explicitly informed of the relation between them. When the stories and critical problem were presented in different contexts, no spontaneous noticing of their analogous structures occurred. Catrambone and Holyoak (1985) and Keane (1985) have recently reported results using the radiation problem that support this conclusion, as do results from studies using other target problems (Reed, Ernst, & Banerjii, 1974). Thus remote analogy in and of itself may not provide a basis for memory search in uninformed subjects.

In conclusion, results from research using several different problems support the conclusion that during problem solving only a very limited search is made of memory. Information that can be shown to be available in memory and potentially relevant to some problem may not be accessed if the connection of that information to the problem is not explicit and/or direct. Human thought seems not to be of great range and flexibility during laboratory problem solving.

Broader implications: problem solving and creativity

The research on problem solving just discussed can provide an organizational framework for an initial examination of the literature on creativity in science and the arts. Although the present viewpoint is nowhere near a theory of creativity, the analysis just presented can serve to generate some expectations about what one should expect to find in examining individual examples of creative thinking. First, if creativity begins with a match between a new situation and one's knowledge, then one should see creative products beginning with rather prosaic variations on old themes. These old themes may come from the work of others, or from the work of the individual in question, depending on circumstances to be elaborated later. Second, novel products evolve in small steps out of these initial attempts. No leaps of creativity should be found for even the most creative outcomes if detailed information concerning the individual's work is available. Third, this evolution does not come about in a vacuum. That is, some prosaic initial product will not be modified into something new unless two factors come into play: The individual must see some inadequacy in the initial product, and the individual must know how to overcome this inadequacy.

The examples to be considered come from science, technology, and the arts. It is relatively obvious that a framework based on research in problem solving might have relevance to work in science and technology, because the production of a scientific theory or an invention usually is a "solution" to some "problem." The case in the arts is less clear, but in order to see how far the present point of view can go, I shall assume that artistic creativity can also be looked on as problem solving. This issue is discussed further by Weisberg (1986, chaps. 7 and 8).

Double helix

Watson and Crick's double-strand helical model of the DNA molecule set off the ongoing revolution in molecular genetics. The importance of this discovery has led some to assume that it must have come about in a burst of creative insight, independent of everything that came before (Adams, 1979, pp. 60–61):

Watson and Crick relied heavily on inspiration, iteration, and visualization. Even though they were superb biochemists, they had no precedent from which they could logically derive their structure and therefore relied heavily on left-handed [non-logical] thinking.

However, contrary to Adams, Watson's own autobiographical account of their discovery (Watson, 1968) indicates that although the model was revolutionary in its effects, it evolved in a relatively straightforward way out of the backgrounds of Watson and Crick, in interaction with the circumstances in which they found themselves (Judson, 1979). There almost certainly were precedents available, and they used them.

Both Watson and Crick had, during their separate training, become impressed with the importance of solving the problem of the structure of DNA. In addition, Crick was a PhD student in the Cavendish Laboratory at Cambridge University, which had for a long time been involved with using X-ray crystallography to analyze the structures of molecules. Watson had seen an X-ray photograph of crystalline DNA and had been impressed with the fact that DNA formed a crystal, as well as with the potential of the X-ray technique to provide information concerning the structure of DNA. Thus, when Watson came to work at Cavendish in the fall of 1951, he and Crick were kindred spirits, and they decided to try to build a model of DNA. Data obtained from X-ray crystallography would provide one of the bases for their work. Much important work on X-ray analysis of DNA was being carried out by a group at King's College, London, and Watson and Crick were familiar with this work and in contact with those scientists before they began their own theorizing. This, then, is one precedent.

A much more important precedent was the work of Pauling, who was world-famous for developing models of molecular structures. Furthermore, he had recently published a model of a protein, helical in shape, that had greatly impressed both Watson and Crick. Therefore, they decided to use Pauling's work as the basis for their own, and they developed a helical model of DNA. Two specific problems arose in constructing this model: How many helical strands should it contain, and where should the bases be located? The DNA molecule looks something like a spiral staircase. There are two helical strands, or backbones, held together by pairs of bases, which form the "stairs." In Watson and Crick's initial model, however, there were three strands, rather than the final two, and the bases projected outward from the backbones, rather than being between them. Watson and Crick chose a three-strand structure for their initial model for several reasons. First, the available X-ray evidence indicated that the molecule was thicker than a single strand. Second, evidence reported by Franklin, from the King's College group, also pointed to three strands. Watson and Crick put the bases on the outside because at that time they could not see a way to put them inside the backbones while maintaining the regular structure shown in the X-ray pictures. Putting the bases on the outside did away with this problem. These first steps in the discovery of the structure of DNA were relatively straightforward: Watson and Crick took an already available model and modified it to solve their specific problem. Nothing in the way of an intuitive leap of creative insight is seen here.

However, Watson and Crick ran into an immediate snag when the group from King's College came to see their three-strand model and told them that it surely was incorrect, based on the King's College data concerning the amount of water DNA contained, among other things. Thus, Watson and Crick were forced back to the drawing board, but not all the way to the beginning. They retained the helical structure, but changed it in response to new information that became available, in an example of a "local search." Two large changes took place in the structure: The bases were moved between the backbones of the helix, and the number of strands went from three to two.

Several pieces of evidence led to a bases-inside, backbone-outside model. First of all, Watson and Crick could not devise a backbone-inside model that did not violate basic laws of chemistry concerning distances between molecules. Second, Watson saw a new X-ray photograph made by Franklin, and he could see that the backbones were on the outside. As far as the number of strands were concerned, again there was information that led Watson and Crick from three strands to two. First, a number of other investigators, including Pauling himself, were working on three-strand models, and none of them showed signs of success. Second, information in a report by Franklin indicated that the backbone chains came in pairs and ran opposite to each other, which led to two strands as the simplest place to begin. Thus, over about a year, Watson and Crick moved away from their initial incorrect model to one that turned out to be correct. This movement to the new model came about as a result of pushes from information that made clear not only that the early model was wrong but also in what direction the solution lay.

There was now one last element to fit in: How were the bases to be paired to connect the backbones? As mentioned earlier, one reason that the original model had the bases on the outside was that there seemed to be no way to fit the bases inside without making the structure too irregular to produce the patterns shown in the X-ray photographs. However, when Watson and Crick built their first two-strand bases-inside model, the models of the bases were not yet available from the machine shop, so they could begin their work with the backbones, without worrying about the bases.

Once the two-strand backbone structure was completed, and the base models became available, attempts were made to pair up the bases in various ways, so that they could serve to hold the two backbones together. The initial attempts involved pairing bases of the same type, called "like-like" pairings, but this led to pairings of different sizes, which would produce an irregular structure, which was unacceptable. According to Watson (1968, pp. 123–125), this failure using like-like pairings led him to try various other combinations, basically by trial and error, until the correct combinations were hit upon.

In conclusion, we have here one of the great discoveries of modern science, and it seems to have come about in a manner very different from the romantic view of the scientist working alone in the laboratory until a sudden insight leads to the creative solution to the problem. In the case of Watson and Crick, their initial work grew directly out of the work of others, and when it was shown to be wrong, they modified it in straightforward ways, until a satisfactory solution was arrived at.

Darwin's theory of evolution

If one reads Darwin's autobiography concerning the events that led to the development of the theory of evolution through natural selection, one gets the impression of a sudden insight (Gruber, 1981, p. 172–173):

In October 1838, that is, fifteen months after I had begun my systematic enquiry, I happened to read for amusement Malthus on *Population,* and being well prepared to appreciate the struggle for existence which everywhere goes on from long and continued observation of the habits of animals and plants, it at once struck me that under these circumstances favorable variations would tend to be preserved and unfavorable ones to be destroyed. The result of this would be the formation of a new series. Here, then, I had at last got a theory by which to work.

Darwin's reading of Malthus allowed him to formulate in essentially complete form the theory of evolution through natural selection. Soon after reading Malthus, Darwin wrote the following in his notebook (Gruber, 1981, p. 173):

Three principles will account for all 1. grandchildren like grandfathers, 2. tendency to small change especially with physical change, and 3. great fertility in proportion to support of parents.

On the basis of this report it would appear that Darwin had simply collected facts in a neutral manner, without any theory, until a passage from Malthus brought everything into place. However, Darwin's notebooks present a very different picture of how the theory developed (Gruber, 1981). As was the case with Watson and Crick, Darwin's work was based on that of others (Eiseley, 1961), and the final form of the theory only gradually evolved.

Interest in the question of how species developed obviously predated Darwin. Indeed, the various components of Darwin's theory had been proposed as separate fragments by others, in some cases many years earlier (Eiseley, 1961). Religious orthodoxy of the time assumed that all the species had been created at once, in final perfect form, by God, and that no evolution had occurred. However, in liberal circles, many scientists and philosophers believed that a strict interpretation of the biblical view was incorrect and that evolution of some sort must have occurred. In addition, there was specifically in Darwin's family great interest in questions concerning evolution, because Darwin's grandfather, Erasmus Darwin, had proposed a theory of evolution based on the inheritance of acquired characteristics. Thus, interest in the questions that occupied Darwin during his adult years probably was stimulated early in his life.

Darwin's higher education, at the University of Edinburgh and Cambridge University, also contributed to his development. At these institutions, Darwin met many scientists who were actively thinking about problems in evolutionary theory and who believed in one or another variant of the then current views, such as Lamarck's theory of inheritance of acquired characteristics. After graduating from Cambridge, Darwin left on a 5-year voyage aboard HMS *Beagle,* whose ports of call provided him with firsthand evidence of the remarkable variety and adaptability of species. In summary, when Darwin returned from the voyage on the *Beagle,* he was a sophisticated scientist who was thoroughly familiar with current theorizing concerning evolution and who possessed a unique collection of facts culled from his observations during the voyage.

Contrary to the report in Darwin's autobiography, he had developed a theory of evolution in July 1837, 15 months before reading Malthus (Gruber, 1981). The early theory is based on the concept of the "monad," an idea that was not original to Darwin. Monads were believed to be simple living particles that were constantly springing spontaneously into life: Each monad develops into a whole group of related species, and when the monad dies, all its species die at once. The monad's developing species respond to environmental forces with adaptive changes, in a variation on the theorizing of Darwin's grandfather. Thus, contrary to Darwin's claims, he had a theory long before reading Malthus, and this early theory was firmly rooted in the scientific theorizing of the time. As with Watson and Crick, Darwin's theorizing had precedents, and he used them relatively directly. Only gradually over the next 15 months did Darwin develop the theory of evolution based on natural selection. This theory evolved out of the monad theory, as it gradually became apparent to Darwin that the monad theory would not do the job of explaining evolution of species.

As one example of the ways in which Darwin's thinking changed, in the monad theory it was assumed that variation among members of a species was in response to environmental change. In the theory of natural selection, variation is assumed to occur independent of the environment, with some of these variations being better adapted than others, and so on. This shift in Darwin's view may have been brought about in part by his analysis of the results he observed during the voyage of the *Beagle,* which showed that great variation came about in nature independent of environmental change. Therefore, rather than being a result, variation became a given.

Thus, when Darwin read Malthus, his ideas had been changing for over a year, to the point that Malthus could make a crucial impression on him. Malthus triggered no great leap of insight, but rather provided the capstone on a reasoning process that had moved in small steps from a theory that was a rather simple variation on already known themes to a theory that would change the world.

Edison's invention of the kinetoscope

Edison's technological creativity produced thousands of inventions, two of the most important of which were a device for storing and reproducing sound (a phonograph) and a device for storing and reproducing moving visual information (the kinetoscope – the first moving pictures). The documentation surrounding these two inventions, including sketches in Edison's notebooks as well as his early patent applications, indicates that Edison's thought processes also may have followed the pattern outlined earlier (Jenkins & Jeffrey, 1984).

The phonograph was invented in Edison's laboratory in 1877, and its demonstration in the next year made Edison world-famous. One preliminary sketch of the phonograph, made on November 29, 1877, shows a cylinder with its long axis horizontal as the central piece of the apparatus. The sound information was carried in a spiral groove impressed into the surface of the cylinder, and a moving stylus was used to retrieve that information from the rotating cylinder. A second sketch, made a few days later, indicates that Edison and his associates had been considering at least three possible mechanisms for storing sound information: a cylinder, a flat disk, and a narrow tape. The final phonograph was one of these possibilities.

About 10 years later, Edison produced the kinetoscope, a machine that enabled a viewer to see moving images. The kinetoscope served a purpose very different from that of the phonograph, and the kinetoscope was very different in design and appearance from the earlier invention. The kinetoscope consisted of an upright cabinet with a viewing peephole at the top. The viewer looked down into the cabinet and saw the moving image. Film was wound on many rollers inside the cabinet, allowing it to be drawn under the peephole, to provide the moving image for the viewer.

Although on the surface the phonograph and the kinetoscope appear to be entirely different devices, analysis of Edison's preliminary work on the kinetoscope indicates that in reality the former served as the basis for the initial development of the latter. Edison's earliest preliminary patent application (called a "caveat"), made in October 1888 for the kinetoscope, contained a sketch that looked nothing like the final version. Rather, this sketch contained an apparatus that had as its central piece a single cylinder that rotated around its horizontally oriented long axis. On the cylinder was a spiral of images that were viewed through a moving eyepiece as the cylinder rotated. Thus, the earliest version of the kinetoscope seems to have been based directly on the phonograph. The written text of the caveat, of which the sketch described was a part, makes clear the relationship between the two inventions (Jenkins & Jeffrey, 1984, p. 5):

I am experimenting upon an instrument which does for the Eye what the phonograph does for the ear, Which is the recording and reproduction of things in motion. . . . The invention consists in photographing continuously a series of pictures occuring [sic] at intervals which intervals are greater that [sic] eight per second, and photographing these series of pictures in a continuous spiral on a cylinder or plate in the same manner in which sound is recorded on the phonograph.

In sum, there is little doubt that the kinetoscope evolved directly out of the phonograph, as Edison took the idea of the horizontal rotating cylinder and tried to use it in a different domain. Although the finished products were entirely different in form, the documents provide evidence concerning the intermediate steps that led from one to the other. Furthermore, there is evidence that Edison was forced to abandon his early phonograph-based kinetoscope because of problems in fashioning the needed spiral of images, which led to the use of film on rolls.

In a historical analysis of Edison's notebooks, including many drawings, Jenkins

(1983) has noted that Edison used a small number of ideas or forms in attacking many problems. Perhaps the most frequent example is the use of the cylinder, as we have just seen, and other such forms were the tuning fork and curved ratchet pawl. Jenkins traces the importance of the cylinder in Edison's inventions to his early work experience as an operator in telegraph offices, which contained mechanical devices using cylinders. In addition, Edison's work on newspapers exposed him to printing presses using rotating cylinders. Finally, his work in machine shops gave him much experience with the lathe, which involves a rotating piece of material being cut into cylindrical form by a cutting tool directly analogous to the stylus in Edison's inventions.

In conclusion, this analysis indicates that Edison's approach to the problem of reproducing moving visual images was based on his earlier work in a related area, which in turn was based on his earlier work experience. Furthermore, the changes in direction that led him away from the initial conception of the kinetoscope seem to have been responses to problems that developed as he attempted to bring his early conception to reality.

The pattern shown in Edison's work on the kinetoscope is somewhat different from that seen in the discoveries of Watson and Crick and of Darwin. In these latter cases, the initial conception was based relatively directly on the work of others. In the case of Watson and Crick, Pauling's work with helical models served directly as the basis for their work, and Darwin's monad theory was also rather directly based on ideas of others. In the case of Edison, on the other hand, the kinetoscope was based on his own earlier work on the phonograph. This earlier work can in turn be traced back to Edison's earlier experiences with cylinders employed in designs by others, but by the time Edison started to work on the kinetoscope he already had available a stock of his own ideas, which he then used as the basis for attacking new problems. However, although Edison had another layer of experience to work with, his own extensive experience, the same basic principles are exemplified in all the work discussed so far. Another example of the development and use of one's own work as the basis for dealing with a new problem can be seen in Picasso's painting of his great mural *Guernica*.

Picasso's Guernica

In 1936, during the Spanish civil war, Picasso was commissioned by the Spanish government-in-exile to produce a work for the government's pavilion in an international exposition to take place in Paris in June 1937. The bombing by the Nazis of the Basque town of Guernica on April 27, 1937, stimulated Picasso to fulfill this commission by producing one of his most famous works, the large mural *Guernica*. This work is particularly important to students of artistic creativity, because Picasso catalogued all of his preliminary work for *Guernica,* some 40 pieces, and he also had the mural photographed four times as he painted it. If one examines this information concerning *Guernica* as work-in-process, one sees the gradual development of the final form of the work (Arnheim, 1962; Blunt, 1969).

Guernica is painted on a large scale – it measures over 25 feet by 11 feet high. There is no color; the painting is done in shades of gray, ranging from white to almost black. The central figure is a horse with its head raised in a scream of agony. Above the horse's head is a sun with a light bulb superimposed on it. A bird flies up toward this sun. On the left is a large bull, whose body faces the middle of the scene, but whose head is turned away. Beneath the head of the bull is a mother, her head tilted back and her mouth open in a scream, holding a dead baby. To the right of center, a woman leans out of a burning building, holding a lamp. On the upper far right, a woman with burning clothes is falling out of a building, while below a woman rushes into the scene. Along the bottom left are the head and arms of a statue of a warrior, in whose hand is a broken sword.

Picasso began to work on sketches for the mural almost immediately after receiving news of the bombing. The first few sketches contain some of the main characters in the final mural (the bull, horse, and woman holding a light), but their organization changes greatly from one sketch to another, and some of them (e.g., the woman holding the light) are not present in all the sketches. In addition, the main characters, as well as several of the other characters, are subjects of separate paintings and drawings, in what seem to be Picasso's attempts to determine exactly how each character should look. In addition, there are elements that are introduced in the middle of the work, but are then removed before completion. One gets the feeling from this work that Picasso had some idea of what he wanted to include in the work, but the specifics were not clear to him when he started. For example, when he began to put paint to canvas, the center of the mural was dominated by a defiant upraised arm, with clenched fist, that was not present in the preliminary sketches. However, Picasso gradually modified it until it disappeared from the final version, as he kept revising things. Indeed, Picasso was making revisions even after the mural was hung in the Spanish pavilion in the Paris exposition, and Blunt believes that one of these revisions was stimulated by another work on display in that pavilion.

It is also of note that the characters and their organization in *Guernica* are closely related to much other work done by Picasso at about the same time, as well as earlier. The horse and bull, for example, appear again and again in works on the bullfight, among others. A girl or woman holding a light, while confronting a bull or minotaur, is also present in many of Picasso's works. Also, an etching, *Minotauromachy,* produced a few years before *Guernica,* contains essentially all the characters that later appeared in *Guernica,* and in a very similar organization. Thus, Picasso developed *Guernica* out of themes that had appeared in his earlier works. Furthermore, Blunt has traced some of the specific gestures and configurations used in *Guernica* to specific sources in the works of earlier artists with which Picasso was familiar.

In conclusion, Picasso's production of *Guernica* parallels closely Edison's production of the kinetoscope. In both cases the initial conception of the work came from earlier work of the individual, and the initial conception evolved into the final version. In addition, the early work of the individual can be seen to have sources in the work of others.

Conclusions

These examples, though highly selective, are still of great importance for theories of creativity. They are cases of creativity of the highest sort, and they are also cases in which some documentary evidence exists concerning the thought processes involved. In all these cases, and in others not discussed because of lack of space (Weisberg, 1986, chaps. 6 and 7), one sees nothing like the creative leaps postulated by the genius view. Rather, in all these cases, some new product – a painting, a scientific theory, or an invention – began as a rather straightforward extension of earlier work. The initial conception then underwent modification, until something new emerged. The important point is that in these cases there is some sort of evidence available that goes beyond the creator's statements concerning the processes involved, and in each case nothing particularly extraordinary occurred from a psychological point of view. This is not to say that these cases do not involve extraordinary occurrences from a scientific, technological, or artistic point of view, but that the cognitive processes involved were not extraordinary.

Sternberg and Davidson (1982, 1983; Davidson & Sternberg, 1984) have recently argued that intellectual giftedness may depend in part on a special set of skills that constitute what they call insightful thinking. According to their view, major intellectual advances, in the sciences and the arts, involve insights, and the ability to carry out insightful thinking may be independent of IQ. Sternberg and Davidson have examined this ability by having subjects attempt to solve problems of various sorts, and then examining the relationships between performance on these problems and other measures of intellectual functioning. The components of this hypothesized insight ability are selective encoding, selective combination, and selective comparison.

Selective encoding involves the ability to pick out the relevant information from a problem and to ignore the irrelevant. According to Sternberg and Davidson, most interesting problems involve large amounts of information, most of which is irrelevant to the solution. Insight involves the ability to determine just which information will be useful in the long run. Fleming's discovery of penicillin is presented as an example of selective encoding, because it depended on Fleming's selectively encoding the information that bacteria had been destroyed by a mold that had accidentally come into contact with the dish in which the bacteria were growing. Rather than encoding the result as a failed experiment, Fleming encoded it as destruction of bacteria, which resulted in a new and valuable way of conceiving of the result.

Selective combination involves putting relevant pieces of information together in just the right way. That is, once the relevant information has been selectively encoded in some problem, it is still necessary to develop the solution out of this information. Sternberg and Davidson cite Darwin's formulation of the theory of evolution as an example of selective combination. According to Sternberg and Davidson, Darwin had available all the facts that ultimately were to form the theory. What was needed, according to Sternberg and Davidson, was a coherent way of putting the facts together.

Finally, selective comparison involves relating some new information to one's preexisting knowledge in just the right way. One uses one's knowledge to understand the new information, and productive use of one's knowledge depends on realizing just how the new information can be matched with what one already knows. As an example of selective comparison, Sternberg and Davidson cite Kekulé's discovery of the benzene ring through the use of the image of the snake biting its tail. Presumably, if Kekulé had not used just that metaphor, he would not have had his insight.

Sternberg and Davidson base their discussion of insight at least in part on their analysis of several great discoveries, discoveries that presumably were based on insight. From my perspective, the situation is much more complicated than Sternberg and Davidson acknowledge. As one example, it does not seem to be the case that Darwin was in possession of all the relevant information years before he produced the theory of natural selection. Gruber (1981) presents a strong case that before he could produce the final theory, Darwin's thinking had to change in crucial ways. These changes were such that it does not seem to be true that everything was in place and simply waiting for a framework to come along. As will be seen shortly, Kekulé's discovery of the benzene ring also may have been more complicated than Sternberg and Davidson's analysis would lead one to believe.

In sum, although Sternberg and Davidson's research may have isolated a mode of thinking that could be called insight, it is not clear to me that this sort of thinking is involved in creative discovery of the sort discussed in this chapter.

Experience and creativity: influences and practice

The present point of view assumes that creative products begin with an individual using personal experience as the basis for approaching some problem. Past experience often is seen in the form of "influences," in which one can see traces of the work of some earlier individual in the work of a creative artist or scientist. Examples of this have already been seen in the case studies just discussed. Watson and Crick were influenced by Pauling, and Darwin was influenced by several of his teachers, among others. Needless to say, case studies of great musicians, artists, and scientists are filled with examples of even the greatest individuals being influenced by the work of others. Specific compositions of Bach, Beethoven, Haydn, and Mozart can, for example, be traced to earlier works by others (Weisberg, 1986, chaps. 6 and 7). Another sort of influence can be seen especially in literature and drama, where specific life experiences serve as the basis for the artist's work. Again, examples abound, ranging from Dostoyevsky's use of his prison experience in *Crime and Punishment* to F. Scott Fitzgerald's use of his life experiences in *Tender Is the Night*. (Weisberg, 1986. chap. 7).

The development that leads from dependence on the work of others to the production of original work of one's own may extend over a significant period of time in the life of the creative individual. A recent study of musical composition by Hayes (1981, chap. 10) estimated that it takes approximately 10 years of composing experience (10 years of practice) before one will produce a masterwork. The early compositions of even the greatest composers often are of value only historically, because musically they are derivative of the work of others. Even Mozart, who began his musical studies around the age of four, did not, according to Hayes's criteria, produce a masterwork until he had been working for 12 years. Thus, an evolution away from the prosaic seems to occur even in the work of the greats.

Creativity and myth

This chapter began with three self-reports from individuals of acknowledged creativity: Coleridge, Mozart, and Kekulé. These are but a small sample of many such reports, all of which are remarkably similar in content (Ghiselin, 1952). These reports obviously contradict the present evolutionary view of creative thinking, and therefore a brief discussion of their validity will be of value. It should first be noted that those three self-reports are contradicted by the case studies discussed in the last section. In the case studies, in which detailed information was available, it was found that the thought processes involved were not of the sort postulated by the genius view. No great leaps of thought were found to occur. As mentioned earlier, there are other case studies available that also do not support the genius view. From this perspective, then, uncorroborated self-reports must be brought into question. Even greater damage to the genius view comes about when these self-reports are examined in detail, because questions can be raised about the validity of all three of them.

Coleridge and "Kubla Khan"

Coleridge claimed that "Kubla Khan" came to him complete, with no effort on his part, in an opium-induced dream or stupor. He was able to commit only a fragment of the poem to paper before he was interrupted, which caused him to lose the rest of the poem forever, or so he claimed. There is other evidence that leads one to believe that almost nothing Coleridge reported about the genesis of "Kubla Khan" is true (Schneider, 1953). Most important, another version of the poem exists, and evidence indicates that this other version is earlier than the version actually published. This, of course, leads to the conclusion that Coleridge worked on the poem before publishing it, which belies his claim that he simply set down the lines that spontaneously came to him in his stupor. Schneider also argues that opium would not have induced the sort of visions that Coleridge claimed to have experienced. In addition, Coleridge was notorious for not telling the truth concerning his work. Finally, I find it difficult to believe that a poet in the throes of writing down a miraculously given poem would allow himself to be interrupted for an hour by a visitor on some "business" errand. Surely Coleridge would have asked the man to wait until he was finished transcribing the two to three hundred lines that had come to him.

Schneider has proposed that Coleridge fabricated the account of the composition of "Kubla Khan" in order to make what was in reality only a fragment of a poem more interesting to his public. If Coleridge could not complete the poem, argues Schneider, then transforming the essentially worthless fragment into all that remained of an interrupted burst of inspiration might make it something valuable. Whether or not Schneider's speculations are correct, there is no doubt that Coleridge's report is of little value to students of creative thinking.

Mozart's letter

The excerpt from Mozart's letter is similar in content to Coleridge's report, in that Mozart claimed that his compositions grew into completed works without his conscious participation. He then wrote down the complete works. Again there is evidence that this report should not be believed. First, there is strong evidence that "Mozart's letter" was not written by Mozart (Deutsch, 1964). This conclusion, though long accepted by musicologists (Anderson, 1966), has not penetrated into the psychological literature. Also, and more important, recent analyses of Mozart's original manuscripts do not indicate that he simply committed to paper already complete works (Sloboda, 1984, pp. 112–114). So here again the validity of the self-report is called into question.

Kekulé's "dream"

The final self-report was that of Kekulé, concerning an alleged dream in which he hit upon the circular structure of benzene through the medium of the image of a snake biting its own tail. In this case also, questions can be raised about the ordinary interpretation of this report. First, there is a question concerning whether Kekulé was even dreaming (Rothenberg, 1979, pp. 395–396). The original report is in German, and Kekulé used the term "habschlaft" (half-sleep) to describe his state, which may mean more that he was daydreaming, perhaps sitting transfixed in front of the fire, rather than truly dreaming. There is also a question concerning whether or not Kekulé was imagining snakes during this incident. In his report, he says that he saw the strings of atoms in "snakelike motion." The use of the term "snakelike" indicates that the strings of atoms had not become transformed into snakes, because he would then simply have referred to snakes. His use of "snakelike" indicates that he was distinguishing between the strings of atoms and snakes. If this analysis is correct, then Kekulé's saying that one snake had seized hold of its tail must only be figurative. Because he had called the motion of the strings snakelike, then when one of the strings formed into a ring, he described it as biting its own tail.

Thus, although Kekulé may have used visual imagination to think about the structure of benzene, he may not have been imagining snakes, and he may not have been dreaming. This analysis is relevant to Sternberg and Davidson's (1983) discussion of Kekulé, cited earlier.

Conclusions

Although this critical review of the three self-reports is no less selective than the earlier analysis of case studies, once again this does not diminish the main point. The self-report examples chosen are among the most often cited in support of the genius view of creativity. The fact that the validity of these examples can be called into question, combined with the earlier analysis of better-documented case studies, indicates that the genius view of creativity may be based on myth rather than fact.

Can one's creativity be increased?

A helpful way to provide a summary of the main points raised in this chapter is to consider the problem of increasing an individual's creativity. There is a great industry built on the premise that many people need help in order to think creatively. Many books provide hints as to how to increase creativity (Adams, 1979; de Bono, 1967), and many methods are taught in courses and seminars that are attended by thousands of individuals each year; see Nickerson, Perkins, and Smith (1985) for a review. The discussion in the present chapter, on the other hand, has led to the conclusion that the thought processes involved in great creative acts are no different than those involved in the things we all do every day. This means that creative thinking must be omnipresent in all of us, which means that it is neither necessary nor possible to increase anyone's capacity to be creative. Therefore, in order to consider the question whether or not one's creativity can be increased, one must reformulate the question, in order to put it into a form that can lead to an answer.

Why would one approach an expert in creative thinking in order to have one's creative capacity increased? One reasonable possibility is that one has had problems dealing with some aspect of one's life, an aspect that presumably could benefit from "creative thinking." I might be concerned that students find my lectures boring, and so I wish to become more creative in thinking of ways to make my lectures interesting. A salesperson might be interested in thinking of new ways to convince prospective buyers to purchase some product. A scientist might be concerned because of having made little progress in solving some important scientific problem. If we now focus on these sorts of specific questions, there may be some information from the earlier discussion that might be helpful.

Great innovations in science and the arts were almost invariably produced by individuals who possessed strong motivation and persistence. Such individuals as Darwin, Picasso, Edison, Einstein, and Beethoven, among many others, spent lifetimes working in their chosen fields, and their genius came about at least in part as a result of this lifetime of work. Commitment provides sufficient time for the small changes that occur as one gathers experience in some domain to evolve into something truly original and innovative. Commitment also brings with it a tendency to spend much time thinking about one's work, which also raises the possibility that something novel will develop. Time spent thinking about one's work can also increase the likelihood that a potentially relevant external stimulus will be noticed (Weisberg, 1986, chap. 1).

A second important conclusion in the present chapter is that creative products are firmly based on what came before. True originality evolves as the individual goes beyond what others had done before. This might mean, perhaps paradoxically, that in order to produce something new, one should first become as knowledgeable as possible about the old. This serves to provide the background so that the individual can begin to work in an area and also serves to provide ways in which to modify early products that are not satisfactory.

These two aspects of creative work, commitment and expertise within one's own area, are neither profound nor novel. All scientists and artists have extensive training, either formally or informally, and very few individuals make a mark in the world without a relatively long commitment to an area beyond their actual training. It might be hoped that something more exciting could be presented concerning the teaching of creative thinking, but the issues are too complex to permit straightforward answers. Consider one personality characteristic that is sometimes cited as inhibiting creativity: fear of taking risks. In a popular book that surveys various ways of increasing creativity, Adams (1979, chap. 3) discusses fear of taking risks as a factor that may interfere with creativity. An individual may come up with a novel and possibly adequate solution to a problem, but fear of being incorrect stops the individual from making it public. Thus, one way to increase one's creative capacity would be to increase one's capacity for taking risks. Adams attempts to do this by trying to convince the reader that nothing really awful will occur if one is wrong, and so taking a risk and failing is better than doing nothing.

Reconsideration of some of the case studies from this chapter, however, indicates that risk taking may not be related in a simple way to producing a creative product. Watson and Crick seemed to take a risk, choosing a helical structure for their model, and it paid off in their being first to develop a model of DNA. On the other hand, such a way of approaching a problem probably would not have helped Darwin develop his theory. In the case of the theory of evolution, the final theoretical structure seems to have required a number of components coming together, and all of them were needed before anything coherent could emerge. Therefore, one cannot simply say: Take more risks. Whether or not one should take a risk may depend on the problem on which one is working. There may be as many ways to be creative as there are problems, in the broadest sense, that humans can ponder. If that is so, then there may be no simple way to change people to make them more creative.

In summary, this chapter has attempted to take seriously several implications arising from laboratory research in problem solving, to provide a framework for analyzing creative thinking in science, technology, and the arts. Laboratory research in problem solving indicates that, contrary to the genius view, creative thinking may require neither extraordinary individuals nor extraordinary thought processes. Analysis of several case studies also shows that, perhaps surprisingly, several great creative achievements also seemed to involve rather ordinary thought processes. This convergence of the results from two such disparate domains indicates that the genius view of creativity, although it has broad and deep roots in our culture, may be basically misdirected.

References

Adams, J. L. (1979). *Conceptual blockbusting* (2nd ed.). New York: Norton.

Anderson, E. (1966). *The letters of Mozart and his family* (2nd ed.). New York: St. Martin's Press.

Arnheim, R. (1962). *Picasso's Guernica: The genesis of a painting.* Berkeley: University of California Press.

Blunt, A. (1969). *Picasso's "Guernica."* New York: Oxford University Press.

Bourne, L. E. Ekstrand, B. R., & Dominowski, R. L. (1971). *The psychology of thinking.* Englewood Cliffs, NJ: Prentice-Hall.

Bransford, J. (1979). *Human cognition. Learning, understanding and remembering.* Belmont, CA: Wadsworth.

Burnham, C. A., & Davis, K. G. (1969). The 9-dot problem: Beyond perceptual organization. *Psychonomic Science, 17,* 321–323.

Catrambone, R., & Holyoak, K. (1985, August). *The role of schemas in analogical problem solving.* Paper presented at American Psychological Association convention, Los Angeles.

Coleridge, S. T. (1816). Prefatory note to Kubla Khan. In B. Ghiselin (Ed.), *The creative process* (pp. 84–85). New York: Mentor.

Davidson, J. E., & Sternberg, R. J. (1984). The role of insight in intellectual giftedness. *Gifted Child Quarterly, 28,* 58–64.

de Bono, E. (1967). *New think: The use of lateral thinking in the generation of new ideas.* New York: Basic Books.

DeGroot, A. (1966). Perception and memory versus thought: Some old ideas and recent findings. In B. Kleinmuntz (Ed.), *Problem solving: Research, method, and theory* (pp. 19–50). New York: Wiley.

Deutsch, O. E. (1964). Spurious Mozart letters. *Music Review, 25,* 120–123.

Duncker, K. (1945). On problem-solving. *Psychological Monographs, 58,* No. 5, Whole No. 270.

Eiseley, L. (1961). *Darwin's century. Evolution and the men who discovered it.* New York: Anchor Books.

Ghiselin, B. (Ed.). (1952). *The creative process.* New York: Mentor.

Gick, M. L., & Holyoak, K. (1983). Schema induction and analogical transfer. *Cognitive Psychology, 15,* 1–38.

Gilhooly, K. J. (1982). *Thinking. Directed, undirected and creative.* London: Academic Press.

Greeno, J. G. (1980). Trends in the theory of knowledge for problem solving. In D. T. Tuma & R. Reif

(Eds.), *Problem solving and education: Issues in teaching and learning*. Hillsdale, NJ: Lawrence Erlbaum.

Gruber, H. (1981). *Darwin on man* (2nd ed.). University of Chicago Press.

Guilford, J. P. (1950). Creativity. *American Psychologist, 5*, 444–454.

Guilford, J. P. (1959). Traits of creativity. In H. H. Anderson (Ed.), *Creativity and its cultivation* (pp. 142–161). New York: Harper.

Hayes, J. R. (1981). *The complete problem solver*. Philadelphia: Franklin Institute Press.

Jenkins, R. V. (1983). Elements of style: Continuities in Edison's thinking. *Annals of the New York Academy of Sciences, 424*, 149–162.

Jenkins. R. V., & Jeffrey, T. E. (1984). Worth a thousand words: Nonverbal documents in editing. *Documentary Editing, 6*, 1–8.

Judson, H. F. (1979). *The eighth day of creation: Makers of the revolution in biology*. New York: Simon & Schuster.

Keane, M. (1985). On drawing analogies when solving problems: A theory and test of solution of generation in an analogical problem-solving task. *British Journal of Psychology, 76*, 449–458.

Koestler, A. (1964). *The act of creation*. New York: Macmillan.

Kohler, W. (1976). *The mentality of apes*. New York: Liveright.

Luchins, A. S., & Luchins, E. H. (1959). *Rigidity of behavior*. Eugene: University of Oregon Press.

Lung, C.-T., & Dominowski, R. L. (1985). Effects of strategy instructions and practice on nine-dot problem solving. *Journal of Experimental Psychology: Learning, Memory, and Cognition, 11*, 804–811.

Martindale, C. (1981). *Cognition and consciousness*. Homewood, IL: Dorsey.

Metcalfe, J. (1986). Feeling of knowing in memory and problem solving. *Journal of Experimental Psychology: Learning, Memory, and Cognition, 12*, 288–294.

Mozart, J. C. W. A. (1964). A letter. In B. Ghiselin (Ed.), *The creative process* (pp. 44–45). New York: Mentor.

Newell, A., & Simon, H. (1972). *Human problem solving*. Englewood Cliffs, NJ: Prentice-Hall.

Nickerson, R. S., Perkins, D. N., & Smith, E. E. (1985). *The teaching of thinking*. Hillsdale, NJ: Lawrence Erlbaum.

Osborn, A. (1953). *Applied imagination* (rev. ed.). New York: Charles Scribner's Sons.

Perfetto, G. A., Bransford, J. D., & Franks, J. J. (1983). Constraints on access in a problem solving context. *Memory and Cognition, 11*, 24–31.

Perkins, D. (1981). *The mind's best work*. Cambridge, MA: Harvard University Press.

Reed, S. K., Ernst, G. W., & Banerjii, R. (1974). The role of transfer between similar problem states. *Cognitive Psychology, 6*, 436–450.

Rothenberg, A. (1979). *The emerging goddess*. University of Chicago Press.

Scheerer, M. (1963). Problem-solving. *Scientific American, 208*, 118–128.

Schneider, E. (1953). *Coleridge, opium, and Kubla Khan*. University of Chicago Press.

Simon, H. (Ed.) (1979). *Models of thought*. New Haven, CT: Yale University Press.

Sloboda, J. (1984). *The musical mind*. New York: Oxford University Press.

Spencer, R. M., & Weisberg, R. W. (1986). Context-dependent effects on analogical transfer. *Memory and Cognition, 14*, 442–449.

Sternberg, R. J., & Davidson, J. E. (1982). The mind of the puzzler, *Psychology Today, 16*, 37–44.

Sternberg, R. J., & Davidson. J. E. (1983). Insight in the gifted. *Educational Psychologist, 18*, 51–57.

Watson, J. (1968). *The double helix*. New York: Signet.

Weisberg, R. W. (1980). *Memory, thought, and behavior*. New York: Oxford University Press.

Weisberg, R. W. (1986). *Creativity. Genius and other myths*. New York: Freeman.

Weisberg, R. W., & Alba, J. W. (1981). An examination of the alleged role of "fixation" in the solution of several "insight" problems. *Journal of Experimental Psychology: General, 110*, 169–192.

Weisberg, R. W., & DiCamillo, M. A. (1986). *Multiple memory searches as the basis for restructuring in an insight problem*. Unpublished paper, Temple University.

Weisberg, R., DiCamillo, M., & Phillips, D. (1978). Transferring old associations to new problems: A nonautomatic process. *Journal of Verbal Learning and Verbal Behavior, 17,* 219–228.
Weisberg, R. W., & Suls, J. (1973). An information-processing model of Duncker's candle problem. *Cognitive Psychology, 4,* 255–276.
Wertheimer, M. (1959). *Productive thinking.* New York: Harper & Row.

7   A computational model of scientific insight

Pat Langley and Randolph Jones

Creativity lies at the heart of the scientific process. Although much of science involves the dreary application of well-worn methods, true progress requires an act of discovery. In some cases, these discoveries take the form of *insight,* in which previously unseen and unexpected connections suddenly reveal themselves to the mind.

Introspectively, the moment of insight often has a "mystical" quality, and this has led many to assume that the process lies outside the realm of human understanding. Early theories of scientific insight shared in this opinion, relying heavily on notions of unconscious (and thus noninspectable) processing. But in the past few dacades, cognitive psychology and artificial intelligence have made significant strides in understanding the nature of human cognition. It seems only natural to apply their methods to develop a "process" explanation of this intriguing phenomenon.

In this chapter we present just such a computational theory of scientific insight. We begin by recounting some well-known examples of the process, along with some early theories that attempted to account for the phenomenon. We also review some more recent attempts to explain insight in process terms, but our reservations about these models have led us to develop an alternative theory. Our framework builds on two separate lines of research in cognitive science: on reasoning by analogy and on qualitative mental models. Thus, we also review some work in these areas before moving on to the details of our model.

The advantages of cognitive simulation

Before addressing the substantive issues, we should briefly consider our methodological assumptions. One of our basic tenets is that the construction of *cognitive simulations* can improve our understanding of human behavior. A cognitive simulation is simply a computer program that is intended to model human cognitive processes in some area. This approach has proved successful in a wide variety of

This research was supported by Contract N00014-84-K-0345 from the Information Sciences Division, Office of Naval Research. We would like to thank Bernd Nordhausen, Donald Rose, Rogers Hall, and Jaime Carbonell for discussions that led to the ideas in this chapter.

domains, including problem solving (Newell & Simon, 1972), vision (Marr, 1982), natural language (Schank & Abelson, 1977), and memory (Anderson & Bower, 1973).

The cognitive simulation approach has a number of advantages over more traditional psychological methods. First, the act of constructing a running computer program ensures that one's theory is internally consistent. Second, one can determine the consequences of changing a theory by adjusting the computational model and observing the new behavior. Most important, it forces one to think in terms of specific representations of knowledge and to specify explicitly processes for manipulating those representations. This leads to more specific – and thus more testable – models of cognitive behavior. We refer the reader to Newell and Simon (1972) and Anderson (1976) for additional discussion of this methodology.

The goal of our research is to construct a running cognitive simulation of scientific insight. Although we have not yet achieved that goal, we believe the very act of thinking in process terms has revealed aspects of insight that we otherwise would have missed.

The problem space hypothesis

Much of the research within the cognitive simulation approach has relied on what Newell (1980) has called the *problem space hypothesis*. This states that all cognitive behavior involves search through some problem space. A problem space is composed of a set of *problem states,* including the initial state from which search begins. New states are generated by applying *operators* to existing states, letting one systematically explore the space until the goal state has been reached.

As an example, suppose we wanted to solve some problem in linear algebra. The initial state might be a set of n equations in n unknowns, such as

$$2x + 3y = 8$$
$$3x - 6y = -9$$

In this case, our goal would be to find some value for each unknown. There are two operators for generating new states – adding two equations together and multiplying an equation by a constant. An intermediate state for the foregoing problem might include the equations

$$4x + 6y = 16$$
$$3x - 6y = -9$$

By applying the right operators in the right order, we would eventually reach the goal state, which would tell us that $x = 1$ and $y = 2$.

Unfortunately, the problem spaces for most interesting tasks are combinatorial in nature, so that many alternative paths present themselves. One response is to carry out an exhaustive search of the problem space, but this rapidly becomes unmanageable for even simple domains. A more reasonable approach is to carry out a *heuristic* search of the problem space, using rules of thumb to suggest likely states to expand and likely operators to select. This approach is not guaranteed to find an optimal solution, but it is likely to produce an acceptable solution in reasonable time. Human problem solvers appear to rely heavily on heuristic search methods.

The problem space hypothesis has been quite successful in studies of artificial intelligence and cognitive science, and we shall see later that most explanations of insight have been formulated within this framework. In fact, the problem space approach has become so popular in some circles that many view it as "truth" rather than as a hypothesis. Nevertheless, one can imagine competing frameworks for describing cognition, and, as we shall see, our theory of scientific insight incorporates such an alternative approach, based on the joint notions of mental models and reasoning by analogy.

The phenomenon of scientific insight

The popular view of science assumes that progress occurs through methodical collection of data and careful inferences from those observations. Although certain scientific work occurs in this mode, real progress often seems to require a "leap of intuition" or a "flash of insight" in which an old problem is suddenly seen in a different light. Let us consider some examples of this phenomenon.

Probably the most famous instance of scientific insight is Archimedes' discovery of the principle of displacement (Dreistadt, 1968). The Greek scholar had been given the problem of determining if the king's crown was pure gold or if the gold was mixed with silver. Knowing the density of gold and the weight of the crown, he needed only to find its volume in order to check for purity. But the crown's shape was irregular, and he could not measure its volume without melting it down. Archimedes worked on the problem for some time without finding a solution. Then, as he lowered himself into a bath, he noticed that the water level rose simultaneously. With this came the realization that any object displaces its own volume when submerged in a liquid and that this provided the means for measuring irregular volumes.[1]

Another well-known example of scientific insight is Louis Kekulé's discovery of the ring structure of the benzene molecule. Kekulé tried for some time to identify a structural model that would account for benzene's chemical makeup. Finally, he sat down by the fire and began to doze (Dreistadt, 1968; Farber, 1966). In his sleepy state he watched the smoke rising from the fire, "twisting in a snakelike motion." At this point, one of the snakes took its own tail in its mouth, creating a ring. In a sudden flash, Kekulé realized the molecule must be structured as a ring.

Insights seem to be fairly common in mathematics, and the eminent French mathematician Henri Poincaré (1952) reported a number of his own insights in a lecture at the Société de Psychologie in Paris. In one particularly striking example he detailed his discovery of an expression for Fuchsian functions (Poincaré, 1952, p. 53):

At this moment I left Caen, where I was then living, to take part in a geological conference arranged by the School of Mines. The incidents of the journey made me forget my mathematical work. When we arrived at Coutances, we got into a [bus] to go for a drive, and, just as I put my foot on the step, the idea came to me, though nothing in my former thoughts seemed to have prepared me for it, that the transformations I had used to define Fuchsian functions were identical with those of non-Euclidean geometry.

This case differs from our earlier examples in the lack of any obvious external stimulus that is closely related to the insight. We shall return to this issue later, because it bears on our theory.

Hadamard's theory of scientific insight

Hadamard (1949) gives us a splendid discussion of the phenomenon of insight. In addition to reviewing numerous instances from the history of science, he identifies four distinct stages that seem to occur in every documented case of scientific insight: *preparation, incubation, illumination,* and *verification.* These stages and their characteristics constitute a set of empirical generalizations relating to insight, and any successful theory must account for their existence.

The preparation phase involves intense effort in attempting to solve a given problem. In some cases this attempt leads directly to a solution, but for especially difficult problems one eventually "gives up." This abandonment constitutes the entry into the incubation stage, during which one devotes one's conscious processing to other issues. Depending on the situation, incubation can last anywhere from seconds to years, but eventually the solution "proposes itself" during the illumination stage, which occurs both unexpectedly and very rapidly. This is the "Aha" experience that produces exclamations like the "Eureka!" of Archimedes. However, these "leaps of intuition" are not always valid and sometimes lead to "false insights." Thus, one still must check the details during the final verification phase.

In addition to describing these four stages and their relation to one another, Hadamard proposes a theory of insight that gives a major role to unconscious reasoning. His explanation assumes three levels of the mind that work together during the process of discovery: the fully conscious, the fringe conscious, and the unconscious. The first refers to our everyday mode of thought, in which we are aware of the mental steps we traverse. The unconscious refers to thought processes that are not available to introspection, of which we are not even aware. The fringe conscious occupies the gray area between these two extremes, in which we are aware of ideas but are not focusing on them. One can view this as the "peripheral vision" area of the mind.

Hadamard's theory states that the preparation stage involves only conscious thought. However, the mental activity during preparation serves to "stir up" ideas relevant to the problem at hand. During the incubation phase, the unconscious mode takes charge and considers alternative solutions that incorporate the ideas produced during the earlier preparation. When the unconscious encounters an especially promising combination, it deposits the result into the fringe conscious. The mind seizes on this new idea and experiences the flash of insight as it enters full consciousness. Finally, one continues in the conscious mode while the result is checked.

Clearly, most of the action in this theory is occurring at the unconscious level, and it is natural to ask how this mechanism manages to sift through so many ideas and distinguish the profitable ones from others. Hadamard argues that the unconscious is able to generate combinations of ideas that are specific enough to be fruitful and yet general enough not to miss the solution completely. This process is likened to firing a shotgun. The pellets spread sufficiently that one does not miss the target, but not so much that it is useless to aim. Hadamard concludes that great mathematicians differ from ordinary people in the selective ability of their unconscious, which lets them generate ideas that are aesthetically pleasing or interesting.

Ohlsson's restructuring theory

Ohlsson (1984a, 1984b) has proposed a computational model of insight by attempting to integrate ideas from gestalt psychology with the problem space framework. In the gestalt paradigm, every situation was characterized by some *structure* in the mind. These structures were influenced by *forces* that could become unbalanced and introduce gaps. An unsolved problem was viewed as some situation in which gaps existed between one's current state and the goal state. When forces became unbalanced enough, *restructuring* occurred, and some new configuration was produced. Gestalt psychologists claimed that these restructuring events were more likely to occur when the problem solver had carefully analyzed the problem, carefully analyzed the goal, and made a series of unsuccessful attempts at solving the problem.

According to the problem space hypothesis, normal problem solving involves a search througt a problem space. Ohlsson claims that restructuring requires search through the *description space* for a problem. That is, restructuring involves finding a different way to *look* at the problem, rather than trying to solve the problem in a straightforward manner. He further assumes that problem solvers are able to "look ahead" a few steps and that this lets them know when they are near their goal. When one encounters an impasse, one attempts to view the problem in a different light. This can lead to a new representation of the problem, which constitutes restructuring. In some cases, this representational shift leads to a state that is only a few steps from the goal; the shift combines with the look-ahead ability to produce a flash of insight.

As an example, Ohlsson presents the problem shown in Figure 7.1, in which one must compute the sum of the areas of a square and an overlapping parallelogram. The straightforward solution is to calculate the area of the square and the area of the parallelogram (which requires calculating the base of the parallelogram) and add them together. Most people do not know the formula for the area of a parallelogram

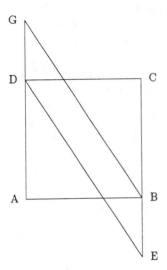

Figure 7.1. Find the sum of the areas of square *ABCD* and parallelogram *EBGD*, given $\overline{AB} = a$ and $\overline{AG} = b$.

and thus cannot solve the problem with the information provided. This causes an impasse, and this in turn leads to restructuring.

One such alteration lets the problem solver view the picture as two overlapping triangles (*DCE* and *GAB*). Given this representation, one can calculate the areas of the two triangles and add the results. These operations are simple, because the base and height of the triangles are given in the problem statement. The feeling of insight might or might not occur in this case, depending on whether or not the problem solver can look ahead the required three steps.

Another restructuring simplifies the problem even further. If one notices that the triangles can be "slipped apart" to form a rectangle, then one need only calculate the area of that rectangle, using the base and height already given. In this case, the feeling of insight is almost certain to occur, because the goal state is only two steps away from the initial state in this new space.

Simon's theory of familiarization and selective forgetting

Simon (1977) has proposed a computational explanation of Hadamard's four stages of insight. The theory combines models of human memory with information-processing models of problem solving. Research on human short-term memory has shown that its capacity is severely limited, but it has also shown that this limitation can be offset by experience. When asked to remember "artificial" input such as digits or letters, people can hold only about seven symbols in memory at one time.

However, given sufficient experience in a domain, humans form *chunks* to describe regularities in that domain. Simon calls this the process of *familiarization.* Memory experiments show that subjects can hold approximately the same number of chunks in short-term memory, regardless of the complexity of the chunks. Thus, one can remember around seven letters, seven familiar words, or even seven familiar sentences. An extreme example is the Gettysburg Address, which is composed of sentences, which are in turn composed of phrases, which are themselves composed of certain words, and so forth.

Simon proposes that familiarization occurs during conscious problem solving of the type that characterizes Hadamard's preparation stage. As one carries out a heuristic search through the problem space, one also builds up higher-level structures that describe regularities in that space. The goals and states that are generated during search are held in short-term memory, and these chunks are stored in long-term memory. On difficult problems, one can easily get lost and be forced to start over from the beginning. Meanwhile, one is becoming more familiar with the structure of the space and its components. Eventually, one may decide that the problem is too difficult and abandon the efforts. At this point, the structures in short-term memory will fade rapidly, but the chunks that have been stored in long-term memory will remain. Simon terms this process *selective forgetting.*

Later, one may reexamine the troublesome problem. However, this time one has a powerful repertoire of chunks available in long-term memory, and these lead the search down a path quite different from those on earlier occasions. These chunks may allow one to move directly to the goal, and in some cases this may occur so rapidly as to produce the experience of illumination. The process of familiarization, combined with the mechanism of selective forgetting, gives the problem solver a new approach, thus transforming a difficult problem into a straightforward problem.

Commentary

Let us consider the similarities and differences among Hadamard's, Ohlsson's, and Simon's theories of the insight process. All assume that Hadamard's four-stage model provides a reasonable description of the phenomena, and they concentrate on explaining the processes that underlie the different stages. Furthermore, all agree that the preparation and verification stages involve conscious problem solving, though Ohlsson and Simon give more detail, because they can build on the results of modern cognitive psychology.

The theories differ in their treatment of the incubation and illumination stages. Although he does not cast it in quite these terms, Hadamard argues that incubation involves a search through the space of idea combinations. This search is carried out by unconscious mechanisms that employ measures of interestingness or elegance, both to select promising candidates and to decide when a likely solution has been found. Illumination is secondary in this framework, serving only to notify the conscious mind of the solution. Most of the interesting action occurs in the unconscious during incubation, though the preparation stage also serves to "stir up" the ideas that are used by the unconscious.

However, developments in cognitive psychology strongly suggest that search of this kind requires conscious attention. Thus, Simon rejects the notion of an unconscious that can selectively search large problem spaces of the sort required for many scientific discoveries. He replaces Hadamard's unconscious search scheme with two much simpler unconscious processes: familiarization and selective forgetting. The first of these occurs during the preparation stage, and the second occurs during incubation. Together, they clear the way for conscious problem-solving mechanisms to find a solution during illumination. This stage occurs so quickly because the chunks acquired in the preparation phase make the search process trivial. This explanation is much more distributed than Hadamard's, assigning significant roles to each stage.

In Ohlsson's theory, the major action occurs during illumination, when the problem solver restructures the problem description so that its solution becomes obvious. This explanation does not attempt to account for the role of incubation, and in fact this stage is not even mentioned in the theory. Presumably, Ohlsson would argue that in some cases restructuring does not occur until some time after an impasse is reached, but this does not explain what causes restructuring when it does occur.

Although each of these theories of insight has its attractions, we are not satisfied that any provides an adequate explanation of the phenomena. Hadamard attributes powerful search capabilities to the unconscious that contradict the findings of cognitive psychology. Simon involves the more plausible mechanisms of familiarization and selective forgetting, but he does not explain why one returns to the problem when one does. Finally, Ohlsson posits a restructuring process that generates a new, simpler problem space. Like Simon's theory, this framework is consistent with our knowledge of the human information-processing system, but it does not explain the incubation stage.

In the following pages we propose an alternative theory of scientific insight that diverges from the existing theories along a number of dimensions. One difference is that it does not rely on the problem space hypothesis, as do the approaches of Simon, Ohlsson, and even Hadamard. Rather, we assume that insight is a memory-related phenomenon that centers on mechanisms of indexing and retrieval. Another distinguishing feature of our framework is the central role played by analogy. Given the importance of this mechanism to our work, we shall diverge slightly to review some earlier work on the topic.

Research on reasoning by analogy

Looking back on our examples of scientific insight, it becomes apparent that all involved some form of *analogy*. Archimedes formed an analogy between his body submerged in the bath and the king's crown submerged in a container of known volume. Kekulé formed a mapping between a snake biting its own tail and the benzene ring. Finally, Poincaré's insight was based on an analogy between the Fuchsian transformations and non-Euclidean transformations.

Polya (1945), Sternberg (1977), and others have argued for the importance of analogy in human cognition. Thus, it would not be surprising to find analogy occurring in scientific discovery. We shall argue that this mechanism plays an important role in many (though not necessarily all) cases of insight, and analogy occupies a central position in our theory of that phenomenon. But before describing this theory, let us first review some previous work on analogy itself.

Dreistadt's analogy-based theory of insight

Dreistadt has noted the role of analogy in historical examples of insight. He summarizes his own theory of insight in the following words (Dreistadt, 1968, p. 111):

This writer explains insight as occurring when one finds a stimulus pattern (the analogy) in which parts of the form or structure are like the structure of the problem-situation and the rest of the structure of this stimulus pattern (the analogy) indicates how to organize the unintegrated materials of the problem or how to recognize the problem by putting the parts that are out of place into their correct place, or both, thereby completing the whole which is then the solution of the problem.

In other words, an insight occurs when the problem solver finds some similarity to the current problem, and this analogy suggests a different view of the problem that makes its solution clear. In this framework, most of the action occurs during the illumination stage, which involves the discovery of a suitable analogy.

To test this hypothesis, Dreistadt (1969) performed a number of experiments to determine the influence of analogies and incubation periods on subjects' ability to solve problems. One group of subjects was given 20 min in which to solve a set of tricky problems. A second group was given the same amount of time to solve the same problems, but was also presented with pictures that contained analogical hints to help find the solution. However, this group was not told the purpose of the pictures. A third group was allowed 5 min to concentrate on the problem, then was given an 8-min incubation period (involving a distracting activity), and finally was given 7 min more to solve the problem. A final group was presented with the pictorial analogies and was given an incubation period.

Dreistadt measured both the number of correct solutions in each group and the closeness of their incorrect answers. He also interviewed subjects about their impressions of the problem-solving task. He found that pictorial analogies significantly aided the solution process, even though subjects were not always aware they had been given a hint. Incubation alone did not seem to help in problem solving, but there was some evidence that incubation enhanced the effect of the pictorial analogies. These results lend credibility to the belief that analogies are important in scientific insight, and we shall return to this view later in the chapter.

Hall's framework for analogy

Although Dreistadt presented evidence that analogy plays a role during insight, he did not suggest details for this process. However, several researchers in the fields of artificial intelligence and cognitive science have described computational models of analogy. Hall (1986) provides an excellent review of these alternative approaches and suggests an organizing framework for research on analogy. This framework includes four components: recognition, elaboration, evaluation, and consolidation.

Reasoning by analogy involves mapping from some existing structure, the *source,* onto some new structure, the *target.* One typically begins with an incomplete description of the target. The first step involves retrieving a plausible source from long-term memory; this is the *recognition* process. Once a likely source has been identified, one must *evaluate* the analogy to ensure that it is reasonable. Assuming the mapping is acceptable, one then carries over relevant aspects of the source to fill out the target description; this is the *elaboration* stage. Finally, for successful analogies, one may want to store an abstract description in memory to simplify retrieval in future situations; this is the *consolidation* process.

We shall use this framework in our discussion of the three particular computational models of analogy that we consider here. We should note that much of the work on analogy focuses on learning tasks, and the consolidation stage plays an important role in this context. However, our focus is on scientific discovery and insight, and consolidation seems less relevant for this domain. Also, Hall's framework downplays the need to store and index experiences in long-term memory before recognition/retrieval can occur. We shall include this earlier step in our treatment of analogy.

Gentner's structure mapping theory

Gentner (1983) has put forth a *structure mapping theory* that attempts to distinguish useful analogies from poor ones. This framework assumes that memory contains representations of objects linked together by predicates. Some predicates accept only one argument, whereas others relate two or more arguments. The attribute *red* is an example of the former; the relation *larger* is an example of the latter. Gentner makes a further distinction between first-order predicates, which relate objects, and second-order predicates, which relate other predicates. The relation *larger* is an example of the first, and *cause* is an example of the second.

The structure mapping theory claims that single-argument attributes are useful when noting *similarities* between two situations, but relations are more important for drawing *analogies.* For example, the statement "the X12 star system in the Andromeda galaxy is like our solar system" involves a similarity, implying that the X12 star is yellow, hot, about the same size as Sol, and so forth. In contrast, the statement "the hydrogen atom is like our solar system" involves an analogy. In this case, we certainly do not mean that the hydrogen atom is hot and yellow, but we do

(a)

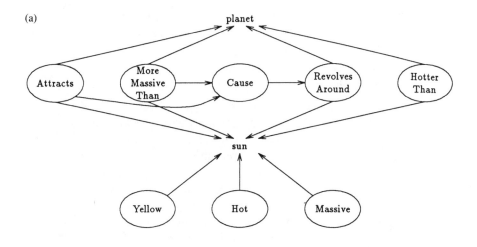

(b)

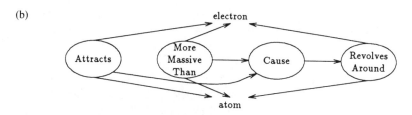

Figure 7.2. Creating a representation for the atom from the statement "The atom is like the solar system." Higher-order relations are carried over, and simple attributes are ignored.

mean that certain objects (electrons) revolve around its nucleus, more or less as planets revolve around the sun.

Gentner's theory does not address the issue of retrieving or recognizing analogies, but it does provide criteria for evaluating their quality, and it does suggest principles for carrying out elaboration. The theory can be summarized by three mapping rules:

1. Disregard attributes of objects, such as size or color.
2. Try to preserve relations between objects.
3. In deciding which relations to preserve, select those that retain consistency among higher-order relations.

Gentner refers to the third rule as the *systematicity principle*. The reasoning behind this principle is that the best analogies retain the highest-order relations.

As an example, consider the partial representation of the solar system shown in Figure 7.2(a). If we state that "the atom is like the solar system," the structure mapping theory predicts that only those relations presented in Figure 7.2(b) will be carried over. In this case, the sun corresponds to the nucleus of the atom, and the planet maps into the electron. Notice that none of the sun's attributes are carried along, nor is the fact that the sun is hotter than its planet, because this relation is not involved in the higher-order *cause* relation.

Winston's theory of analogy

Winston (1980) has proposed an alternative theory that focuses on different aspects of the analogical reasoning process. As in Gentner's framework, memory consists of objects linked together by relations, and together these form schemas describing some connected set of events. But Winston provides much more than this; his theory also addresses the issues of indexing and retrieval.

When a new event or description is stored in memory, it is indexed by the type of object it contains. For example, if one reads a story about a wicked stepmother and a beautiful girl, the schema summarizing the story will be indexed through those concepts. Later, when one reads another story involving a wicked stepmother or a beautiful girl, one will be reminded of the earlier schema. The actual process is both more complex and more general than this account suggests. Winston organizes concepts in "is-a" hierarchies, so that "wicked stepmother" will be stored as a subtype of "stepmother," "stepmother" will be stored as a subtype of "parent," and so forth.

Thus, a story involving any type of parent might remind the reader of the original schema, though to a lesser extent. But this extension means that, potentially, any new experience can remind one of any earlier experience. Winston responds to this issue by preferring connections that are more discriminating during the retrieval process. For instance, fewer stories will be indexed by "wicked stepmother" than by the more general "parent" concept. As a result, a new story containing a wicked stepmother will be more likely to remind one of an earlier story with a wicked stepmother than will new stories containing other kinds of parents. This approach has some similarities to "spreading activation" models of retrieval.

Once a plausible source for the analogy has been established in this manner, Winston's model compares all possible mappings between the source and the target and then evaluates them according to their degree of match. This evaluation process gives preference to higher-order relations, but it also takes objects into account. The approach also differs from Gentner's in that the elaboration process carries over both relations *and* attributes. Finally, the method consolidates its analogically based findings by transforming them into production rules, but this process need not concern us here. Winston has tested his mechanism in a number of domains, including story understanding and electric circuits.

Carbonell's theory of derivational analogy

Carbonell (1986) has explored the use of analogy in problem solving. When one encounters a completely novel problem, the only choice is to employ weak problem-solving methods such as heuristic search or means–ends analysis. However, when the current problem shares features with an earlier problem for which the solution is already known, one can use this knowledge to direct search on the current task.

But Carbonell argues that superficial similarities in problem structure and solution path are less important than the *reasons* why particular steps were taken. He suggests that weak problem-solving methods lay down a derivational trace in memory. This trace not only contains the final solution path but also includes failed paths and the reasons why those paths did not lead to a solution. It also includes subgoals and the reason for their creation.

When a problem solver encounters a new problem, the first step is to apply weak methods to search for a solution. If the initial reasoning steps are similar to those used in another problem, then one retrieves the earlier problem and its derivational trace. Once a plausible analogy has been identified, the mapping is elaborated by "replaying" the derivations from the earlier problem and checking to see that similar derivations carry over to the new problem. In cases in which the same reasoning holds for both problems, the analogous path is followed. In other cases the analogous derivation does not hold, and some different justification must be found for problem solving to proceed. As in Gentner's theory, the emphasis here is on evaluation and elaboration, though Carbonell also addresses the problems of indexing, retrieval, and consolidation.

Commentary

Before moving on, we should attempt to extract some useful lessons from the earlier work on analogy. One immediate observation is that these theories are weak on the side of indexing and retrieval. Gentner does not even address this issue, and Carbonell must carry out some search before being reminded of an earlier problem. Winston provides the most coherent model of retrieval, employing a mechanism similar to Anderson's (1983) spreading activation theory. This simple mechanism has two interesting properties. First, it seems quite plausible that activation could spread in parallel, and that this process could occur at unconscious levels. Second, the mechanism may sometimes suggest very poor analogies, because it focuses on the types of objects shared by two situations, not on their relations. Later we shall see that these features of spreading activation play an important role in our theory of insight.

All three theories share a concern with the elaboration process, in which one constructs a detailed mapping between source and target and carries over relevant structures. However, they disagree significantly on methods for determining relevance. Winston uses causal relations to select an optimal mapping, but once this has been established he carries along all consistent structures. In contrast, Gentner explicitly abandons single-argument predicates and retains only those relations that occur as arguments of higher-level relations. This naturally leads to a more abstract description of the target than does Winston's approach. However, Gentner's emphasis on the number and nature of arguments seems somewhat ad hoc. Carbonell's claim is more elegant – that one carries over only those structures that were used in *deriving* the source structures. We shall reinvoke this idea later as well.

An alternative theory of insight

We are now ready to present an alternative theory of scientific insight. In many ways, our framework is an extension of Dreistadt's analogy-based scheme, with computational ideas borrowed from Carbonell, though Gentner and Winston have also influenced our thinking. We present an overview of the theory and its differences from earlier frameworks. Then we consider the details of the theory and the phenomena it covers.

An overview of the theory

The basic tenet of our theory is that insight does not result from search through a problem space, but rather is a *memory-related* phenomenon. Moreover, the process of insight often involves the recognition, evaluation, and elaboration of analogies. We do not claim that all insights can be explained in this manner, but we believe that many examples from the history of science have this quality.

However, one can instantiate this general view in different ways. One argument, following Hadamard's line of reasoning, is that unconscious processes lead to the recognition of analogies during incubation. These mechanisms would search the space of possible mappings and, when a suitable analogy had been found, would deposit the result in the fringe consciousness. Presumably this search would be directed by heuristics of elegance (or even by Gentner's notion of systematicity). This scheme is identical with Hadamard's, except that his "combination of ideas" has been replaced by the recognition of useful analogies.

We shall argue instead that the process of analogical retrieval occurs entirely during the illumination stage and that this retrieval usually is cued by some external event. This explanation requires a very rapid mechanism, presumably one that occurs in parallel. A spreading activation process (like that used by Winston) has precisely these characteristics, and this will form another cornerstone of our theory of insight.

But if analogies are formulated during illumination, what purpose is served by the incubation stage? Our theory provides a simple answer to this question: There is *nothing* occurring during incubation. There are no unconscious processes selectively searching a problem space, as Hadamard suggests, nor is there even significant forgetting, as Simon proposes. Instead, the memory system is simply biding its time, waiting for some cue to initiate retrieval of a promising analogy.[2] When this occurs, it takes place very rapidly, giving the flash of insight that so many scientists have experienced.

Note that we are not rejecting the notion of unconscious processes. Both indexing and retrieval are unconscious in that the problem solver has no conscious control over them. We have rejected (along with Simon) only the concept of unconscious

Table 7.1. *A comparison of four theories of insight*

Stage	Hadamard	Ohlsson	Simon	Current
Preparation	"Stirring up" of ideas	Generation of impasse	Familiarization	Indexing of useful structures
Incubation	Unconscious search for ideas	Nothing	Selective forgetting	Nothing
Illumination	Noticing a solution	Restructuring, look ahead	Informed problem solving	Retrieval of analogy
Verification	Checking solution	Checking solution	Checking solution	Checking solution

reasoning. Such a process is inconsistent with currently accepted theories in cognitive psychology, which assume that problem solving requires conscious attention. We have replaced it with the much weaker mechanism of unconscious spreading activation. This component is completely consistent with recent work, and some widely recognized theories (Anderson, 1983) rely heavily on such a mechanism.

Our theory makes less controversial claims about the preparation stage. There is little doubt that conscious problem solving occurs during this period and that this lays the foundation for the later illumination. Like Simon, we believe that preparation serves to index useful structures in memory, and we depart from his view only in the purpose to which these structures are later put. Our emphasis on analogy makes the particular form of indexing very important; we shall have more to say about this later.

The verification stage also clearly involves conscious checking of the insight's validity, but our model of this stage also differs from earlier theories. Recall that Hall's framework distinguishes between evaluation and elaboration. The first of these components is closest in spirit to traditional notions of verification, because it involves checks on the quality of the proposed analogy. But the process does not stop there. One must also decide which aspects of the source one should carry over to the target situation; this is the elaboration process. As we shall see later, our model of elaboration incorporates Carbonell's notion of derivations.

Table 7.1 presents the major differences between our theory and earlier models. To summarize, we claim that insight is a memory-based phenomenon, in contrast to the search-based theories of Hadamard, Ohlsson, and Simon. The theory further states that insight is a form of reasoning by analogy, requiring indexing during the preparation stage, retrieval during the illumination stage, and elaboration during the verification stage. Finally, the theory states that no significant processes occur during the incubation period.

Process models and behavioral descriptions

We have seen that structures are indexed in memory during the preparation stage and that this lays the foundation for retrieval during illumination. However, we have not yet stated what types of structures are stored, nor what indexing scheme is used. There are many possible responses to these questions, but the one we have taken builds on Forbus's (1984, 1986) *qualitative process* theory. Thus, we should review this framework briefly before moving on.

Like other researchers[3] in the area of qualitative physics, Forbus has noted that people often reason about physical processes in a qualitative manner. For example, if asked to describe the process by which water boils, one might say, "If you heat water, its temperature will increase until it reaches the boiling point; after this the water turns into steam." Note that this statement does not mention specific quantities of heat, temperature, or rates of change. Instead, it focuses on the *qualitative* changes.

Forbus's framework centers on the notion of *processes* that produce changes over time. Heating, boiling, evaporation, and fluid flow can all be described as such qualitative processes. Each process can be described in terms of the objects involved, the conditions under which it occurs, and its influences or effects. When a set of objects meets the conditions on a process, that process becomes "active" and leads to changes in those objects. Consider the process of boiling water as an example. In this case, the objects consist of a heat source, a container, and some water in the container. The condition on this process states that the water's temperature must be greater than the boiling point of water. When this occurs, two changes result: The amount of water decreases, and the amount of steam increases.

Given a set of processes and an initial state, Forbus shows how one can generate an *envisionment* for that physical system. An envisionment specifies all possible qualitative states that the system can enter, along with the order relations between those states. Each state contains only qualitative information, such as whether a quantity is increasing, decreasing, or remaining constant. In some situations an envisionment will contain nondeterministic branches, and in these cases one cannot predict which behavior will actually occur.

For instance, the envisionment for heating water in a closed container will include three possibilities. First, if the temperature of the heat source is less than the boiling point, then the water will get hotter until it reaches this temperature and then remain constant. Second, if this temperature is greater than the boiling point, then at some point the water will begin turning into steam, and this will continue until all the water is gone. In the third case, the pressure within the container will build up sufficiently to cause an explosion. Each of these situations corresponds to a different path in the envisionment, which we present graphically in Figure 7.3.

In summary, Forbus's qualitative process theory describes physical systems at two levels – a *theoretical* level in terms of processes and structures and a *behavioral* level in terms of envisionments. We shall see that this distinction has important implications for our theory of insight.

The task of theory formation

Now that we have explained the distinction between process structural models and envisionments, we can clearly describe a task that commonly confronts the scien-

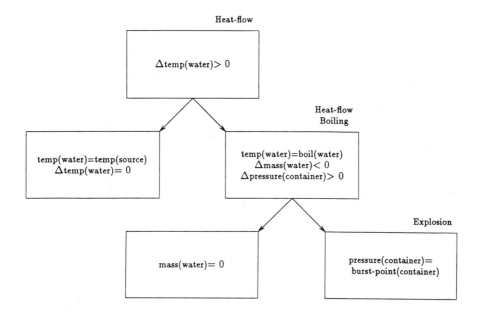

Figure 7.3. An envisionment for boiling water.

tist. Because one can use a process structural model to *derive* an envisionment, we can view the former as an *explanation* of the latter. But in many cases the scientist can induce a behavioral description for a physical system by observing its behavior and must then infer some process model that accounts for that envisionment. We shall call this the task of *qualitative theory formation*.[4]

This problem lends itself readily to analogy-based solutions, as can be seen from Figure 7.4. Let M_S represent the process structural model for some known phenomenon, such as the flow of fluid through a pipe, and let E_S stand for the envisionment derived from that model. Given some new behavioral description E_T that has been induced from observations, such as the behavior of an electric circuit, one can form an analogy between E_S and E_T. Once this mapping has been established, we can use M_S to infer an analogous process structural model M_T. If we have been careful in the mapping process, then M_T will constitute an explanation of E_T in the same sense that M_S explains the behavioral description E_S.[5]

We shall limit our model of scientific insight to the task of qualitative theory formation. This means that it will not account for Poincaré's insight about the Fuchsian transformations, because this did not involve the construction of a qualitative process model to explain observed behavior. However, many examples of scientific insight (including Archimedes' and Kekulé's discoveries) do take on this form, and we shall focus on these in the remainder of the chapter. We believe that our theory can be extended to cover other aspects of insight, but we have no firm evidence to present in defense of that claim. Now that we have defined the class of phenomena that we hope to model, let us turn to the details of our theory.

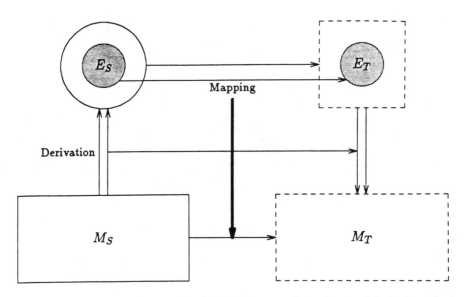

Figure 7.4. The mappings found in E_S to E_T are applied to M_S, thus inferring M_T. New objects and relations are inferred in E_T and M_T based on the derivation of E_S from M_S.

Indexing, spreading activation, and retrieval

According to Hall's framework, the first step in reasoning by analogy involves retrieving a candidate structure. However, before this can happen, such structures must have been stored in long-term memory, and they must be indexed in ways that allow their retrieval. Scientists undoubtedly index their domain knowledge in many ways, but our theory states that the most important indexing scheme for analogical retrieval centers on behavioral descriptions or envisionments.

For example, consider a situation in which two containers have different levels of liquid. If we connect these containers with a pipe, fluid will flow from the one with a higher level of liquid to the one with a lower level. This process will continue until the system has reached equilibrium. One very important aspect of this system is that it began with two unequal quantities of the same type, and these quantities changed over time until they became equal. Thus, one could index this envisionment through the concept of *equilibrium,* though certainly other features would also come into play.

One promising mechanism for explaining retrieval centers on the notion of *spreading activation.* In this framework, memory is viewed as a large semantic network (Quillian, 1968) consisting of nodes connected by labeled links. Some nodes correspond to general concepts such as *water* and *height.* These may be *activated* by interaction with the environment, and when this occurs, activation "spreads out" from the source nodes in concentric rings.[6] Theoretically, this process occurs unconsciously and in parallel.

Anderson (1976, 1983) incorporated the notion of spreading activation in his

ACT theory to model human fact retrieval. In this framework, the semantic network played the role of long-term memory. As new symbols entered short-term memory, activation spread out from these symbols through the semantic network, causing portions to enter short-term memory. In order to explain various memory phenomena, Anderson hypothesized that as one spread out from a given source node, the initial activation was split between the links emanating from that node. Thus, a node with a large "fan" would have less impact on retrieval than a node with a smaller fan. In addition, activation was divided proportionally according to the *trace strength* of the links involved. This trace strength increased the more often a link was stored or accessed.

Now let us see how the spreading activation approach can be used to model the illumination process. As before, assume that the scientist already has stored knowledge of many physical situations as schemas in long-term memory and that he has indexed these situations through features of their envisionments. Now the scientist encounters a new situation and constructs an envisionment from his observations. Activation will spread out from this description, possibly pushing the activation of an existing schema above threshold and depositing the structure into short-term memory. Presumably, human memory contains thousands of such schemas, many having features in common with the new situation. But if we assume that activation is divided proportionally according to trace strength, then well-stored schemas will be greatly preferred. And schemas that have been given significant attention in the recent past – during the preparation stage – will have very high trace strengths indeed.

This explanation accounts for insights like that of Archimedes, in which some new experience itself becomes the source of the analogy. But it does not explain another form of insight, in which the analogy maps between two structures already in long-term memory. In such cases, the scientist already has the necessary schema E_S in memory during the preparation stage, but he does not retrieve it until later, after some appropriate cue occurs. At first glance this seems odd, but the explanation becomes apparent on closer inspection. During the preparation stage, the scientist's attention is focused on the current schema E_T, which is gradually being laid down in memory with ever higher trace strengths. Activation spreads out from this structure, but because of the high fan and low trace strengths of analogous schemas, none rises above threshold. Finally the scientist gives up on the problem.

Later, some cue enters memory from the environment that reminds the scientist of the older, better-understood schema E_S. If the cue itself has little fan, this schema will be retrieved even with its low trace strength. Once E_S enters short-term memory, activation spreads from it to associated schemas. This time the fan is large, but one schema among the many competitors has a very high trace strength: E_T. Illumination occurs as this schema enters short-term memory and the mapping between E_S and E_T becomes apparent. Insight occurs at this moment, rather than during preparation, because activation does not spread away from schemas with high trace strengths; rather, it spreads *toward* them.

Consider the situation in which two objects with different temperatures are brought into contact. Over time, the temperature of one object will increase, and the other decrease, until the temperatures stabilize when equilibrium is reached. Suppose we spread activation out from the resulting envisionment through indices such as having two objects in *contact* and two quantities reaching *equilibrium*. One promising analogy for explaining the behavior of the temperatures is the envisionment for fluid flow that we described earlier. This mapping would not suggest itself during preparation because there are many schemas that share some features with the temperature situation. But later, some environmental cue such as a waterfall might cause retrieval of the fluid flow schema, and this in turn would retrieve the temperature schema.

This explains the nature of the retrieval process and its sudden character, but presumably such retrievals occur in everyday life without the ''Eureka!'' experience. Yet the rarity of such events follows naturally from the notion that activation occurs at different levels. In normal situations, we retrieve relevant schemas and deposit them in short-term memory, but at a relatively low level of activation. In true cases of insight, the retrieved schema has been stored so strongly that when finally retrieved, it receives a major influx of activation. If we assume limited amounts of such activation, then the retrieved schema effectively becomes the center of attention, flushing all other structures almost instantaneously. This rapid reorganization of the contents of short-term memory gives us the ''Aha'' feeling we associate with true illumination.

Elaboration through derivation

In Hall's framework, once a potential analogy has been recognized and evaluated, the mapping must still be elaborated. But how does one decide which aspects of the source to carry over to the target? Examples from the history of science provide some constraints on this process. When Dalton proposed the atomic theory of matter, it was presumably based on an analogy with macroscopic objects that could be decomposed into parts. Yet notice that although macroscopic objects have features like color and smell, Dalton did not endow atoms with these attributes. Similarly, the caloric theory of heat was based on a fluid analogy, but its authors did not carry along aspects of fluids such as taste or viscosity.

The point here is that, at least in scientific analogies, the elaboration process is quite selective. Only certain characteristics of the source situation are carried over into the target description. This is one of Gentner's main arguments for her structure mapping theory; in her framework, higher-level predicates determine which structures will be elaborated and which will be ignored. Although we could simply have borrowed this solution from Gentner, the presence of Forbus-style qualitative processes in our theory suggests a more elegant way to achieve the same effect.

Recall that Carbonell's theory of analogy relied heavily on the notion of *derivations*. A structure from the source (e.g., portions of a search tree) was carried over to the target only if an analogous derivation held for that structure in the target. What is interesting about Forbus's qualitative process theory is that it provides mechanisms for *deriving* behavioral descriptions (envisionments) from process and structural descriptions. We can then use these derivations to decide which process components and structural aspects of the source situation should be elaborated in the target situation.

For instance, suppose we have a qualitative process model of fluid flow toward equilibrium, as described earlier. The structural description of this situation may contain many features, such as the color of the liquids, their taste, their relative heights, and so forth. However, only some of these attributes are used to derive the environment that predicts that the fluids will move toward equilibrium. Now suppose we form an analogy between this envisionment and the observation that adjacent objects with different temperatures also move toward equilibrium. We would like to infer some structural description of the new situation, but which attributes and objects should we carry over?

Our theory states that one should carry over only those aspects that were actually used in the original derivation. In this case, the heights of the liquids were used, and so their analog (temperature) would be included in the new description. Features like taste and color were not used in the derivation, and so these would be omitted from the new model. Note that new objects as well as attributes may be inferred. One cannot have the height of a fluid without first having the fluid, and so one cannot have temperature without having some analogous fluid. Early heat theorists called this substance *caloric*.

Returning to Figure 7.4, we can see the relation between derivational elaboration and the other mechanisms in the theory. A Forbus-like derivation process is used to explain the source envisionment (E_S) given the source model (M_S). The entire structure is indexed by characteristics of this envisionment, and these links are used by the spreading activation process during retrieval. Given an envisionment (E_T) for the target (presumably inferred by observation), this retrieval mechanism suggests the source envisionment as a likely analogy. If this mapping is consistent, then the elaboration process plays the source derivation "in reverse" to determine the relevant objects and attributes of the target model (M_T).[7] When this stage is complete, the scientist has generated an abstract process structural model that explains the observed behavior by analogy with another situation.

Predictions of the theory

Let us examine how our theory accounts for some insight-related phenomena. First, recall that the duration of the incubation stage can vary widely. According to the theory, this occurs because the problem solver must wait until an appropriate cue appears. This might be readily available (as in Dreistadt's experiments), or it might take weeks or months to present itself. In the former case, illumination will occur almost immediately; in the latter, illumination will be delayed until the cue arises.

In some cases, no useful cue ever appears, and the problem remains unsolved. Presumably this is a common occurrence, but we seldom hear about failed insights because they are not very newsworthy.

A second phenomenon is that different people have different levels of ability in problem solving and discovery. At first glance our theory cannot explain such individual differences. If cues appear randomly, then anyone should be able to make great discoveries by simply being in the right place at the right time. However, this analysis ignores the importance of the indexing that occurs during the preparation stage. Appropriate indexing is all-important to the process of analogical retrieval, and different levels of domain knowledge can lead to quite different indexing schemes. Thus, experts in a given domain are more likely to store problems in ways that will let them be easily retrieved later. And the more attention given to a problem during the preparation stage, the more ways in which it will be indexed and the more firmly will its links be established. This explanation contrasts sharply with that given by Hadamard, which attributes differences in creativity to differences in unconscious reasoning processes.

We have seen that dreams play an important role in some insights, and this also seems to cause difficulty for the theory. If insights rely on external cues to initiate analogical retrieval, then they should never occur during dream states. However, this objection also disappears on closer inspection. There is no inherent reason why the retrieval cues must be *external;* they might also be internally generated during periods of free association, and this is exactly what dreams provide. But because the chains occurring in dreams are semirandom, they provide little more direction than chance external cues. Thus, dream-based illuminations may be delayed as long as those based on interactions with the environment. Kekulé did not dream of a snake because his unconscious mind was gnawing at the benzene problem. Rather, he dreamed of a snake by chance, and this cued a useful mapping to the problem.

The theory does not provide a satisfactory account of the Poincaré episode. In this case, illumination came to the mathematician as he was stepping onto a bus, and he did not report any external cue that seems related to the problem. However, this does not mean that such a cue was not present. Recall that the retrieval process itself is unconscious; so it seems quite plausible that some cue was available and reminded Poincaré of the non-Euclidean transformations, even though he was not aware of it. Dreistadt's (1969) experiment suggests that this situation is relatively common. Many of his subjects did not think they had been aided by the analogies, and those who did were not clear as to how the pictures had helped.

The final phenomenon predicted by the theory is the occurrence of "false insights." These tend to be overlooked in the discovery literature because usually they are rejected soon after generation. But most scientists will admit that some of their most promising insights have failed to stand up under scrutiny. Recall that the spreading activation process responsible for retrieval in our theory is not very selective. In many cases it will propose analogies that will not carry through when examined more closely. Nor would we expect more than this from such a rapid, unconscious recognition process. Of course, the ratio of false insights to useful ones will depend on the indexing scheme and the particular connections formed, and this will depend on the problem solver's level of expertise and the effort spent during preparation. In general, we would expect expertise and hard work to increase the proportion of true insights.

Conclusions

In the previous sections we reviewed some examples of scientific insight and Hadamard's four-stage description of this process. We examined some earlier theories that have attempted to account for the roles played by Hadamard's stages: preparation, incubation, illumination, and verification. However, we found these search-based explanations lacking and proposed an alternative theory that views insight as a memory-based phenomenon. The new theory is based on the dual notions of analogy and qualitative mental models; it draws heavily on concepts developed by earlier researchers in these areas, but links them together in a new organization. Finally, we saw that this theory accounts for many of the features normally associated with insight.

Although our focus has been scientific insight, we should briefly consider our framework's implications for other forms of creativity. We shall not argue that analogy is the only path to creative thought, but we find it plausible that this mechanism does underlie many forms of original thinking. To the extent that this holds, many of the mechanisms contained in our theory of scientific insight will carry over into these other areas. These include our two main biases: that insight is explained better in terms of memory processes than search methods, and that retrieval mechanisms such as spreading activation account for illumination effects without the need for unconscious reasoning processes. Although we place significant limits on our theory as a whole, we believe that these two claims have great generality and can profitably be applied to explain other forms of creative behavior.

Before closing, we should address two traditional concerns of the literature on creativity. The first involves methods for measuring creative ability. On this count, our theory takes an extreme stance: Humans possess no general creativity factor; so no such component exists to be measured. Instead, humans possess a wealth of knowledge structures indexed by concepts that a person judges important. The level of creativity that one exhibits will depend on one's knowledge, one's indexing scheme, and the particular situation in which one finds oneself.

But this claim suggests a useful response to the second traditional concern of creativity work: methods for improving creative ability. We have seen the important role that preparation plays in scientific insight, and presumably any creative act must have substantial knowledge structures on which to build. One cannot expect to be creative in any domain until one has achieved knowledge of that domain. Knowledge of an area may also improve retrieval abilities by leading one to index structures through concepts useful to that domain. Creativity is more than simple retrieval, involving the application of old ideas to new situations, but retrieval plays an essential part in the creative experience.

At this point, we have presented only the vague outline of a theory. The next step is to specify enough details to let us implement the framework as a running cognitive simulation. Whether or not our theory will hold together against this harsh test, only time and experience will tell. Most likely, the process of constructing this model will reveal many problems and inconsistencies, but these should lead us to refine and improve the model, until we achieve a real understanding of the nature of scientific insight.

Notes

1 It is said that Archimedes' joy at this insight was so great that he leaped from his bath and ran naked through the streets of Syracuse, exclaiming "Eureka!" (I have found it!).

2 This suggests the need for a fifth group in Dreistadt's experiment, which would be supplied with pictorial analogies only *after* the incubation period. Our theory predicts that this group's problem-solving ability would be comparable to that for the group that had analogies for the entire time.

3 We refer interested readers to de Kleer and Brown (1983), Kuipers (1984), and Iwasaki and Simon (1986) for alternative approaches to qualitative physics. We find Forbus's framework the most consistent with our goals, but we do not have the space to discuss the reasons here.

4 Of course, there are many other facets to scientific discovery, but we do not have the space to consider them here. We refer interested readers to Lenat (1983) and Langley, Simon, Bradshaw, and Zytkow (1986) for computational studies of some other aspects of discovery.

5 This framework for analogical scientific theory formation was developed independently by Falkenhainer (1987) in his work on *verification-based analogical learning*.

6 Quillian focused on finding intersecting paths between source nodes. Recently, Charniak (1986), Granger, Eiselt, and Holbrook (1986), and Norvig (1985) have reinvoked this mechanism to model natural language understanding and inference. We have not used this particular approach in modeling insight, though it may provide a plausible alternative.

7 Note that one can also infer missing components of the envisionment. However, this process is purely structural and does not rely on the notion of derivations.

References

Anderson, J. R. (1976). *Language, memory, and thought*. Hillsdale, NJ: Lawrence Erlbaum.

Anderson, J. R. (1983). *The architecture of cognition*. Cambridge, MA: Harvard University Press.

Anderson, J. R., & Bower, G. H. (1973). *Human associative memory*. Washington, DC: V. H. Winston.

Carbonell, J. G. (1986). Derivational analogy: A theory of reconstructive problem solving and expertise acquisition. In R. S. Michalski, J. G. Carbonell, & T. M. Mitchell (Eds.), *Machine learning: An artificial intelligence approach* (Vol. 2, pp. 371–392). Los Altos, CA: Morgan Kaufmann.

Charniak, E. (1986). A neat theory of marker passing. In *Proceedings of the Fifth National Conference on Artificial Intelligence* (pp. 584–588). Philadelphia: Morgan Kaufmann.

de Kleer, J., & Brown, J. S. (1983). Assumptions and ambiguities in mechanistic mental models. In D. Gentner & A. L. Stevens (Eds.), *Mental models* (pp. 155–190). Hillsdale, NJ: Lawrence Erlbaum.

Dreistadt, R. (1968). An analysis of the use of analogies and metaphors in science. *Journal of Psychology, 68*, 97–116.

Dreistadt, R. (1969). The use of analogies and incubation in obtaining insights in creative problem solving. *Journal of Psychology, 71*, 159–175.

Falkenhainer, B. (1987). Scientific theory formation through analogical inference. In *Proceedings of the*

Fourth International Workshop on Machine Learning (pp. 218–229). Irvine, CA: Morgan Kaufmann.

Farber, E. (1966). Dreams and visions in a century of chemistry. In R. F. Gould (Ed.), *Kekulé centennial* (pp. 129–139). Washington, DC: American Chemical Society.

Forbus, K. D. (1984). *Qualitative process theory* (Technical Report No. 789). Cambridge, MA: Massachusetts Institute of Technology, Artificial Intelligence Laboratory.

Forbus, K. D. (1986). *Interpreting observations of physical systems* (Technical Report No. UIUCDCS-R-86-1248). University of Illinois at Urbana-Champaign, Department of Computer Science.

Gentner, D. (1983). A theoretical framework for analogy. *Cognitive Science, 7,* 155–170.

Granger, R. H., Eiselt, K. P., & Holbrook, J. K. (1986). Parsing with parallelism: A spreading-activation model of inference processing during text understanding. In J. L. Kolodner & C. K. Riesbeck (Eds.), *Experience, memory, and reasoning* (pp. 227–246). Hillsdale, NJ: Lawrence Erlbaum.

Hadamard, J. (1949). *The psychology of invention in the mathematical field.* Princeton, NJ: Princeton University Press.

Hall, R. P. (1986). *Understanding analogical reasoning: Computational approaches* (Technical Report No. 86-11). University of California, Irvine, Department of Information and Computer Science.

Holland, J. H., Holyoak, K. J., Nisbett, R. E., & Thagard, P. R. (1986). *Induction: Processes of inference, learning, and discovery.* Cambridge, MA: MIT Press.

Iwasaki, Y., & Simon, H. A. (1986). *Theories of causal ordering: Reply to de Kleer and Brown* (Technical Report No. CMU-CS-86-104). Pittsburgh: Carnegie-Mellon University, Department of Computer Science.

Kuipers, B. (1984). Commonsense reasoning about causality: Deriving behavior from structure. In D. G. Bobrow (Ed.), *Qualitative reasoning about physical systems* (pp. 169–203). Amsterdam: Elsevier Science.

Langley, P., Simon, H. A., Bradshaw, G. L., & Zytkow, J. (1986). *Scientific discovery: Computational explorations of the creative processes.* Cambridge. MA: MIT Press.

Lenat, D. B. (1983). The role of heuristics in learning by discovery: Three case studies. In R. S. Michalski, J. G. Carbonell, & T. M. Mitchell (Eds.), *Machine learning: An artificial intelligence approach* (pp. 243–306). Los Altos, CA: Morgan Kaufmann.

Marr, D. (1982). *Vision.* San Francisco: Freeman.

Newell, A. (1980). Reasoning, problem solving, and decision processes: The problem space hypothesis. In R. Nickerson (Ed.), *Attention and performance VIII.* Hillsdale, NJ: Lawrence Erlbaum.

Newell, A., & Simon, H. (1972). *Human problem solving.* Englewood Cliffs, NJ: Prentice-Hall.

Norvig, P. (1985). Frame activated inferences in a story understanding program. In *Proceedings of the Ninth International Joint Conference on Artificial Intelligence* (pp. 624–626). Los Angeles: Morgan Kaufmann.

Ohlsson, S. (1984a). Restructuring revisited: Summary and critique of the gestalt theory of problem solving. *Scandinavian Journal of Psychology, 25,* 65–78.

Ohlsson, S. (1984b). Restructuring revisited: An information processing theory of restructuring and insight. *Scandinavian Journal of Psychology, 25,* 117–129.

Poincaré, H. (1952). *Science and method* (F. Maitland, Trans.). New York: Dover.

Polya, G. (1945). *How to solve it.* Princeton, NJ: Princeton University Press.

Quillian, M. R. (1968). Semantic memory. In M. L. Minsky (Ed.), *Semantic information processing.* Cambridge, MA: MIT Press.

Schank, R. C., & Abelson, R. P. (1977). *Scripts, plans, goals, and understanding.* Hillsdale, NJ: Lawrence Erlbaum.

Simon, H. A. (1977). *Boston studies in the philosophy of science: Vol. 54. Models of discovery.* Boston: Reidel.

Sternberg, R. J. (1977). *Intelligence, information processing and analogical reasoning: The componential analysis of human abilities.* Hillsdale, NJ: Lawrence Erlbaum.

Winston, P. H. (1980). Learning and reasoning by analogy. *Communications of the ACM, 23,* 689–703.

8   Freedom and constraint in creativity

Philip N. Johnson-Laird

> One's own free and unfettered volition, one's own caprice, however wild, one's
> own fancy, inflamed sometimes to the point of madness – that is the one best and
> greatest good, which is never taken into consideration because it will not fit into
> any classification, and the omission of which always sends all systems and theories
> to the devil.
>   – Dostoyevsky (1864)

Creativity is a mystery, and many people believe that it should remain a mystery. It should not be scrutinized too closely, says the anxious Romantic, because there is a danger in knowing too much about it. If we discover its sources, they may dry up. The cynical Realist asserts a different proposition: Those who cannot create study those who can. Critics and historians have assessed acts of creation by the canons of their day. Artists and scientists have reflected on their own and others' inspirations. And, above all, psychologists have carried out tests to measure creativity, experiments to explore it, exercises to enhance it, and investigations to reveal it in the lives of gifted individuals. Contrary to Romantic and Realist alike, a remarkable amount of imagination has been exercised in studying imagination, and we are none the worse for it. Alas, we are not too much wiser, either.

Few students of creativity have stopped to define what it is that they are studying. On the whole, a priori definitions do not advance science, but impede it. The advance of science, however, enables us to frame superior a posteriori definitions. My goal in this chapter is to arrive at such a definition of creativity. To reach that goal, I shall first analyze the nature of free will – for to be creative is to be free to choose among alternatives. Next, I shall consider constraints on creativity – for what is not constrained is not creative. These considerations will enable me to propose a computational theory of creative processes. The theory postulates a relation between computational power and the temporal demands of creating new ideas. I shall explore this idea in a particularly tractable domain – musical creativity – and establish certain existence proofs in the form of computer programs that generate bass lines and tonal chord sequences. The theory is computational because

I am grateful to my colleague Roy Patterson for encouragement and for developing the
software that turns raw numbers into musical sounds.

I want to avoid a defect that has been common to theories of creativity from Wallas (1926) to Bateson (1979): an amalgam of vagueness and incompleteness that takes too much for granted. If quantum electrodynamics and meteorology can be modeled computationally, then it should be possible to do the same for theories of creativity. It seems a sensible strategy to start with the hypothesis that the processes of creation are computable. If they are not, then they may be beyond the scope of science, or else the foundations of computability theory may be wrong.

A working definition

The best recent dictionary of psychology (Reber, 1985) offers the following definition:

> creativity   A term used in the technical literature in basically the same way as in the popular, namely, to refer to mental processes that lead to solutions, ideas, conceptualizations, artistic forms, theories or products that are unique and novel.

With one caveat – to which I shall return presently – I applaud this definition. But I fear that its emphasis on mental processes may win few adherents in certain quarters, and so let me first defend it.

In a fascinating historiometric project, Simonton (1984) has analyzed many sorts of data and showed that there are systematic relations between such data and the chances of an individual becoming an acknowledged genius. Simonton defines genius in terms of fame and influence and makes no distinction between creativity and leadership. He writes: "when the most famous creators and leaders are under scrutiny the distinction between creativity and leadership vanishes because creativity becomes a variety of leadership." No one can doubt that certain creators may become leaders, or that certain leaders may exercise a high degree of creativity. But not all great creators have their schools of followers or are even judged to be great within their lifetimes. In his day, J. S. Bach was known primarily as an organist, and his compositions were neglected until his genius was recognized by Mendelssohn and other nineteenth-century composers (on whom his techniques had little influence). Conversely, a political or military leader may be a leader by exercise of force, and a spiritual or religious leader may be a leader by virtue of asceticism. Leadership need not depend on imagination, and there is no warrant, other than Simonton's fiat, for identifying it with creativity. The mind of a successful leader may work in quite a different way from the mind of a successful creator, and the danger in equating the two is that the difference between them will be overlooked.

A focus on genius and exceptional acts of creativity also has its dangers. On the one hand, there may be many intangible social factors at work in the creation of major works of art and science. Of course, one should like to understand them, but it is difficult to investigate scientifically what it was about Periclean Athens, Renaissance Florence, Elizabethan London, or fin-de-siècle Vienna that made them such outstanding forcing grounds for the intellect. On the other hand, such a focus leads naturally to the view that there is some sort of discontinuity between prosaic acts of imagination and products of genius. There may be such a discontinuity – indeed, I shall make such a case later in this chapter – but unless we investigate both the mundane and the marvelous we shall never discover its nature.

At this point, let me make my one objection to Reber's definition. It asserts that the products of creation should be "unique and novel." Uniqueness and novelty are, of course, matters that can be determined only by considering what else has been created in other places and in other times. Two astronomers working independently in the middle of the nineteenth century predicted within a year of each other that there was a further planet beyond Uranus. The discovery of Neptune confirmed their prediction. Are we to say that only one of them, the one with priority, exercised a creative process of thought? By no means. I shall assume that the critical factor is that the product of a creative process should be novel *for the creator*, not merely remembered or perceived. If Pierre Menard, the eponymous hero of Borges's (1970) story, rewrites *Don Quixote* word for word, not by copying it but by becoming Cervantes (or, with more difficulty, by remaining himself), then by my criterion he does not fail to be creative. Nor do we fail to be creative, as is Borges's point, when we reread the novel with a deliberately anachronistic attribution to a twentieth-century author.

Choice and freedom of will

Many mental processes deliver products that are novel to those who entertain them. If I ask you to multiply two numbers together, or to reverse the order of words in a sentence, then the result may be something that you have never experienced before. Yet both of us, I suppose, would be disinclined to judge your performance as creative. We would not withhold the judgment because you merely did as you were told – Bach merely did as he was told in composing the *Musical Offering* on a theme given to him by Frederick the Great. We withhold it because, unlike musical composition, the tasks I gave you can be performed by rote. That is to say, they can be carried out as a result of a calculation, or deterministic procedure, that gives no freedom whatsoever to the imagination. Of course, you could do these tasks imaginatively. The point is that you do not have to; you will succeed perfectly well using procedures that leave no room for choice.

The concept of freedom that I have invoked refers, of course, to freedom of will – a puzzle that philosophers have agonized over for centuries (see Dennett, 1984, for some avuncular comfort on the topic). The problem of free will and the problem of creativity are, in some respects, one and the same. They can both be solved together.

If a task can be carried out by a process that at no stage calls for a choice to be made, then I shall say, in the parlance of computer scientists, that it is "deterministic." Thus, long multiplication is deterministic, because what is done at each stage is, in principle, wholly determined by the numbers to be multiplied and the current state of the calculation. Human beings, of course, have certain deterministic behaviors, such as the protective blink of the eyelid. They can also choose to carry out deterministic procedures – as when they choose to carry out a long multiplication. But human beings are also able to behave in ways that are not deterministic. By this claim, I do not mean that they violate the laws of nature, nor do I mean that their behavior is necessarily governed by indeterminate quantum events in brain cells. What I mean can be illustrated by asking the reader a simple question:

What are you going to do next?

You could choose – rational individual that you are! – to continue reading this chapter (if only to find out my solution to the riddle of free will). But you could equally well decide that you have had enough of creativity for the time being, and go out for a walk. There are many, many other possibilities. (Indeed, the problem of life is solved if you always have an answer to my question.) Normally, we decide what to do next either in response to events in the world (such as ringing telephones) or in response to mental states (such as boredom). And, normally, the decision is made tacitly: We decide what to do without reflecting on *how* the decision should be made. Such tacit decisions are likely to reflect a number of factors, both conscious and unconscious, that folk psychology refers to as "intuitive" or as "gut reactions." But if we do reflect on the matter, we can decide how to make the choice. We can even decide – should we so wish – to make an *arbitrary* choice.

If we are confronted with two equally appealing alternatives, then, rather than deprive ourselves of both as a result of indecision, we can plump for one alternative, not on the basis of any further rational evaluation but as a result of an arbitrary decision. Buridan's ass is said to have starved to death as result of being unable to decide which of two equally attractive bales of hay to eat. This dilemma seems implausible, because the slightest movement toward one bale or the other is likely to break the conflict. Approach–avoidance conflicts, however, are more likely to have a paralyzing effect. Animals that are arrested by them lack freedom of will. Human beings, however, are wont to say to themselves, "This is ridiculous: I'll have to do something." They may then, as a result of this higher-order reflection about the choice, make an arbitrary decision.

When someone makes a seemingly arbitrary decision, and has no idea on what it was based, psychologists often suppose that it was, in fact, determined by some minuscule aspect of the environment. Psychoanalysts emphasize the role of the internal environment; behaviorists emphasize the role of the external environment. If we knew the state of the individual's unconscious mind, or bank balance, they say, then we could account for the decision, which was entirely determined by such factors. It is merely our ignorance that forces us to treat it as nondeterministic. There are some splendid experimental demonstrations of how factors outside the individual's consciousness can influence the outcome of a decision (Nisbett & Wilson, 1977). Nevertheless, there are decisions that are truly nondeterministic. You may resolve – at a meta level – to make a deliberately arbitrary decision and to ensure its arbitrary nature by recourse to external means. You spin a coin, toss a die, or, if you are a psychologist, consult random-number tables.

What gives us freedom of will is the ability to reflect about *how* we shall make a decision, and thus to choose at a meta level a method of choice. We may decide to set out the pros and cons for the alternatives and attempt to make a rational decision, perhaps by seeking to minimize our maximum regret (cf. Pascal's wager on the existence of God, and Darwin's decision to marry); or we may decide to make a tacit intuitive choice on the basis of a "gut reaction" and without further reflection; or we may decide to make a decision based on some factor outside our control (e.g., consulting the Bible, I-Ching, or the Delphic oracle, or following a spouse's advice, whatever it may be); or we may decide to make an arbitrary choice, either plumping at random for one alternative or selecting an external randomizing mechanism. We may even decide not to decide, but to wait to see how the spirit moves us at the last moment.

The meta-level choice of a decision procedure may itself be made in the usual tacit way. But we can confront the question explicitly and make a conscious decision (at the meta-meta level) about how to choose (at the meta level) the method of choice. Should you continue reading or go out for a walk? You decide to spin a coin to decide whether to choose by minimaxing or by tossing a die. And how did you make *that* decision? There is potentially no end to the hierarchy of decisions about decisions about decisions, and so forth. Similar hierarchies form the basis of consciousness, intentional behavior, metacognition, and the development of an understanding of meaning and inference (Johnson-Laird, in press-a). They seem to depend on the ability to embed mental models within themselves recursively (Johnson-Laird, 1983).

Fortunately, there are at least two constraints likely to curtail the hierarchy of meta-level decisions from towering ever upward. First, the business of life demands that we reach decisions rather than get lost in speculation about how to reach them. The buck must stop somewhere. The decision at the highest level is always necessarily tacit. It can never be made explicitly, for if it were, there would, of course, be a still higher level at which a decision was taken to use the particular explicit technique, and this higher decision must have been tacit (on pain of an infinite regress). Second, there are constraints between the levels. If we decide to choose at random between alternatives at one level, and one of these alternatives is itself a random method of choice, then we might as well go straight to the latter. It can be rational to decide to make a random decision (in certain games, for example), and it can be rational to decide to make a rational decision (in certain other games, for example). But can it be rational to decide (at a meta-meta level) to decide at random (at a meta level) between making a rational or random decision? I think not.

We are free not because we are ignorant of the roots of many of our decisions, which we certainly are, but because we know that we can choose how to choose, and we know that among the range of options are those arbitrary methods that free us from the constraints of any ecological niche or any rational calculation of self-interest. This fact lies behind Dostoyevsky's deepest beliefs, epitomized in the quotation at the beginning of this chapter, and behind the Existentialists' fascination with gratuitous acts. One demonstrates freedom (if not imagination) in acting arbitrarily.

Freedom in creation

Freedom of choice occurs par excellence in acts of creation. When an artist paints a picture, at each point there are several possible brush strokes that could be made. When a musician improvizes a melody, at each point there are several possible notes that could be played. When a scientist imagines how a phenomenon might be explained, at each point there are several lines of thought that could be explored. When a speaker expresses an idea, at each point there are several possible forms of expression. In every case, the set of choices is constrained by largely tacit mental criteria that determine the genre and the individual's style. Sometimes, perhaps, these criteria reduce a particular set of possibilities to just a single item, but in general there is a range of options.

How is the choice among options made? Sometimes it depends on principle. But if the principles by which an individual creates were to completely determine every choice, then apart from the first stroke on the canvas, the first note on the piano, the first line of thought or word in the sentence, everything would be inevitable. There would be only as many works as there were beginnings. It follows that some choices are arbitrary. Among them are those occasions on which the individual explicitly exercises freedom of will and knowingly makes – or attempts to make – an arbitrary choice from among the set of viable possibilities. The mind certainly contains a system for making arbitrary choices. Nondeterminism in a deterministic device, such as a computer, is simulated by borrowing a technique from the casino at Monte Carlo and choosing at random. However, people tend to be rather poor at making genuinely random choices when they are asked to do so in the psychological laboratory. The departures from true randomness do not count against the existence of a mental system for arbitrary decisions, but rather imply that the mechanism lacks access to anything like a random-number generator and that perforce one such decision may influence others. Evidently, if the brain is governed by quantum indeterminacies, it is unable to exploit them.

In short, creativity depends on arbitrary choices and thus on a mental device for producing, albeit imperfectly, nondeterminism. Unlike calculation and other deterministic procedures, which yield the same response in the same situation, a genuine process of imagination could deliver a different response the second time around if the same stage of the process could be reinstated exactly. At each step, there may be more than one possible continuation. What determines the set of possible continuations is a matter that I shall take up next.

Criteria, genres, and the paradox of creativity

Creativity is like murder – both depend on motive, means, and opportunity. Society has, as I have already noted, dramatic effects on the creation of works of the imagination. There are grounds for supposing that these effects can be loosely divided into (a) diffuse global factors that affect motivation and opportunity and (b) specific cultural factors that influence the means of production – genre, paradigm, and style. The former are indeed the province of historiometricians. For instance, Simonton (1984, p. 170) observes that political instability in one generation depresses in the next the likely number of major creators in discursive fields such as science, philosophy, and literature. Specific cultural factors are the province of critics and historians. Cultural practices lead to the crystallization of artistic genres and scientific paradigms. These frameworks are the products of earlier creative processes, which are transmitted, often with significant modifications, from one generation to the next.

As Reber's definition allows, people create solutions, ideas, conceptualizations, artistic forms, theories, and products. I want to distinguish, however, between creation within an existing genre or paradigm and the creation of a new framework itself. Creation within a framework depends on access to its principles – the criteria or constraints of the framework – and ultimately these principles must be embodied within the mind of the creator. Even the invention of a new framework (i.e., new principles) must meet certain other criteria – not everything goes – but, as we shall see, these criteria are unlikely to be embodied in the mind. The creative process therefore depends on criteria. Conversely, any outcome that lies outside all frameworks is likely to be judged as uncategorizable rather than as creative.

When I talk of criteria, it is natural to think of the sorts of principles that are spelled out in theoretical treatises and in works on aesthetics and the philosophy of science. In fact, I have a different and broader notion in mind that I can bring out by reminding the reader of the central paradox of creativity (Perkins, 1981, p. 128). People are better critics that creators. The paradox, of course, is that if they have the knowledge to judge the products of a creative process, then they ought to be able to use it to generate such products in the first place. The resolution of the paradox depends on two factors. First, the explicit knowledge that is consciously accessible to a critic is by no means sufficient for the generation of ideas, which depends on other tacit forms of knowledge. Second, this tacit knowledge is not automatically available to consciousness.

The mind appears to depend on a set of separate processors that communicate data one from another, but that are not privy to each other's internal operations or representations; there are various versions of this hypothesis (Fodor, 1983; Johnson-Laird, 1983; Rumelhart, McClelland, and PDP Research Group, 1986). Hence a particular form of mental representation may be used by one ability, but not by another. Consider, for example, whistling a tune. It depends on a mental representation of a sequence of musical intervals. The ability to transcribe the tune in a musical notation also depends on a mental representation of a sequence of musical intervals. You can whistle a tune, but can you write it down? Most people can whistle, but even among those who can cope with musical notation, only a few can write down a tune as a result of being able to whistle it. The task is difficult because the melodic representations for whistling are not available to the symbolic process of writing.

In the same way, the tacit criteria for generating ideas are not available to conscious critical processes. Because critical criteria are easy to communicate to other people but insufficient for creation, whereas generative abilities are unconscious and ineffable, critical judgment tends to be considerably in advance of the ability to create works of the imagination. The paradox of creativity therefore leads ineluctably to the view that there are many criteria on which the creator must rely and that by no means all of them are available to overt inspection. Some of these criteria are common to many practitioners; they constitute the genre or paradigm. Other criteria are unique to individuals; they constitute an individual style of thought within the more general framework.

The principles that I have described amount to a theory of creativity at the computational level (Marr, 1982) – a theory of *what* has to be computed, namely, nondeterministic choices among the options characterized by a set of criteria. A theory at the algorithmic level must specify *how* the choices are made. In fact, I shall argue that, depending on the demands of the creative task, there are three possible classes of procedures. The crucial determinants of which sort of procedure is used are whether creation occurs within a framework or is intended to produce a new framework, and whether or not there is any opportunity to revise the creative product. I shall consider the resulting types of creativity in the next three sections of this chapter.

Creation within a genre in real time

If it is necessary to work rapidly within a framework – typically an artistic genre – with no opportunity for revision, then a sensible procedure is for the principles governing the genre and the individual's style to be used at each point in the process of *generating* ideas. They will constrain the set of options as tightly as possible. If they still leave open several options at any point, then a rapid arbitrary choice can be made from among these alternatives.

This procedure is likely to be used whenever there is time pressure on the creator. Thus, I hypothesize that it is used in all extemporaneous performances, including the making of artifacts in media that allow no second chances, the spontaneous use of natural language in discourse, and the improvisation of music, dance, and other art forms. As a test case, I shall consider musical improvisation because it can be treated largely as the syntactic organization of sounds into patterns, without having to worry about what, if anything, those patterns might represent.

Musical improvisation is governed by principles that must be in the musician's mind and that must suffice for the generation of music in real time. There is no opportunity to go back and revise an improvisation, and the musician cannot afford to make mistakes (i.e., to choose notes that do not make up a satisfactory melody of the appropriate variety). Many great composers – Bach, Mozart, and Liszt, for example – were consummate improvisers. Beethoven is another particularly interesting case, because he improvised with such fluency and brilliancy that his extemporaneous works were considered by some of his contemporaries to be better than his compositions (Sonneck, 1967). Yet his notebooks show that he composed with the greatest of difficulty. The two skills evidently depend in part on different underlying processes, as is borne out by the existence of composers who cannot improvise and improvisers who cannot compose.

What is common to most forms of improvisation is a reliance on two quite separate mental components: first, a long-term memory for a set of basic structures, such as the chord sequences of modern jazz or the ragas (scalic patterns) of Indian music; second, a set of tacit principles that underlie the improvisatory skill. We know that these two components exist because the basic structures are accessible to consciousness, and musicians can talk about them, write them down in a suitable notation, and teach them to neophytes. But, this explicit knowledge is not sufficient to enable a musician to improvise. Hence, there is a second component, which is relatively inaccessible to consciousness. Some musicians are aware of a few of its principles, but no one has complete access to them. Musicians learn to improvise by imitating other virtuosos and by experimenting with various possibilities. They learn to improvise by improvising, and they thereby develop their own particular styles within a genre.

A jazz musician can make up melodies that fit a large variety of different chord sequences. These chord sequences are known by heart, and the same basic sequence is used over and over throughout a piece. The computational problem in improvisation is therefore to produce in real time an acceptable melody that fits the chord sequence, and the tempi of modern jazz may call for melodies to be extemporized at an extremely rapid rate (e.g., 10 to 12 notes per second). A plausible conjecture about the solution to this problem can be based on the differences between the basic structures and the tacit principles.

The chord sequences are not made up during performance, and they may be the work of several musicians over a long period of time. Hence, it is expedient to do as much work as possible in the construction of the chord sequences so that they provide a rich structure that is latent with possibilities for the improviser. I shall presently outline a theory of this process.

The tacit skills have to run efficiently in real time. They govern the choice of notes to fit the harmonic implications of the chord structure and to make a good melody. I conjecture that these principles embody as little *computational power* as possible. What this conjecture means, in practice, is that the principles should place a minimal load on memory for the results of intermediate computations. In other words, the principles should take as input the basic chord sequence and deliver an

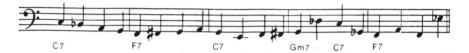

Figure 8.1. A fragment from an improvised bass line.

improvised melody as directly as possible without any internal representation of an intermediate form.

As an initial test of this conjecture, I have established an existence proof of the feasibility of such a computational architecture, because I have shown that it is possible to produce passable improvised bass lines without using intermediate representations.

The double bass player in modern jazz improvises a bass line to fit a given tonal chord sequence. Figure 8.1 presents a fragment from a typical bass line, together with the chords on which it is based. The bass line is rhythmically simple, just a steady four beats to the bar, though other styles are more complex. The actual timing of the notes depends on an exquisite sense of the metrical pulse of jazz. Nevertheless, the bass line allows us to approach the improvisation of a melody without the complications of rhythm; for a discussion of rhythm, see Johnson-Laird (1987).

There are several theories of how a bass player decides what note to play next. The player might merely choose any note in the range of the instrument that is among those making up the current chord. But this procedure would leap wildly around from a low note to a high note in a most unmelodic way, and it would fail to use "passing" notes, that is, notes that are not in the current chord but that pass from one such note to another (e.g., the second bar of Figure 8.1, which contains two passing notes to the chord of F7: the chromatic F♯ and the more consonant G that leads back to a major note of the chord, A).

A second method was suggested by Ulrich (1977). He argued that the melodic improvisations of jazz musicians are made up from existing motifs – fragments of melody – that are woven together to form a new melody. The musician does not make up new melodies, but rather modifies existing motifs to fit the current harmonic situation. This idea was implemented in a program devised by Ulrich and in a more sophisticated program developed by Levitt (1981). Levitt's program takes as input both a chord sequence and an existing melody. It divides the melody into units of two bars, which are then reused in a different order and in variant forms that fit the current harmony. The program is deterministic; that is, given the same input melody and chord sequence, it produces the same improvisation. Jazz musicians, however, do not perform in this way. They use motifs some of the time, but no one, apart perhaps from a complete beginner, uses them all of the time. It is easier, in the long run, as any competent performer will attest, to make up new melodies than to remember a vast array of motifs and to modify them to fit the chord sequence; see, for example, the reminiscences of David Sudnow, 1978, a well-known sociolinguist

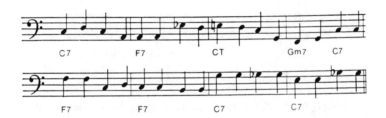

Figure 8.2. A fragment from the output of the program generating bass lines.

who learned to play jazz piano. There is no more evidence for creation solely by motif than there is for conversation solely by cliché.

Perhaps the most plausible hypothesis is that bass players choose their notes in order to meet two sets of criteria. The first set reflects the player's tacit knowledge of harmony, including both the notes that are concordant with chords and those that may be used in passing. The second set reflects a tacit knowledge of the appropriate "contour" underlying successful melodies. Here, the general idea is likely to be that after a series of small steps in scale, a step of a rather larger interval, and vice versa, makes for a pleasing melody. These principles are embodied in the two sets of criteria used by my computer program.

The program takes a chord sequence as input and delivers a viable bass line as its output. To produce each note, it first generates a small step, a large step, or the same note again, according to the rules of a grammar for contours derived from a corpus of improvisations. The grammar is "regular"; that is, it can be used with the minimum of computational power, which does not need any memory for the results of intermediate computations. The program then selects a pitch that meets the constraint of the step size and a set of harmonic principles. Where more than one possible note meets the various constraints, a random choice is made between them. Figure 8.2 presents a fragment from an entirely typical output of the program. The output, which also contains a rudimentary accompaniment based on the chord sequence, is played by a further program, devised by Roy Patterson and Rob Milroy, that synthesizes the sound of the double bass and the accompaniment.

The program is quite competent, but it lacks two abilities of the jazz player. It makes no specific use of chromatic runs of several passing notes (see the second bar of Figure 8.1), and it makes no use of motifs, which occasionally are featured in bass performances. Likewise, the program commits a minor solecism that revealed the existence of a special category of passing notes of which the author was previously unaware. The modifications to rectify these shortcomings do not require a larger memory for intermediate computations, but merely a slightly larger buffer for what has just been played.

The reader may be worried about the use of a grammar. It is often claimed that a creator "breaks the rules" in order to produce a more original work of art. Likewise, although a grammar may capture a genre, individuals have their own unique styles. Both these objections are instructive, but not decisive. If a creative process breaks the rules, then either it must make a choice at random regardless of the consequences or it must be governed by yet further criteria. These criteria can in turn be captured in a grammar. Hence, the breaking of a rule can be described by yet another rule (or else it is merely an arbitrary infraction). If an individual has a unique style, then it must depend on idiosyncratic biases in choosing alternatives. A grammar can likewise be framed to capture this style.

The procedure used by the bass program exemplifies a computational architecture in which criteria are used directly in the generation of a creative product. Because the criteria suffice to define a genre, the output is guaranteed to be at least viable, and the procedure can also be of weak computational power, which requires a minimal memory for the results of intermediate computations. Hence, the generative stage yields only a relatively small number of possible options, all of which meet the desired characteristics. Where there is more than one possible continuation, an arbitrary choice can be rapidly made. The choice has to be arbitrary because all the criteria are used in the generative process. The procedure can also rely on a long-term memory for structures produced using a greater degree of computational power. They enable the finished product to have more intrinsic interest than could be generated solely by an ''on-line'' procedure. The procedure as a whole is highly efficient, but it is feasible only if there is some way for previous experience to yield a mental representation of the criteria that govern the generative stage. I have elsewhere likened this computational architecture to Lamarck's theory of evolution (Johnson-Laird, 1987). He proposed that what an organism acquires by adapting to its environment can be conveyed to its progeny, and thus acquired constraints can guide the process that generates species.

Creation within a framework in stages

The generation of ideas by tacit principles does not always yield a product that meets the creator's critical criteria. In the case of improvisation, there is nothing to be done about such shortcomings. But in many genres there is no pressure to produce a performance in real time, and consequently there is an opportunity to revise unsatisfactory works. This possiblity is indeed the norm for most forms of creativity.

There is a corollary; if there is time to revise or to reject the products of a generative process, then the ultimate results are likely to rely on a high degree of computational power. That is, they can be produced making considerable use of a memory for intermediate results. It does not follow that the creators must make greater use of their working memories; if it is possible to leave a permanent record of the product in some external medium, then that record is itself a form of memory for an intermediate result. In certain artistic forms, such as painting and sculpture, the incomplete work is itself such a record. In science and other forms of art, it is possible to record incomplete or tentative ideas in some notation. Writing enhances

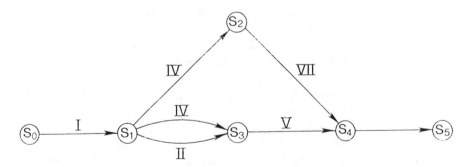

Figure 8.3. A device for generating chord sequences.

the computational power available to a creator by providing an external memory for intermediate results.

We saw in the previous section that jazz improvisations are based on chord sequences that are developed "off line" (i.e., without the need to make them up in real time). Hence, the theory predicts that the development of such chord sequences will demand rather more computational power than the spontaneous improvisations based on them. In order to test this prediction, I have examined a corpus of such chord sequences and have written a computer program to model – in rather abstract terms – the processes that might be responsible for their generation.

There is a large body of musical theory concerning the structure of tonal chord sequences (of the sort that includes those used in jazz). Most of these theories are too vague and incomplete to be directly modeled in computer programs, but they are sufficiently clear to establish their degree of computational power. Thus, theorists from Rameau (1722/1971) to Forte (1979) spell out systems that do not need intermediate representations. Ironically, these theories are equivalent in computational power to "regular" grammars of the sort that I used in accounting for improvisations in real time. A typical fragment from such a theory of chord sequences is illustrated in Figure 8.3. The Roman numerals denote the root of the chord: I = the tonic, V = the dominant, and so forth. (Nonmusicians need not worry about the interpretation of these symbols, but should treat them as strings in an abstract symbolic language.) A chord sequence is generated by starting in the initial state, S_0, and making transitions from one state to another. As each transition along an arrow is made, the symbol above the arrow is generated. Thus, the device produces, for example, the following sequence of symbols: I II V I, which corresponds to the standard tonal sequence of tonic, supertonic, dominant, tonic. A more realistic device would specify the type of chord on each of these roots – say a major triad on I, a minor triad on II, a seventh on V, and a major triad on I. The device shown in the figure is nondeterministic in that in state S_1 there are three different choices available. Some modern theorists have proposed adding probabilities to the different choices in order to model their frequencies of occurrence (Eigen & Winkler, 1983).

Devices that make no use of memory for intermediate results are not powerful enough to generate the tonal chord sequences of modern jazz. They are not powerful enough to generate the chord sequences of classical music, but the case is easier to make for jazz. As any jazz accompanist will attest, a piece has an underlying chord sequence that can be realized in many different superficial variations. Thus, the traditional chord sequence known as the "twelve bar blues" has many alternative forms. Steedman (1982) has outlined a set of rules that generates these alternatives from the underlying basic sequence. His grammar takes for granted the existence of an intermediate representation, namely, for the underlying basic sequence, and it also employs context-sensitive rules that call for intermediate representations in their own right. It might be argued that if the grammar could also generate the underlying sequence, then it would be able to produce variations on it in one pass (i.e., the underlying form would not need to be stored in memory). I have devised a program that produces tonal chord sequences from scratch in order to test this possibility. In fact, the program vindicates Steedman's analysis.

The program takes three stages to generate a chord sequence. Stage 1 employs a grammar containing such rules as

TWO-BARS → | I | Vd |

to generate an *underlying* chord sequence. Many of the rules contain more than one possible expansion, and the program makes a random choice in such cases.

There are many possible variations on the underlying sequence, I Vd, including the following three sequences:

Imj7	VIm7		IIm7		V7	
Imj7	bIII7		bVImj7		bII7	
Imj7	IVm7	bVII7	bIIIm7	bVI7	IIm7	V7

Stage 2 of the program uses context-sensitive rules similar to those of Steedman to interpolate chords into the underlying sequence according to the "cycle of fifths," one of the major dimensions of tonal space (Longuet-Higgins, 1979). Hence, given as input the sequence

| I | Vd |

the program, on detecting a chord containing the symbol d, can transform it into a seventh (symbolized as "7") and insert a previous chord that is related to it by the cycle of fifths:

| I | II7 V7 |

A further step of the same sort can be used to insert a chord in front of II7:

| I | VIm7 II7 V7 |

By working backward in this way – a procedure that requires a considerable memory for intermediate results – the final result of stage 2, depending on the choices of expansion, might be

| Imj   VIIm7 III7 | VIm7 II7   V7 |

Stage 3 employs a further set of context-sensitive rules in order to substitute one sort of chord for another and to make another sort of interpolation. Given the previous string as input, and depending on its choices, it can produce

| Imj7   IVm7 bVII7 | bIIIm7 bVI7 IIm7   V7 |

which is a sequence used by the late Thelonious Monk for one of his compositions.

One of the main features of this program, like the program for base lines, is that even though its principles are well understood, it is impossible to predict its output on any particular occasion. The program is not intended to model directly the mental processes of musicians devising chord sequences. It shows that whatever these processes may be, they call for a considerable degree of computational power, certainly more than is available to the rules implicit in music theory. It would be impossible to capture the superficial variations on underlying forms without exploiting some such degree of power. Likewise, the interpolations must be made one at a time and require a record of the previous state of the chord sequence. Musicians who devise new chord sequences must have access to principles that resemble those embodied in the program. However, they do not have to make up chord sequences in real time. They can write them down and work on them in the same way as composers. There is thus no reason for them to use their memories in the same way as the program; the written chord sequence is available for consultation. Musical literacy has ensured that computational power exerts no psychological price.

The procedure exemplifies a creative computational architecture that depends on several stages. These stages divide the criteria of the genre into those that guide an initial generative process and those that are used to modify its results – to select them, or not, as calling for further work. The generative stage is clearly nondeterministic (i.e., arbitrary choices must be made from among the options defined by the grammar), and the subsequent stages may also be nondeterministic.

The creation of novels, paintings, and other works of art typically is carried out within the conventions of an existing genre. Likewise, the creative processes of a scientist normally occur, as Kuhn (1970) has argued, within the constraints of an existing paradigm. These types of creativity invariably depend on a multistage procedure, though probably of a more complex form than the one I have exemplified. The creator generates ideas making use of some initial constraints, but other constraints may be spread over many stages, or unsatisfactory products may be fed back from an evaluative stage to a generative stage for modification. The reason for this division of labor, as I argued earlier, would be that the generative process has no access to the evaluative criteria. In the case of scientific hypotheses, a major evaluative constraint is a set of empirical observations.

Creation of new frameworks

The invention of a new genre or paradigm is ranked above all other forms of creation, but such events are rare. There appear to be no common principles that account for such transitions within a field – from one genre of art to another, or from one scientific paradigm to another. Moreover, the ultimate success of a major innovation depends on events of which the individual creators (and everyone else) is entirely ignorant. For artistic revolutions, these criteria include both socioeconomic factors and other contemporary developments in the world of the arts; for scientific revolutions, they include the subsequent availability of resources to explore the innovation and, of course, its success in making sense of empirical results – a factor that cannot be foreseen at the time of the innovation. It follows that there are no general criteria or principles that underlie all and only the successful major transitions in a particular domain of art or science.

If there are no principles that govern all major innovations in a domain, then there can be no neo-Lamarckian procedure for this type of creativity. Suppose that there were such a procedure for painting. Given as input the principles of early art, it would have to produce a set of viable alternative developments including the principles of perspective; and given the principles of mid-nineteenth-century painting, it would have to produce those of Cubism among a set of other viable alternatives. Likewise, a neo-Lamarckian procedure for physics would have to produce Newtonian physics from its precursors, and then follow that up with special relativity. Such tasks are obviously impossible if, as I claim, these various revolutionary transitions cannot be accounted for by any common set of principles for the relevant domain.

Because the creation of new genres and paradigms is so difficult, it might depend on an essentially arbitrary or random generative process. New species evolve as a result of the random shuffling of genes, followed by the constraints of natural selection, which eliminate organisms that are not viable. A possible architecture for creativity has the same "neo-Darwinian" design. Its first stage consists of a procedure that combines elements at random to generate a potentially vast number of putative products, and its second stage uses a set of constraints to filter out the products that are not viable. There is a long tradition of such mechanisms for creativity. Some proposals have been satirical, such as Mozart's scheme for musical composition by the shake of a die (O'Beirne, 1971), Swift's machine in the academy of Lagado in *Gulliver's Travels,* and Orwell's machine for writing cheap novels in *1984.* Other proposals are serious, and indeed the generation of ideas at random has been proposed by several authors as the only possible creative process (Bateson, 1979; Campbell, 1960; Skinner, 1953). Yet, shooting first (at random) and asking questions later (in terms of criteria) has a patent and inescapable difficulty. It is grossly inefficient. Most of the products of an arbitrary assembly of elements will not be viable. This point was discovered the hard way in the mid-1960s when computer scientists attempted to build intelligent programs by assembling them at random from simple components (Fogel, Owens, & Walsh, 1966).

The evolution of species is slow, even though there are millions of organisms engaged in the random shuffling of genes. Moreover, species do not evolve in a single step. It was not necessary, for instance, that the complete genetic specification of *Homo sapiens* be assembled as the result of a single random shuffling from an unorganized set of genes – an evolutionary step that is singularly unlikely to have occurred by chance. New species derive from existing species, and complex organisms have gradually evolved by common descent from less complex organisms. Hence, the nature of the elements that are randomly combined can improve the efficiency of the procedure. They should not be simple conceptual atoms, but rather existing sets of interrelated ideas.

Despite its inefficiency, a neo-Darwinian procedure is the only mechanism available if there is no way in which the generative process can be guided by selective constraints. This condition is the basis of modern evolutionary theory, but there is no reason to suppose that it applies to the production of revolutionary ideas. It is more likely that this generative process is guided by some criteria in a multistage procedure. The productive use of knowledge is a central part of genius. Although there are numerous potential heuristics, such as the search for revealing analogies, there are unlikely to be sufficient criteria to yield a tractable computational algorithm for producing successful innovations (Johnson-Laird, in press-b).

Conclusions

If creative processes are computable – and there are, as yet, no grounds for abandoning this hypothesis – then creativity can be defined in the light of the theory that has been advanced in this chapter. Creation yields products with three characteristic properties:

1. They are novel for the individual who creates them.
2. They reflect the individual's freedom of choice and accordingly are not constructed by rote or calculation, but by a nondeterministic process.
3. The choice is made from among options that are specified by criteria.

Although I have not labored the point, there are only three general classes of procedures that meet this definition: a neo-Lamarckian process in which the criteria are used to generate possible products, and an arbitrary choice is made from among them; a multistage process in which criteria are used to generate a work and to modify it, with the possibility of arbitrary choices in either stage; and a neo-Darwinian process in which a wholly arbitrary generation of ideas is followed by selection in terms of criteria. As a source of innovation, however, this last procedure is more likely to be used by nature than by human beings.

References

Bateson, G. (1979). *Mind and nature*. London: Wildwood House.
Borges, J. L. (1970). Pierre Menard, author of the *Quixote*. In D. A. Yates and J. E. Irby (Eds.), *Labyrinths: Selected stories and other writings*. Harmondsworth, Middlesex: Penguin.

Campbell, D. (1960). Blind variation and selective retention in creative thought as in other knowledge processes. *Psychological Review, 67,* 380–400.

Dennett, D. C. (1984). *Elbow room: The varieties of free will worth wanting.* Cambridge, MA: MIT Press.

Dostoyevsky, F. (1972). *Notes from underground.* Harmondsworth, Middlesex: Penguin. (Original work published 1864.)

Eigen, M. & Winkler, R. (1983). *Laws of the game: How the principles of nature govern chance.* Harmondsworth, Middlesex: Penguin.

Fodor, J. A. (1983). *The modularity of mind: An essay on faculty psychology.* Cambridge, MA: MIT Press.

Fogel, L., Owens, A., & Walsh, M. (1966). *Artificial intelligence through simulated evolution.* New York: Wiley.

Forte, A. (1979). *Tonal harmony in concept and practice* (3rd ed.). New York: Holt, Rinehart, & Winston.

Johnson-Laird, P. N. (1983). *Mental models: Towards a cognitive science of language, inference, and consciousness.* Cambridge University Press.

Johnson-Laird, P. N. (1987). Reasoning, imagining, and creating. *Bulletin of the British Psychological Society, 40,* 121–129.

Johnson-Laird, P. N. (in press-a). The development of reasoning ability. In G. Butterworth and P. E. Bryant (Eds.), *Proceedings of Stirling Conference on Human Development.* Cambridge University Press.

Johnson-Laird, P. N. (in press-b). Analogies and the exercise of creativity. In A. Ortony (Ed.), *Proceedings of the Illinois Workshop on Analogies.*

Kuhn, T. S. (1970). *The structure of scientific revolutions* (2nd ed.). University of Chicago Press.

Levitt, D. A. (1981). *A melody description system for jazz improvization.* Unpublished MSc thesis, Department of Electrical Engineering and Computer Science, MIT. Cambridge, MA.

Longuet-Higgins, H. C. (1979). The perception of music. *Proceedings of the Royal Society, Series B, 205,* 307–322.

Marr, D. (1982). *Vision: A computational investigation in the human representation of visual information.* San Francisco: Freeman.

Nisbett, R. E., & Wilson, T. D. (1977). Telling more than we can know: Verbal reports on mental processes. *Psychological Review, 84,* 231–259.

O'Beirne, T. H. (1971). From Mozart to the bagpipe, with a small computer. *Institute of Mathematics and Its Applications, 7,* 11–16.

Perkins, D. N. (1981). *The mind's best work.* Cambridge, MA: Harvard University Press.

Rameau, J. P. (1971). *Treatise on harmony.* New York: Dover. (Original work published 1722.)

Reber, A. S. (1985). *The Penguin dictionary of psychology.* Harmondsworth, Middlesex: Penguin.

Rumelhart, D. E., McClelland, J. L., & PDP Research Group. (1986). *Parallel distributed processing: Explorations in the microstructure of cognition: Vol. 1. Foundations.* Cambridge, MA: MIT Press.

Simonton, D. K. (1984). *Genius, creativity, and leadership: Historiometric inquiries.* Cambridge, MA: Harvard University Press.

Skinner, B. F. (1953). *Science and human behavior.* New York: Macmillan.

Sonneck, O. G. (Ed.). (1967). *Beethoven: Impressions by his contemporaries.* New York: Dover.

Steedman, M. J. (1982). A generative grammar for jazz chord sequences. *Music Perception, 2,* 52–77.

Sudnow, D. (1978). *Ways of the hand.* London: Routledge & Kegan Paul.

Ulrich, J. W. (1977). The analysis and synthesis of jazz by computer. In *Fifth International Joint Conference on Artificial Intelligence* (pp. 865–872).

Wallas, G. (1926). *The art of thought.* London: Cape.

9   Creativity as a mechanical process

Roger C. Schank

What is creativity? In general, laypeople tend to think of creativity as something mystical and unexplainable. But what this means to an artificial-intelligence (AI) researcher is that there seems to be no algorithm behind the creative process. Our premise here is that such an algorithm must exist, in principle. Even though very few people in AI work on creativity *per se,* AI is based on the premise that there is nothing mystical in the processes that underlie thinking. Arguments against the tenets of AI, such as those of Searle (1980) and Dreyfuss (1979), always seem to be based on the idea that, in principle, some things are unknowable about the nature of mind. Philosophers and others often seem to believe, without ever quite saying so, that one cannot simply write down the rules that underlie intelligent processes. Often these arguments get transformed into a discussion of whether or not, once such rules were discovered and a machine built that would embody them, it would be reasonable to claim that such a machine is *intelligent,* is *understood,* is *creative,* or whatever.

What I shall term the *philosopher's question* concerns the issue whether or not simply following rules qualifies as embodying the process that those rules describe. In other words, the issue for them is this: If a machine had all the rules for creativity and it could follow them so as to enable it to create new ideas, things, or whatever, would it actually be reasonable to claim that that machine was creative? Clearly, AI assumes that if a machine creates, then it is creative. So let us leave the philosophical arguments to the philosophers and here address the *AI question:* Can we write a set of rules such that if a machine followed them it would be able to create new things? When the AI question is solved, we then will be able to address the *psychological question:* Assuming that AI has given us a set of rules that enable machines to create, do people use the same (or similar) rules?

How is it possible that there exists a set of rules that embody the method by which ideas are created? This is a difficult problem, but by looking at a particular kind of creativity, namely, the creation of novel explanations, and by dividing that task into reasonable tasks, we can make the problem more tractable.

The model of understanding that I assume here is the Dynamic Memory model of processing (Schank, 1982). The dynamic memory model of processing is an elaboration of the knowledge structure model of processing (Schank & Abelson, 1977).

220

The premise of the knowledge structure model is that an input is processed by reference to a knowledge structure such as a script or a plan. The input is integrated into the structure, which enables the understander to infer events and states to have occurred that normally are part of the knowledge structure that is being used to process the input. Dynamic memory refines this model so that when an event is processed for understanding, it is necessary to interpret that event not only in terms of available knowledge structures but also in terms of relevant previous experiences in memory. Cumulative experience also modifies the knowledge structures. Thus, scripts, plans, and other mental structures are seen as constantly changing, based on the experiences of the system.

The overall premise behind this model is that understanding requires an active memory, full of knowledge based on repeated ossified experiences and also full of novel experiences that are unmerged with other events. In order to understand, one must have a set of knowledge structures and experiences that one can draw on as a kind of reference point. One of these structures is something I call an *explanation pattern* (XP). An XP is a standard explanation that has been used many times before. Creativity depends on the use of such XPs.

My claim is that there are basically two subprocesses that characterize creativity. The first, which is inherently a *search process,* is finding a candidate XP to use when one is in need of an explanation. The second, which is inherently an *alteration process,* is modifying and adapting the XP in such a way as to allow an explanation originally derived from one situation to be relevant to a rather different situation.

We shall discuss XPs later, but first let us consider what it would mean for search or alteration to be considered to be a creative process. In a sense, any creativity that would exist in either of those processes would be with respect to the novel techniques used in that process. And, of course, novelty being relative, the issue becomes one of the lack of usualness of the techniques being employed. This seems like an odd measure of creativity. Or is it? Perhaps creativity means no more than the application of a technique or rule where one would not expect to apply it. Perhaps creativity is, in that sense, purely a relative term.

Scripts and other knowledge structures (Schank & Abelson, 1977) are useful for placing events that are not obviously causally related into preestablished causal chains. The advantage of using such structures is that one does not have to compute everything as if it had been seen for the first time. Understanding relies on our ability to take shortcuts by assuming that what we have just seen is not that different from something with which we were already familiar. All we need do, in many cases, is to say "Yes, A is just like B; so I shall proceed as if it were B." Not all understanding is script-based, of course, but planning mechanisms also exhibit this reliance on past experiences that have been codified and fossilized.

The same is true of explanation. A great many of our explanations rely on explanations that we have previously used. People are inherently lazy in this way, and this laziness is of great advantage, as we shall see. Much of the point behind my earlier work on memory (Schank, 1982) was to show how people use past experiences to help them interpret new experiences. Reminding is one of the key methods by which this is accomplished. Seeing A as an instance of B is helpful in making generalizations and thus in learning about both A and B. The fact that generalizations often are inaccurate does not stop us from making them, nor does it lessen their value.

In explanation, a similar phenomenon occurs. We rely on XPs to create new explanations from old explanations. This makes the process of explanation easier, but susceptible to certain kinds of mistakes. It also makes creativity possible.

Explanation patterns

An XP is a fossilized explanation. It functions in much the same way as a script. When it is activated, it connects an unexplained current event with an explanation that has been used at some time in the past to explain an event similar to the current event.

An XP is a standard, stereotyped answer, with an explanation, to a question. After having received an answer in general terms (the XP) one can begin to try to alter that answer so as to make it relate to the particulars at hand. Thus, the algorithm is as follows: Take a particular question, and generalize from it in order to find a general question under which is indexed a general answer. Then take the general answer and particularize it to find the specific answer to the original particular question.

Finding additional patterns

The key to inventing creative explanations lies in intelligently indexing XPs. One way to explain something unusual is by reference to something different for which there exists an explanation. So one way to find a candidate set of XPs is to change the event that is to be explained into one that is like the original event but sufficiently different that it might bring up a new idea that is relevant. In this way we have the possibility of finding additional XPs that are not connected to the indices at hand but might be relevant. Thus, for example, we might know of an XP that relates to cars or elephants. We might want to test it to see if it might relate to a horse as well. Therefore, we attempt to change the event that needs to be explained into another event that we can explain.

XPs often have a trite and boring form, like that for clichés or proverbs. Normally, such frozen patterns might bear little relation to any creative process. But taken out of context, they often can shed light on new domains of inquiry. That is the philosophy behind the intentional misapplication of XPs. When one applies patterns where they do not obviously belong, interesting things can result. Creativity, then, can result from applying old explanations in places where those explanations were never intended to apply.

Creating new from old

The most interesting applications of XPs, ironically, are not their intended uses. XPs are fossilized reasoning. They represent our intention not to think very profoundly about a subject. When we use an XP in its intended role, we are deciding to forgo complex reasoning of our own in favor of using a well-established reasoning chain that has been useful before. Essentially, the normal use of an XP is of the following form:

1. Identify an event sequence needing explanation.
2. Establish indices that are likely to lead to an XP.
3. Find a relevant XP.
4. Apply the XP to the event sequence.

This is the normal situation, but what is most interesting about XPs is their abnormal use. That is, it is in the misapplication of an XP that possibilities for creativity arise. "Misapplication" is somewhat of a misnomer here, because that misapplication often is quite intentional.

A look at some XPs

Before we can get into the details of how to misapply a pattern correctly, we must specify exactly what an XP looks like. In general, one would expect that any XP would have been used quite frequently by an understanding system in the normal course of processing various commonplace events.

The intent of explanation can be either additive or explaining-away. The additive explanation process has as its goal the addition of a new explanation to one's repertoire of explanations, in other words, to learn something new. The explaining-away explanation process has as its goal to eliminate a confusing situation from consideration by reducing it to a situation that has already been explained. When an uncommon event is being processed, and no applicable knowledge structure is found, an XP is sought. In the additive explanation process, this XP is then a candidate for adaptation, from which a new explanation will result. When explaining away, the XP that is found is assumed to be sufficient to account for the current anomaly.

Let us consider what information must be represented in an XP by examining the normal functioning of an XP. First, there must be indices to be used in calling up an XP. Second, there must be relevance conditions for verification of the applicability of an XP. Because creative explanation involves "tweaking" an XP that we do not believe to be precisely relevant, we also need to have some information about the potential usefulness of tweaking a given XP that does not apply directly. For this, we need to know some key features, features whose presence will indicate that it is worthwhile to tweak the XP. To make this assessment, we need to know the belief-support relationships between the parts of the packaged explanation. That is, when we are dealing with a situation that is not quite what the XP explains, we must know which parts of the XP's explanation are inviolate and which can be modified.

The next part of an XP is the set of episodes for which it has previously been used. As we have seen when considering reminding, explanations revolve around the expectation failures they explain; so particular episodes are stored under an XP. These episodes indicate where the XP has been previously applied. Finally, we should be able to apply the knowledge from an XP when we are planning, as well as when we are correcting failures. This is done by storing a stereotyped summary of the explained situation in the XP. This summary tends not to be stated in the language of expectation failures or explanations; instead, it is often a proverb or rule of thumb. Thus, the parts of XPs must include the following:

> Indices
> Relevance conditions
> The explanation chain
> Belief-support relations
> Prior episodes explained by the XP
> A stereotyped description of the XP

Thus, an explanation pattern might have the following parts:

1. An anomaly that the pattern explains (which is the main index into the XP)
2. A set of relevant indices under which it can be retrieved
3. A set of states of the world under which the pattern is likely to be a valid explanation
4. A set of states of the world under which the pattern is likely to be relevant, even if it is not immediately applicable
5. A pattern of actions, with the relationships between them, showing how the event being explained could arise
6. A set of prior explanations that have been made possible by use of this pattern
7. A reason that stereotypes the behavior being explained

As an example, consider a classic XP: *killed for the insurance money*. This pattern is useful when it is necessary to explain why someone was killed. If the person who is dead is "worth more money" dead than alive, then it is not uncommon for an understander to assume that the person may have been killed for the insurance money. The pattern is as follows:

1. An anomaly that the pattern explains: *untimely death*
2. A set of relevant indices under which it can be retrieved: *untimely death; death heavily insured*
3. A set of states of the world under which the pattern is likely to be a valid explanation: *one of the conditions from 2, and one of the conditions from 4*
4. A set of states of the world under which the pattern is likely to be relevant, even if it is not immediately applicable: *deceased was rich; relatives did not love him; beneficiary is suspicious character*
5. A pattern of actions, with the relationships between them, showing how the event being explained could arise: *beneficiary dislikes policyholder; dislike makes beneficiary want to harm policyholder; beneficiary has goal to get a lot of money; inheriting is a plan for getting inheritance; insurance means that inheritance will*

include a lot of money; inheriting requires that the policyholder die; beneficiary kills the insured to harm him and to get money
   6. A set of prior explanations that have been made possible by use of this pattern: *deaths seen in movies; Mafia killings*
   7. A reason that stereotypes the behavior being explained: *a good way to get rich and simultaneously get rid of the disliked policyholder*

This XP is what we can call a *culturally shared pattern*. That is, we would expect that many people might have such a pattern and that talking about that pattern would not require a great deal of explanation in itself. In other words, it is like a restaurant in the sense that one need not think much about it in order to operate with it.

Another type of XP might be called an *idiosyncratic pattern*. These patterns are quite prevalent in human reasoning processes, and thus it is rather important to study them and to employ them in any explanation system. Idiosyncratic patterns are often ill-formed in that they may not constitute a coherent or rational explanation. Examples of such patterns must come from real live individuals; so here are two, one gathered while I was politicking against the Vietnam War, and one gathered from a friend:

When I was collecting voters for an antiwar candidate, one of the people I contacted began to argue with me about the war. He said that the reason that I was against the war was that I was a coward and was just trying to avoid fighting in it. I argued my point of view, but he just ended up saying: "I fought in World War II when I was your age, and now it is your turn to fight in your war."
A friend of mine told me his views on how to "pick up" women. He claimed that it was absurd to even try to pick up a woman who was under the age of 28. He had a complex series of reasons for this, most having to do with the shaky reasoning abilities of young people, but in the end it became clear to me that he simply had not had any success with women under the age of 28.

There are two XPs here. The first: This generation should fight a war because past ones did. The second: Older men cannot pick up women under 28 because the women are too immature to appreciate them. Now, clearly, both of these patterns are irrational. Nevertheless, they are in use by at least two real people. Let us take a look at how the second one looks in the format given earlier for XPs:

   1. An anomaly that the pattern explains: *failures with younger women*
   2. A set of relevant indices under which it can be retrieved: *chance meetings; failures with women; singles bars; loneliness*
   3. A set of states of the world under which the pattern is likely to be a valid explanation: *the man is successful with older women; he fails with younger women*
   4. A set of states of the world under which the pattern is likely to be relevant, even if it is not immediately applicable: *problems with relationships; questions of maturity*
   5. A pattern of actions, with the relationships between them, showing how the event being explained could arise: *woman has chance meeting with man; quick meeting means she has to evaluate him immediately; she is not experienced enough to see his good qualities immediately; bad impression means she does not want to continue with him*
   6. A set of prior explanations that have been made possible by use of this pattern: *all past failures with younger women*

7. A reason that stereotypes the behavior being explained: *younger women expect too much from a new relationship*

A key point is that the summary need not be a rational conclusion from the conditions, nor is there any reason that the XP has to have the correct explanation of the situation. It is also important to note that in the pattern of actions, the relationship between steps that we are representing is belief-support, not deduction. In most people's picture of the world, there is seldom an absolute causal link between a supporting fact and what it supports; it may be necessary to accumulate a lot of independent evidence for a condition before we believe it. For example, in the killed-for-the-insurance-money XP, either the desire of the beneficiary to hurt the policyholder or his desire to inherit money is support for his killing the policyholder, and for some people, either would be sufficient motivation for murder. We would not normally believe that either alone would result in a murder, whereas the two together are fairly convincing evidence.

Even when a pattern is idiosyncratic and ill-formed, it is useful for reasoning. That much is obvious, because people do use such rules to explain the behavior for which the rules were concocted. The question with respect to XPs, however, is whether or not and how those patterns can be applied to situations other than those for which they were originally intended. The issue for creativity in the use of XPs is how to misapply them.

The issue in misapplication must be embodied in the notion of a partial match. It is all well and good to establish that someone has been killed and that he had a large estate that is to go to his evil son-in-law, and thus to suspect his son-in-law. Such a suspicion comes from matching the pattern "killed for the insurance money," and there is really no more to say about such a match other than such patterns must exist in memory in order for such matches to occur. But the really interesting case is when "killed for the insurance money" is used to explain a set of circumstances that are superficially quite different from those of son-in-law, rich man killed, and so on.

There are at least three important issues to explore about XPs:

1. What culturally shared XPs exist in memory?
2. How are these patterns accessed for normal application?
3. How are these patterns accessed such that they can be misapplied to generate novel or creative explanations for events that have no obviously applicable pattern?

The relevance of culturally shared patterns and idiosyncratic patterns for creativity comes in their adaptation to novel situations. The next question is how this adaptation takes place. We call this process "tweaking" and shall now explore how it might function.

There are two separable processes in the creative misapplication of an XP. The first is finding a candidate XP for consideration. The second is altering the constraints of that XP so that it applies to the current problem. Each of these processes requires its own kind of creativity.

The creativity inherent in proposed explanations depends critically on the questions on which the search is based. The novelty of the search process depends on the novelty of the question asked. Could there be a standard set of questions that, when asked, might cause creative thoughts to occur? Does applying a standard set of questions and thus obtaining a set of new answers constitute creativity? Where is the creativity in that process?

The explanation process begins by taking a standard set of questions, which can be seen as specifying a standard set of search techniques, and attempting to determine which of these questions make sense, given the issue at hand. Some questions may be found to be silly or irrelevant, and others may be found to be quite useful. It is not particularly creative to take a standard list of questions and apply them. It also is not creative to decide that certain questions are silly or irrelevant. It may be creative to perceive that a given question that on the surface seems irrelevant ought to be considered. That could lead to an unusual reminding and the potential for a creative analogy.

The issue here, it should be clear, is a kind of intentional reminding. When we are faced with the problem of explaining something, and no existing XP provides an obvious explanation, the adaptation of another, superficially unsuitable XP to the current situation is attempted. The first step is to find a reasonable XP to modify. The next step is to try to adapt the XP to fit the current situation without violating its belief-support relations. During the process of adaptation, it may be found that alternative XPs will suggest themselves as more suited to the adaptation. Adaptation of XPs found by intentional reminding is controlled by a set of tweaking heuristics. This suggests that creativity depends on two primary factors, namely, a set of methods for getting reminded, and a set of methods for adapting remindings in such a way as to fit the new situation. Plus, one must also have a creative attitude. This attitude manifests itself in the ability to keep alive obviously errant remindings or obviously irrelevant XPs long enough to see if they can be made more useful.

If this is true, what does it tell us about computers and their possible creativity? The creative attitude is easy. All we need do is be willing to compute a great deal. Of course, we might do nothing else; so some heuristics for knowing when to abandon a hypothesis might be nice. Thus, we are left with the notion that creativity in a computer means supplying the computer with three types of heuristics, namely:

Creativity heuristics
1. Heuristics for the intentional reminding of XPs
2. Heuristics for the adaptation of old patterns to the current situation
3. Heuristics for knowing when to keep alive seemingly useless hypotheses

The understanding cycle

The critical issue in learning and creativity is expressed by what I call the *understanding cycle*. The understanding cycle starts with a failure to understand. This is followed by a question about why that failure occurred, followed by an explanation of the failure. This is followed by a question about the generality of the explanation that was found, which in turn is followed by a reminding of a similar type of failure. The end result is a new generalization, a new fact, that has been learned. This is how creativity flows from failure. The cycle of understanding is simple enough:

> We fail.
> We wonder why.
> We find an explanation.
> We get reminded of similar situations in which we found similar explanations.
> We wonder if this new reminding ought to be considered as presenting us with a new generalization.
> We make the new generalization and add it to memory, thus creating another prediction that possibly can fail.

Constructing explanations is the essence of creativity, because explanations are, in essence, predictions about how things will happen. They are the start of a kind of mental scientific method that gathers data and draws conclusions, albeit unconsciously most of the time.

What is the difference between this kind of creativity and the kind we usually find more impressive? Often this difference manifests itself in the belief that some domains of inquiry are prone to creativity, whereas others are not. Nothing could be further from the truth. Creativity is simply coming up with an idea one did not have before one started to think. The ultimate novelty of that idea is solely a question of how creative everyone else has been about the original subject. Individual creativity is absolute. If one thinks it up on one's own, it is creative. Creativity within a society is relative to whether or not what one thought up on one's own has been thought up by others as well.

The goal of explanation: generalization

All efforts at explanation should, and inevitably do, tend toward the goal of generalization. World events and human behavior are highly complex, which is why creating explanations and theories is such a challenge. This complexity means that much of the work of explaining will have to involve generalizations. We do not simply seek to know why a given person does what he does (although we settle for that if it is the best we can do); we also want to create a generalized explanation or hypothesis that will hold true in similar cases or situations. We try to make rules of thumb for the outcomes of events, especially events involving human motivation, in such a way as to create rules that will hold in circumstances other than the particular situations we have encountered.

How explanation starts

Before we try to explain something, we have to determine what needs explaining. We need to realize that something is wrong, or that something does not work the way we think it should. We need to recognize failure and anomaly. When we have an expectation failure, the attempt to explain that expectation failure usually will bring to mind other expectation failures with similar explanations.

The explanation process is an inherently creative process that tends to correct itself, unless, of course, a person inhibits or turns off the other parts of the expectation failure–question–explanation–reminding–question–generalization cycle.

But what is it that we must explain? It seems obvious that we try to explain what we do not understand. But there is a sense in which most of the time we understand very little. We do not have complete models of the people with whom we interact. We do not have a fully developed model of the physical world from which we can always make accurate physical predictions. We most definitely have only incomplete models of how and why the social institutions that control our lives behave the way they do. It seems fairly obvious that we do not attempt to explain everything that we do not understand, nor should we.

Explanation begins with failure

In order to learn, we must fail and then explain why we or our previous explanations have failed. We tend to look for an explanation when we do not understand something. When do we not understand something? When our expectations fail, or when our previous explanations fail.

The most important part of the creative process is the ability to notice that something is wrong, that somewhere our expectations are not being met. Creativity and learning derive from the need to correct failures and understand anomalies in the world. We can create solutions, correct failures, and explain anomalies only by identifying where we have been wrong.

Learning thus requires *expectation failure,* followed by explanation. A curious or anomalous situation may require that we reevaluate a tremendous number of expectations, rules, theories, and beliefs that relate to the situation. People are constantly questioning themselves and each other to find out why someone has taken a certain action and what the consequences of that action are likely to be. In order to find out how we learn, we must find out how we know that we *need* to learn. How do we discover anomalies? How do we know that something does not work?

Critical in the understanding cycle is the ability to ask questions. Once an anomaly has been found, posing the right question about that anomaly can lead to finding an interesting answer. A question such as "Why did that anomaly happen?" may not be very useful. Thus, in the clever posing of questions, we may find clever answers.

The idea, then, is that to make computers creative, we must equip them with the ability to detect anomaly, to formulate the right questions about an anomaly, to accumulate and utilize a large store of XPs, and to find them when needed in order to apply them to a situation for which no standard explanation is known.

Solving Terrorism

One way to see how the whole process works is to try to solve an inherently difficult or unsolved problem, by computer. Of course, we have not yet fitted a machine with all the heuristics necessary for creativity; so we shall first do this as a *thought experiment*. Consider the problem of international terrorism. If a person came up with a novel solution to this problem, we would consider that person creative indeed. Could we get a machine to suggest solutions? Of course, I am going to suggest that we can, by supplying that machine with a great many XPs, with the heuristics to find reasonable candidates to adapt to the current situation, with the heuristics to do the adaptation, with the ability to recognize a viable solution, and with the patience to try. Of these, the ability to recognize viability is probably the most difficult, because it depends on a more or less complete world model. Nevertheless, recognition of viability is not something one ordinarily considers to be all that creative.

The first step in creative explanation is to find the thing that needs to be explained, of course. Here we shall attempt to explain why the terrorists are fighting and how it can be stopped.

In order to attempt to answer this question, we must begin the process of *question transformation*. That process takes in a question such as ours and transforms it into one or more questions for which XPs are known to exist. The claim here is that this process of question transformation can be taught – to people or to a computer. The premise is that there exists a standard set of *explanation questions* (EQs) that are asked whenever an anomaly is found. We have determined that the following set of EQs is quite useful:

EQ1: What caused an unexpected event?
EQ1.1: How will an unexpected event benefit others?
EQ2: What factors caused this event and can they happen again?
EQ3: What were the underlying causes of this bad event?
EQ4: How did the victim enable this bad event?
EQ5: What did the victim do wrong in this bad event?
EQ6: What circumstances led to this event?
EQ7: Why did this institution act this way?
EQ8: What are the policies of this institution?
EQ9: What are the goals of this institution?
EQ10: What plans was this institution carrying out?
EQ11: What did this institution decide was most important?
EQ12: What will this institution do next?
EQ13: What caused the actor to behave this way?
EQ14: Is the actor a member of any group that is known to use this anomalous behavior?
EQ15: Why would the group that the actor is a member of use this anomalous behavior?
EQ16: What makes this particular group behave differently from other groups?
EQ17: How does this behavior fit in with a group of behaviors?
EQ18: What plans does this group have?
EQ19: Why does this group have the goals that it does?
EQ20: What counterplan was the actor performing?
EQ21: What previous behavioral change led to this event?

EQ22: How is this action typical for this actor?
EQ23: How is this event a typical counterplan applied to this actor?
EQ24: How is this apparently ineffective plan in reality a good plan for some unseen goal?

After bringing these questions to mind, the next task is to attempt to adapt these questions to the current situation, eliminating those that are irrelevant:

EQ1: too general
EQ1.1: How does terrorism benefit people?
EQ2: What motivates the terrorists?
EQ3: What is the reasoning of the terrorists?
EQ4: How do the victims get into the situation in the first place?
EQ5: Do the victims make an error of some kind?
EQ6: What events tend to precede terrorist acts?
EQ7: What are the motives of the institutions that back terrorism?
EQ8: What are the policies of those institutions?
EQ9: What are the goals of those institutions?
EQ10: What plans are those institutions carrying out?
EQ11: What did this institution decide was most important?
EQ12: What will this institution do next?
EQ13: redundant
EQ14: What other groups behave in a similar manner?
EQ15: Why do such groups behave that way?
EQ16: What makes this particular group behave differently from other groups?
EQ17: because we are considering a group of behaviors, this is irrelevant
EQ18: What general plans do groups that the actors belong to have?
EQ19: Why does this group have the goals that it does?
EQ20: What event is terrorism trying to prevent?
EQ21: Why is there so much terrorism now?
EQ22: irrelevant
EQ23: irrelevant
EQ24: Does terrorism support some goal that is not obvious?

The next step is to find the XPs indexed under the foregoing EQs. Of course, some of these will yield fairly standard explanations that we have all learned for explaining terrorism. Because what we are interested in here is creative explanation, we must focus on the EQs that have no XP indexed directly under them, or that ask a question that is unusual enough that one would have to think about it some. Looking at the list in this way yields

EQ1.1: How does terrorism benefit people?
EQ4: How do the victims get into the situation in the first place?
EQ5: Do the victims make an error of some kind?
EQ6: What events tend to precede terrorist acts?
EQ14: What other groups behave in a similar manner?
EQ15: Why do such groups behave that way?
EQ16: What makes this particular group behave differently from other groups?
EQ18: What general plans do groups that the actors belong to have?
EQ20: What event is terrorism trying to prevent?
EQ21: Why is there so much terrorism now?
EQ24: Does terrorism support some goal that is not obvious?

Now let us consider what XPs are indexed under these EQs or what XPs might be brought to mind by transforming these EQs slightly. We shall look at each question in turn, indicating some XPs that might be relevant:

EQ1.1: How does terrorism benefit people?
    war brings plunder; revenge brings happiness; recognition brings importance
EQ4: How do the victims get into the situation in the first place?
    vacations bring risk; travel brings risk; homesickness causes disturbed behavior; change upsets routine
EQ5: Do the victims make an error of some kind?
    bullies pick on cowards; people who are into symbols pick victims who are symbolic
EQ6: What events tend to precede terrorist acts?
    full moon arouses werewolves; revenge
EQ14: What other groups behave in a similar manner?
    nations at war; marital disputes; professional infighting; office politics; children's disputes; revolutionaries
EQ15: Why do such groups behave that way?
    jealousy; inability to share; dominance problems; arrested development; general unhappiness
EQ16: What makes this particular group behave differently from other groups?
    poverty; lack of control of own lives; political oppression; pawns in the games of others; religious differences; true-believer mentality
EQ18: What general plans do groups that the actors belong to have?
    Moslems, kill infidels; Lebanese, fix country; young people, let off steam; young people, be idealistic
EQ20: What event is terrorism trying to prevent?
    violence disturbs status quo; violence brings repression, which brings revolution; fanaticism disrupts boredom
EQ21: Why is there so much terrorism now?
    new breeding grounds; frustration over lost wars; loss of power of Arab block because of oil price drops; new fanatics gain power; religious resurgence in Moslem world
EQ24: Does terrorism support some goal that is not obvious?
    somebody gets rich through terrorism; someone gets power through terrorism

The foregoing XPs all came to mind as I thought about the situation. Obviously, a great deal of the creative process is hidden in the ability to think up XPs at the right time. One method for doing this is to try to see the original issue as if it were something else. For example, in the preceding, by considering irrelevant features that precede events that are dastardly, the idea of full moons and werewolves occurred to me. Such silly ideas are the stuff of which creative explanations are made, of course.

However, my intention here is twofold. I am interested in the creative process in people and in how that process might be applied to machines. Thus, to make machines creative, we shall have to do careful work on the heuristics by which one comes up with candidate XPs, as I have said. Until that complete set of heuristics is gathered, there are other alternatives. For example, simply by seeing terrorism as a member of a class of actions, one can begin to come up with XPs in a fairly standard way. Therefore, let us consider this list again, but this time in a different way.

This time, I have chosen a list of proverbs that have been classified under various major and minor headings. Below are the original EQs again, this time followed by the major and minor headings and the proverbs that correspond to the EQs, the proverbs being those that I found to be relevant from *The Penguin Dictionary of Proverbs*. Not all the EQs had proverbs that were relevant, of course. Here again, one can see that the trick is in the indexing. In this case, the proverbs in this book were classified under headings that forced me to decide whether or not they were relevant to the case at hand. In other words, here again, I had to decide what ideas best related to the issue of terrorism seen from any possible perspective.

EQ1.1: How does terrorism benefit people?
    Adversity value: He that is down need fear no fall.
                        Adversity is the touchstone of virtue.
    Adversity effects: Adversity makes a man wise, not rich.
EQ2: What motivates the terrorists?
    Badness sources: Covetousness is the root of all evil.
                        No mischief but that a woman or a priest is at the bottom of it.
                        When the weasel and the cat make a marriage, it is a very bad presage.
    Crime sources: Poverty is the mother of crime.
                        He that is suffered more than is fitting will do more than is lawful.
EQ7: What are the motives of the institutions that back terrorism?
    Troublemaking: Pouring oil on the fire is not the way to prevent it.
    Peace: The stick is the surest peacemaker.
    Hypocrisy: If you want to see black-hearted people, look among those who never miss their prayers.
EQ8: What are the policies of those institutions?
    Asking effects: Ask and it shall be given to you.
                        He that demands, misses not, unless his demands be foolish.
    Authority advantages: Better to rule than be ruled by the rout.
                        It is better to be the hammer than the anvil.
    War tactics: Cities are taken by the ears.
EQ9: What are the goals of those institutions?
    Corruption religious: No penny, no paternoster.
    Corruption causes: He who squeezes in between the onion and its peel picks up the stink.
                        Keep not ill men company lest you increase their number.
                        Fish begin to stink at the head.
EQ10: What plans are those institutions carrying out?
    Fear power: Fear is stronger than love.
                        There is no remedy for fear but cut off the head.
    Enemies: For a flying enemy make a golden bridge.
EQ11: What did this institution decide was most important?
    Believing value: Faith will move mountains.
    Believing doubt: The more one knows, the less one believes.
    Deeds value: 'Tis action makes the hero.
    Deeds intention: The good intention excuses the bad action.
EQ12: What will this institution do next?
    Danger effects: You may play with the bull until you get his horn in your eye.
                        Danger makes men devout.
EQ14: What other groups behave in a similar manner?

Crime: Show me a liar and I will show thee a thief.
Cowardice: Some have been thought brave because they were afraid to run
                away.

Having been reminded of these proverbs, by whatever method, the issue is
whether or not they can be adapted to be of use in understanding terrorism and
perhaps finding a solution for it. In other words, can one make use of these proverbs
in such a way as to create a new idea from them? The claim is, of course, that one
can, in the following way. Consider the following proverbs taken from the preceding list:

EQ1.1: Adversity makes a man wise, not rich.
EQ2:   Covetousness is the root of all evil.
        No mischief but that a woman or a priest is at the bottom of it.
        He that is suffered more than is fitting will do more than is lawful.
EQ7:   Pouring oil on the fire is not the way to prevent it.
EQ8:   It is better to be the hammer than the anvil.
        Cities are taken by the ears.
EQ9:   No penny, no paternoster.
        He who squeezes in between the onion and its peel picks up the stink.
        Fish begin to stink at the head.
EQ11:   The more one knows, the less one believes.
        'Tis action makes the hero.
EQ12:   You may play with the bull until you get his horn in your eye.
        Danger makes men devout.
EQ14:   Some have been thought brave because they were afraid to run away.

The foregoing proverbs constitute an explanation for a number of things, and
within them lies a suggestion of what to do to fix the situations to which they refer.
Here, then, is where the second part of the creative process comes in. After finding
an XP (and proverbs are very standard and usual XPs), one begins to adapt it. This
may require using it solely as a vehicle for finding other, more relevant XPs. In
other words, an XP is, in one of its most important roles within the process of
creative explanation, a source of indices to remindings or to other XPs. That having
been said, let us look at each of these proverbs to see what they suggest:

From EQ1.1 we found "Adversity makes a man wise, not rich." This was a
reference to the effects on the victims of terrorist acts. Thus, one can come up with
the idea that people who suffer from terrorism become wiser because of it, but
although this may well be true, it is rather useless as is. However, suppose that we
reverse the problem here. One of the goals of explanation is to find rules of the
world that seem to work so as to be able to adapt them to one's own circumstances.
We use the following tweaking rule:

*If a rule applies in a given situation, try reversing its actors and objects and see
what happens.*

We come up with the idea that perhaps if the terrorists should suffer more adversity,
they would get wiser. This brings to mind the idea, using the XP "Divine retribu-
tion," of hijacking or kidnapping some of them for a change.

Using the first XP derived from EQ2, "Covetousness is the root of all evil," we get the simple idea that the reason the terrorists do what they do is because they want something, money and power being two prime things that people tend to want. As we said, one of the prime purposes of the search for XPs is to find appropriate indices to other XPs. In this case, because we are looking for plans of action, those, too, can come to mind. Thus, two plans come to mind here, connected to covetousness, namely, give them what they want, and convince them they cannot have what they want. Thus, we now have the idea of giving a large grant to the PLO, in exchange for an agreement to stop terrorism, or, alternatively, giving Israel nuclear weapons to use in retaliation for terrorist attacks.

The next proverb, "No mischief but that a woman or a priest is at the bottom of it," is of interest because it brings up two rather unusual new indices. We use another tweaking rule:

Whenever there is a character in an XP, try changing the character to a different one within the same set, in order to find a reminding or relevant rule.

We can begin to think of mothers, teachers, and so on, and for priests, we can think about any member of the clergy. This latter attempt to think of a Moslem clergyman might bring up Ayattolah Khomeini, giving us the idea that killing Khomeini would end the terrorism.

This next one, "He that is suffered more than is fitting will do more than is lawful," is simply a realistic explanation. If taken as a call to action, one gets the idea to attempt to eliminate the suffering. From there it is any easy step to come up with the standard solution of a Palestinian state. From there, we use yet another tweaking rule:

Rather than the obvious object, change the obvious into another object that also satisfies the rule.

We can come up with many reasons why they may be suffering: poor housing, lack of sanitary conditions, and so forth. Any one of those will produce some suggestions; for example, perhaps we should build a luxury housing development for them to end their suffering.

From "Pouring oil on the fire is not the way to prevent it," we get the idea that it is the intention of the leaders of the terrorists to incite trouble. Now we need a reason why they would want a constant state of trouble. This is actually quite close to the heart of the matter in reality, and many XPs come to mind, including an XP from the 1960s that I recall, namely, social unrest brings revolution. There is another old standard here: little man benefits from war between two big men. These are not creative explanations, of course, just realistic ones.

Next, we have two attempts to explain the theory under which terrorists operate: the first, "It is better to be the hammer than the anvil," giving a philosophy for downtrodden people, and the second, "Cities are taken by the ears," giving the operating philosophy that underlies propaganda warfare. Again, suggested solutions are to get to the heart of these issues. In the first, one might think of ways to make the Palestinians more proud of their own positive achievements. In the second, one might decide to fight a war of words in Lebanon, using stronger methods than are now used. This latter, which one might call the 1984 XP, is often used as the excuse for creating a totalitarian state.

Those in the next set all deal with who is behind it all. The first, "No penny, no paternoster," suggests that the clergy are behind it all and that they can be paid off in money. The second, "He who squeezes in between the onion and its peel picks up the stink," suggests that the people surrounding the terrorists are so corrupt that one must get them first. Here that might mean Syria, Khaddafi, or the PLO leaders. The third, "Fish begin to stink at the head," implies that the leaders are to blame.

The next, "The more one knows, the less one believes," suggests that the problem with the terrorists is primarily that they are "true believers" and that there is a standard remedy for that, namely, education. So perhaps we should open a free university for them, or else give them all scholarships to U.S. colleges.

" 'Tis action makes the hero" suggests that the terrorists need to be heroes. Thus, one solution would be to give them another opportunity to be heroes. Using the XP that "Opportunity makes heroes," we must provide the opportunity. Perhaps we should start a war in which they can fight and be heroes. Or, on the other hand, using the proverb indexed under EQ14, "Some have been thought brave because they were afraid to run away," we have the suggestion that the terrorists really would like to run away. Perhaps we should launch a rescue operation to liberate them from their leaders.

Finally, we have two rather realistic commentaries on it all. The first, "You may play with the bull until you get his horn in your eye," suggests that it will all go away of its own accord, and the second, "Danger makes men devout," suggests that there is no way to prevent religious fanaticism as long as people feel themselves to be in danger.

Conclusion

In order for people or computers to be creative, they must have many XPs available to them. These will come in two ways: Some will be fed to them directly (something most people are quite willing to do for other people, as parents, teachers, or friends); others they will learn as new XPs through creative misapplication.

If we are interested in creativity by computer, we might go about making an exhaustive list of the XPs with which a creative computer can function. Creativity by machine demands exhaustive data, experiences that can be adapted and used to explain other experiences.

What exactly have we done here? We have looked at a few of the possible types of XPs that might exist. Naturally, there are thousands, maybe even hundreds of thousands, of XPs in existence. (Here, I am not talking about proverbs exactly. I used proverbs here because they can be found in books, and because my own idiosyncratic XPs would need a fair amount of explanation, and explaining my own personal view of the world is hardly the point.) XPs have, as their primary role, the intention of rendering comprehensible what is initially incomprehensible. They have also, as a secondary role, the capacity to be brought to mind somewhat inappropriately, in such a way as to serve as fodder from which creative explanations can be made. The XPs given here are universal in the sense that they are to be found as wisdom from books; so they are not quite expressive of what XPs are really like. Nevertheless, they are useful for illustrative purposes.

Of course, the intent here was not to produce a method by which types of XPs could be generated. One would expect to find XPs that relate to each combination of categories presented, but the fact that that is the case is besides the point. People, by and large, do not generate very many XPs for themselves. On occasion, they see many examples of the same phenomena and find that an explanation will work over and over again, thus creating an XP. Average people use XPs they have been told or taught or have read about somewhere.

I mention this because although it is perfectly fine to go after the problem of finding out how we can create XPs, there is a much more serious problem to be attacked first. Our computers are not yet at the level of the average person, by any means; so it makes little sense to have them attempt to create their own XPs. That having been said, why, then, have we focused on issues of creativity here?

Essentially, the two problems are inextricably tied together. One cannot understand without applying XPs, and one cannot explain something new without misapplying an XP to some extent. Thus, my point is that creativity, in the sense of explaining new phenomena by intentional misapplication of an XP, is not as sophisticated a phenomenon as one might think. Rather, it is easier than the intentional invention of an explanation, starting from scratch. Thus, one method of explanation, the application of an XP, is so much easier than the other, the invention of a new XP, that it is clear which should be studied first and clear which is the first subject to worry about with respect to AI. Now, as it happens, during the normal use of XPs, they are necessarily misapplied and thus create new XPs. This is not the same thing as attempting to create a new explanation from scratch. My claim is that it is the method that people use for explanation and creativity, and thus it ought to be the method that machines use.

To come up with new ideas, start with old ideas. This is straightforward enough and seems hardly worth remarking. However, as I noted earlier, one rarely uses the word ''creativity'' in the same phrase in which one uses ''computers.'' My point is rather simple. Creativity is not such a mysterious process. It depends on having a stock set of explanations and some heuristics for finding them at the right time and for tweaking them after they have been found. These last two steps should not be denigrated with respect to their complexity. Search processes and adaptation of patterns are two of the biggest problems facing AI. I have not attempted to talk about either of them much, because any attempt to do so, in a work on something else, would be rather superficial. They are major problems in their own right.

However, they are not problems of creativity. At least they do not seem so on the surface. We do not think of search and adaptation of old patterns to new situations as being very creative. Surely there is nothing mystical about those processes. Surely creativity lies elsewhere. But, I do not believe that to be the case.

Creative solutions and creative explanations can be found mechanically. Creativity is not mystical. It lies within the provinces of search and adaptation and is heavily dependent on reminding. It should be possible to design mechanisms whose output is creative. Creative machines are possible, in principle. This ought not trouble any humanist. Rather, any further understanding of humans, including demystification, ought to be welcome.

References

Dreyfuss, H. (1979). *What computers can't do: A critique of artificial reason.* New York: Harper & Row.

Schank, R. C., & Abelson, R. (1977). *Scripts, plans, goals and understanding.* Hillsdale, NJ: Lawrence Erlbaum.

Schank, R. C. (1982). *Dynamic memory: A theory of learning in computers and people.* Cambridge University Press.

Searle, J. (1980). Minds, brains and programs. *Behavioral and Brain Sciences, 3,* 417–424.

Part III

The role of the individual–environment interaction in creativity

The study of creative lives

10 Inching our way up Mount Olympus: the evolving-systems approach to creative thinking

Howard E. Gruber and Sara N. Davis

Karl Duncker began his classic monograph "On Problem-Solving" (1945) with this remark: "To study productive thinking where it is most conspicuous in great achievements is certainly a temptation, and without a doubt, important information about the genesis of productive thought could be found in biographical material. But although a thunderstorm is the most striking example of electrical discharge, its laws are better investigated in little sparks within the laboratory."

The familiar metaphor likening the creative moment to a bolt of lightning deserves scrutiny. Taken right, it is apt not only for the mystification of magical moments but also for the demystification of the creative process.

A bolt of lightning is by no means a unitary event. It has inner structure and temporal development. There is a period of preparation in which electrical charge is built up; the charge is not a "trait" of the thundercloud, but a relationship between cloud and ground below, or between cloud and cloud (i.e., a difference in electrical potential). The buildup of potential difference involves a positive feedback mechanism in which myriad collisions of ice pellets or water drops produce the charge; these earlier events, though of low intensity, prepare the way for intensification later on.

In one type of flash, a downward stroke proceeds in branching steps from cloud to ground; when this "stepped leader" comes near the ground, "an upward discharge jumps from the target object to meet it" (Orville, 1977). This upward stroke is the brilliant event that we normally see as lightning – the result of all that preceded it. Usually there are three to four strokes within a flash (sometimes many more) that can be detected not by the naked eye but by high-speed photography. The aftermath of lightning, thunder, comes a little later, involves quite different processes, and lasts much longer.

Not only is the individual lightning stroke complex, it is part of a more complex system – the thunderstorm as a whole. And each storm is part of a still wider worldwide system of storms – a few thousand going on at any given time – thus maintaining a state of dynamic equilibrium, the approximately constant negative charge at the earth's surface.

There is in Duncker's use of the creativity–lightning metaphor a double irony: first, because Max Wertheimer, who was Duncker's mentor, in his classic *Produc-*

tive Thinking (1959/1945) made ample use of historical case materials (Galileo, Gauss, Einstein); second, because Duncker's own work was primarily an exemplary exercise in careful qualitative analysis of problem-solving protocols. Neither Duncker nor Wertheimer made systematic experimental laboratory attempts to manipulate the conditions of creativity or to "measure" the creativity of the solutions arrived at by their subjects.[1]

In our constructionist, evolving systems approach, the creativity–lightning metaphor holds good so long as it is understood correctly. Insights, like lightning strokes, represent not a break with the past but the steady functioning of the creative system at work. By the same token, emphasis is withdrawn from the supposed single great stroke of insight and transposed to the many moments of insight that occur in the course of a creative effort. Elsewhere, Gruber (1981b) has estimated that as many as one or two noteworthy insights per day (or 500 per year, coming to 5,000 in a project taking 10 years) may be characteristic of highly creative people. Moreover, each moment of insight has its own internal structure, its affective and cognitive microgenesis. The fact that it is a process in time means that the creative person has some measure of control over it; as it develops, one can welcome or reject it, shape and steer it. Finally, sudden moments of sharp insight must take their place within the complex, evolving system that is the creative person at work.

Aims

This chapter has three aims. First, we want to describe and illustrate our use of the case study method in the study of creative thinking. Second, we want to present a brief version of the evolving-systems approach to creative thinking as it has been elaborated thus far. Third, we want to discuss some of the major difficulties of the case study method and some next steps to be taken in developing the evolving-systems approach.

We have chosen to take up the case studies first and to sketch the evolving-systems approach at the end of the essay. This reflects the actual course of events, as this approach grew out of the case studies (Gruber, 1981a). But it may help the reader if we make certain points clear at the outset.

Although we emphasize the fact that almost all creative products result from long periods of purposeful work, we do not deny the role of chance events and spontaneous play. We do insist that such occurrences must be incorporated into ongoing enterprises under the control of the creative person.

It would be foolish to deny the role of greatly cultivated skills as part of the creative process. But in our competence-oriented profession, working within a "can do" society, it is all too easy to overemphasize skill. For example, Henri Poincaré probably was Einstein's nearest rival in steps toward the theory of relativity. Einstein was a competent mathematician, but Poincaré was superb. What the latter lacked was the right sense of direction. To take a second example, this one from the arts, the notable forgers of history – individuals whose forgeries have found their way into the great museums of the world – obviously have had skills equal to or even surpassing those of the artists they have copied. Unfortunately, their exercise of these skills has not been mobilized for creative work, but for copying.

This is why we insist that the central problem for the study of creative work is to understand how one organizes and reconstructs a life to form a system of knowledge, purpose, and affect that can do creative work. Of course, this is not one problem, but many, and the name we have given them is the evolving-systems approach to creative work.

The case study method

Our cognitive case studies of creative work, to be reported here, treat the materials of the life histories of our subjects as problem-solving protocols of long duration, requiring probing hermeneutical interpretation in order to reconstruct the events we hope to understand. We have long insisted on three fundamental propositions:

1. Each creative person is a unique configuration.
2. The most challenging task of creativity research is to invent means of describing and explaining each unique configuration.
3. A theory of creativity that chooses to look only at common features of creative people probably is missing the main point of each life and evading the main responsibility of research on creativity.

Nevertheless, there are two sorts of commonality to be considered. First, even investigators interested in the understanding of uniqueness may use similar strategies in their inquiries. Indeed, it is in some degree necessary to do so in order to arrive at the conclusion of uniqueness. Second, even unique creative individuals may share some important characteristics with other unique creative people. Or, perhaps better put, different episodes of creative processes may resemble each other in some interesting respects. These commonalities may be important as the context within which the unique processes appear.

One of the main aims of this chapter is to describe a set of case studies that illustrate a common strategy that for want of a better term we may call the "cognitive case study method." The process of description (i.e., writing this chapter) will, we hope, make more explicit the strategies entailed in the practice of a psychological craft that we have been developing for some 30 years.

We focus on a group of nine doctoral dissertations completed between 1962 and 1985 under Gruber's direction. We omit dissertations now in progress on Erasmus Darwin, Freud, Shaw, Van Gogh, and Piaget. As preparation for writing this chapter, Davis interviewed the authors of seven of the nine dissertations on which we draw.

We have had to face one difficulty that is both methodological and pedagogical. A single teacher cannot have expert knowledge of each of the diverse cases described herein. Accordingly, on each advisory committee someone was included who did have the necessary expertise; we might better say *some* of the necessary expertise, because no one investigator fully knows a case. Probably the best-studied case in the history of science is that of Charles Darwin, partly because of the wealth of documentation he left, and partly because of the general interest of his work for so many different disciplines. It has taken a small army to get as far as we have in Darwin scholarship. And it may well be that the most important work is yet to be done.

This brings up a second methodological-pedagogical point. When this long project began, we used to speak bravely of studying "the cognitive economy as a whole." But it is evident that this is an abstract ideal, not to be forgotten, but honored in the breach. Each case study must choose a few foci and commit many painful omissions. A "few" foci should always mean more than one, for it is in the *interplay* of different aspects of the case that it comes alive.

The case study method in relation to other methods

The merit of the case study method lies in its ability to consider a large number of issues together and in their relationships. The question may well be put: Why not apply the highly developed methods of multivariate analysis? There are four principal reasons. First, we are concerned with process rather than traits. Second, multivariate techniques, with their reliance on measurement, assume that it is appropriate and possible to measure the relevant population on the relevant traits, which seems utterly implausible to us, for reasons given later. Third, we place great emphasis on the need to understand creative people at work in their own contexts; the emphasis on measurement decontextualizes what is being studied. Fourth, the need for large numbers of subjects forces the use of inappropriate populations, such as U.S. Coast Guard trainees or unselected high school students. Although these are certainly valuable and interesting human beings, usually we can have no guarantee that the sample taken includes a single person who is functioning creatively. Better to start with widely agreed-upon cases.

In the study of creative work, each case can be distinguished from the others on some variable for which it makes absolutely no sense to measure the others, and in fact no provision for such a measure could ever be envisaged until that case comes under scrutiny. As the poet Blake wrote in *The Marriage of Heaven and Hell*, "One Law for the Lion and Ox is Oppression." More important, what really counts in each creative life is the *pattern* in which knowledge, purpose, and affect are organized, as well as the fit of the pattern to a set of tasks that do not preexist but are constructed by the creative individual in the course of the work.

For example, when young Darwin set out on the voyage of the *Beagle,* he enjoyed an ample and unprofessional vagueness in his goals (Darwin, 1934). Young Huxley, on the other hand, setting out on the voyage of the *Rattlesnake,* was crisp, professional, and brilliant (Huxley, 1935). Any awards committee would have chosen Huxley for the fellowship and put Darwin on the waiting list – and never would have known enough to regret the choice. We cannot conclude from this that initial vagueness is somehow always better than initial precision, or the reverse. But the two stories can alert us to the relation between early goals and later achievement; understanding how that works out in a given case is a task for the student of the case.

Huxley's brilliance and precision stood him in good stead. His career was brilliant and creative. When in 1858 he finally heard of Darwin's theory, he exclaimed, "How stupid not to have thought of that!" He then became an effective proponent of Darwin's ideas. Although he explained it beautifully and insisted on its plausibility, he never quite espoused the theory of evolution through natural selection, and this fact helps, perhaps, to explain why he did not invent it. He was penetrating enough to see the unsolved problems in the theory – but so was Darwin. Huxley was probably too committed to an early form of positivism (he wrote a biography of Hume) to be comfortable with a theory that was such a web of long-range inferences. This tough-mindedness was a good quality for Huxley and served him well. Although it was Darwin who had the greater impact, we cannot say that Huxley would have been better off to have been more like Darwin.

There have, of course, been numerous attempts to study aspects of the creative process in the experimental laboratory. We refer to our own attempts to do so as "quasi-experimental," and this for two reasons. First, our primary methodological commitment is to the case study method, and we wish to avoid getting so drawn into any particular experimental program as to forget our goal of understanding the person as a whole and in context. Second, the source of the problems taken up in this way is not some ongoing paradigm of experimental research, shared by a number of investigators, but the requirements thrust upon us by the case. The very fact that we are studying an unusual case and trying to understand it as a whole sometimes draws attention to neglected issues that are suitable for experimental or other narrow-beam approaches. By taking up such issues experimentally, we hope both to illuminate the case and to contribute to a wider field.

One example of this kind is Gruber's study of the process of synthesis of different points of view. In his studies of Darwin, Gruber has been quite struck by the point that the same panorama of species looked quite different from different points of view (Darwin, 1859). For example, the Galapagos Archipelago flora and fauna change their aspects if one examines them in their relation to South American species (the nearest continent) or if one examines them only in their island-to-island relationships. In a striking passage, Darwin describes his own puzzlement over such matters. The passage (Darwin, 1859, p. 50) begins, "When a young naturalist" – obviously himself – and goes on to explain the initially paradoxical observations that occur as one moves from place to place, naturalizing, and how the paradoxes of taxonomy can be resolved by altering one's point of view and by making use of the expert knowledge of others with different points of view. This has become, in Gruber's laboratory, a study of the cooperative synthesis of points of view, using quite different materials from those studied by Darwin, but always with an eye cocked for understanding the problems of synthesis (Gruber, 1985; Gruber & Sehl, 1984).

Davis (1985) wished to study the way in which the meaning of a story evolves as one reader encounters the story repeatedly. As part of her method, Davis wanted to use an interruption method in which the reader is stopped from time to time and asked about various issues concerning character, plot, setting, and symbolic meaning. But it was important to know if, or how, the interruption method affected the reader's responses to the story. Davis explored this issue in a subsidiary experiment with other subjects, thus demonstrating the feasibility of the approach.

The case study method as we have practiced it is quite distinct from psycho-analytically oriented psychobiography. Such studies have emphasized the underlying motives of the creative person, their childhood origins, and their neurotic character. Our focus of attention has been on *how* creative people do their work, rather than on *why*, and on the developmental process within the career, rather than on that leading up to it. We are far from denying the importance of unconscious processes. We nevertheless see them as occurring in a person struggling and often succeeding in taking command of them to make them serve the interests of consciously and freely chosen enterprises. By the same token, we take seriously the consciously held systems of belief and intentionality of the creative person. This, in turn, requires us to take a phenomenological stance in reconstructing subjects' experiences from their own points of view. In these matters, our position resembles that of Rothenberg (1979). These methodological questions have been discussed at length by Wallace (1985).

Case studies of creative work as doctoral dissertations

Are case studies of the creative process good subjects for doctoral dissertations? A number of difficulties immediately appear. Training in psychology or other social sciences does not prepare the investigator for this kind of work; for example, the hermeneutical skills of interpretation are remarkably absent from courses in research methods. Each case requires immersion in a highly specialized subject matter, and this takes considerable time. Problems of this kind can be solved if the student is willing to make the necessary investment; it is important that the supervisor not understate the difficulties. At least one question remains unanswered: How can we make "real science" out of studies of unique individuals?

Admittedly, the diversity of cases and treatments poses a problem, but it also presents an opportunity. Consider a certain cartoon in the *New Yorker*. In the first four panels we see a naked man standing on some flotsam in a wide ocean, slowly fitting together the pieces of flotsam in the sea around him like a jigsaw puzzle. Thus he constructs the little island that will have to serve as his terra firma. Then comes dawn, and he discovers all around him an ocean full of other naked figures, all doing the same thing.

We can take this cartoon as emblematic of the diversity of our cases and of their relative isolation from each other. Or we can take it as standing for the next task: fitting the islands together.

To explore these and kindred questions, we have chosen to describe several dissertations, all completed under Gruber's direction. We hope to show that at least a start has been made at solving these problems, and that it is worth the effort. The discussion is organized under three main headings: basic commitments and organizing schemes, the role of metaphors in creative work, and the interactions of creative individuals with their worlds.

Benjamin Franklin's scientific work

Donald Hovey's dissertation was completed in 1962 at the University of Colorado. It then seemed quite daring to introduce data from the history of science into a dissertation done in an experimental psychology program, and so a compromise was agreed on by Hovey and the faculty involved. The case study would be combined with experimental studies of problem solving related to the case. Accordingly, the thesis bore the hybrid title "Experience and Insight: Experiments on Problem-Solving and a Case Study of Scientific Thinking."

Hovey had been struck by some interesting similarities in the way that Benjamin Franklin solved several widely disparate scientific problems. In addition, Hovey was skeptical of the impression given by Franklin's autobiography (1874) and by later biographers that Franklin's interest in the science of electricity had been provoked by a single, rather late encounter that had led quickly, within 4 to 6 months, to his momentous discoveries concerning electricity. From his discerning reading of the documentary evidence, including some material newly available from the work of Cohen (1956) and Labaree (1959), Hovey drew up the following picture:

1. Franklin applied the same schemata in solving disparate problems. It was already well known that when water begins to flow in a canal, the water at the lower end must move first, making way for the water behind it, and so on. This results in the counterintuitive fact that the elapsed time before onset of flow at successive points increases as one moves upstream (i.e., in the direction opposite to that of the flow itself). Franklin applied this model to the time of onset for a storm seeming to move from north to south (wind comes out of the north, storm begins earlier in the south). He also applied it to a more speculative hypothesis on the circulation of electrified "particles of air" in producing the aurora borealis. Franklin's work on the storm-movement problem was set off by an unusual coincidence of a storm and an eclipse of the moon; the careful timing of the eclipse in various places, together with coincidental observations of the advent of the storm, gave rise to the anomalous data that Franklin's model could explain.

Perhaps one should add that Franklin's immersion in problems of air circulation had earlier played a part in his invention of the Franklin stove.

2. Hovey gave a version of the fluid-movement problem to experimental sub-

jects. They were given prior guided experience with the water-in-canal problem, leading to successful solutions. Nevertheless, they were not able to solve the storm-movement problem. Of course, this corresponds to the historical facts, because it required a person like Franklin to take the same step in history. From this, Hovey concluded that having the necessary components for solving a problem does not automatically lead to a solution. Here he was explicitly siding with Maier (1940) in an ongoing debate. He also drew on Birch's (1945) revision of Köhler's work on chimpanzees: Birch showed that even in innovative and insightful problem solving, the apes required a background of experience with the materials involved.

3. Hovey took the next step of examining the hypothesis that Franklin must have had a long-standing commitment to certain scientific ideas. This would at once explain his originality in solving the storm-movement problem and his apparent speed of work after he began his electrical inquiries.

4. The conceptual structure of Franklin's theory of electricity includes the following schema:

    a. Atomism
    b. Conservation
    c. Equilibrium
    d. Circulation
    e. Heat and electricity regarded as material elements
    f. Highly static view of microstructure of atmosphere
    g. Reliance on principles of attraction and repulsion

5. At least some of these ideas, notably *conservation* and *equilibrium,* could be found in Franklin's earlier thinking about these matters. In his pamphlet "A Dissertation on Liberty, Necessity, Pleasure and Pain," Franklin concluded:

1. A Creature when endu'd with Life or Consciousness, is made capable of Uneasiness or Pain. 2. This Pain produces Desire to be freed from it, in exact proportion to itself. 3. The Accomplishment of this Desire produces an equal pleasure. 4. Pleasure is consequently equal to Pain. (Hovey, 1962, p. 76, citing Labaree, 1959)

This was written in 1724 when Franklin was 18 years old. It bears some remarkable formal similarities to Franklin's analysis, over 20 years later, of the Leyden jar.

6. Hovey supplemented this historically based study with some experimental work on general aspects of problem solving. He used materials similar to those used by Maier and Duncker. He made a careful analysis and introduced experimental control of the models available to the subjects, and drew the following conclusions:

The nature of the problem solution is in part determined by the availability of cognitive models to the individual. . . . The initial solution tendencies in a problem are the result of the interaction between the model initiating the problem and the situation characteristics. Whether a solution tendency persists to become the problem solution is dependent upon the degree of functional similarity between the initial solution tendency and subsequently appearing aspects of the problem situation. Problem-solving behavior in these experiments is not a response to objective stimuli within the situation, nor is it the reflection of dominant response tendencies brought into the situation. Instead, the behavior is coordinated to functional relationships arising jointly from the situation and from the individual's models. (Hovey, 1962, pp. iii–iv)

It should be added that Gruber and Gruber (1962) had pointed out that Darwin, too, had applied the same schemata repeatedly. In one striking instance during the *Beagle* voyage in 1834, Darwin had developed a theoretical model of the formation of coral reefs. His theory of evolution through natural selection bears a strong point-for-point resemblance to the coral reef theory. Yet when Darwin became committed to the search for a theory of evolution, his first moves by no means exhibited this formal structure. It seems that even well-developed and well-mastered models and schemata are not automatically applied to new problems.

The thought form of gradualism in Charles Darwin's life work

In writing *Darwin on Man,* Gruber (1981) focused more on the changing structures of belief systems, or of theoretical models, than on the issue of recurrent themes. During the same period, however, Holton's interesting work *Thematic Origins of Modern Science* (1973) appeared. Also, in Ferrara's work (1984) on "networks of enterprise" we found that it is difficult if not impossible to give a good account of the organization of purpose in the form of the person's manifold projects and enterprises without taking into account themes that cut across these boundaries. These developments, together with our group's general concern for ensembles of metaphors and other figures of thought, set the stage for Keegan's efforts.

In a number of areas there has been a persistent search for units of analysis appropriate for description of the organization of knowledge and beliefs. In developmental psychology, in problem-solving research, in work in artificial intelligence, and in research on expert systems, various approaches have been explored. These can be divided into two main categories: the specific and the general. Among the specific kind are schemata, scripts, and plans. Abelson (1981, p. 715) writes that "one simple form of scheme is the script embodying knowledge of stereotyped event sequences."

Among the general kind are to be found principles, structures, themes, and Keegan's candidate, *thought-forms*. As Keegan describes the idea of a thought-form, it is closely related to Holton's effort (1973) to search out the basic themes of modern science, except that "the thought-form can be viewed as the incarnation of a theme *within* an individual" (Keegan, 1985, p. 29).

In order to see one thought-form adequately, it is necessary to situate it in its intellectual context and examine how it functions in the work of the thinker. In his dissertation, "The Development of Charles Darwin's Thinking on Psychology" (Keegan, 1985), Keegan set out to understand Darwin's thought-form of gradualism by means of the following steps:

1. He traced the recurrences of Darwin's use of the thought-form in a variety of contexts.
2. He examined one of Darwin's enterprises in some detail, with particular attention to the thought-form of gradualism. With an intentional allusion to Freud's life, Keegan called this enterprise "Darwin's Project for a Scientific Psychology." Keegan studied Darwin's effort to construct a science of psychology as it evolved over a period of five decades.

Table 10.1. *Varieties of gradual change*

Phenomenon	Cause	Appearance
Earthquake	Migration of fluid magma	Stepwise
Terraces at Coquimbo	Denudation by sea action	Stepwise
"Roads" of Glen Roy	Denudation by sea action	Stepwise
Coral reef formation	Deposition of calcareous material	Insensibly gradual
Formation of vegetable mold	Deposition of excreta	Insensibly gradual

3. He divided Darwin's life into five major periods and examined the recurrences of the thought-form of gradualism within each.
4. He examined the thought-form of gradualism in relation to other important thought-forms.
5. He compared the psychology enterprise to Darwin's other enterprises.
6. He transcribed and analyzed the full text of Darwin's "baby diary," with special attention to its place in Darwin's psychology enterprise and its relevance to the thought-form of gradualism.

Keegan discussed two variants of the gradualism thought-form: stepwise change and change by "insensible" (i.e., infinitesimal) amounts. For Darwin, as long as the steps were small enough, both kinds of change qualified as gradual. This way of thinking inevitably calls into play the idea of *scale,* because a large step on one time scale may be small on another. Earthquakes are good examples of this point, and Darwin had experienced an impressive one in Chile, during the voyage of the *Beagle.* An earthquake that changes the level of the ground by 2 feet is an enormous event from the point of view of momentary human affairs, but on the geological time scale it may be an almost imperceptible part of a process of elevation lasting millions of years, Darwin argued.

Outside the field of psychology, of course, the thought-form of gradualism was widespread in Darwin's thinking (Table 10.1).

Among the other thought-forms Keegan discusses as part of Darwin's thinking are evolutionism, or progressionism, and materialism. For a full development of all of these it was necessary for Darwin to assume that a scientific psychology was possible, and to make that assumption was tantamount to setting to work on its elaboration.

When Darwin began his theoretical efforts (first in geology), his earliest and always his primary commitment was to gradualism, not to any specific mechanism of change, not even to his favorite, natural selection. This point helps to make psychological sense out of some of Darwin's apparent waverings. Rather than switching allegiances from one belief system to another, he was moving around within a hierarchically organized system of beliefs and intellectual commitments.

In *Darwin on Man* (1981), Gruber's main emphasis was on the reconstruction of a series of changes in a belief system: Darwin's successive attempts to construct a workable theory of evolution. As compared with this emphasis, Keegan's special

Table 10.2. *Time scale and perception*

Event	Human perception	Geological effect
Earthquake	Vivid and significant	Trivial
Gradual denudation	Imperceptible	Highly significant

contribution is to examine one mechanism at work in the process of theory construction, the recurrent application of a particular thought-form.

Within Darwin's epistemological framework, this reiteration had two merits. On the one hand, it led to the solution of particular problems, as illustrated in Table 10.1. On the other hand, by solving diverse problems *in the same way,* it helped to establish general laws and to lend credibility to a coherent view of natural change, summed up in Darwin's thinking in the phrase "nature makes no jumps" (Table 10.2).

Keegan traces the development of the thought-form of gradualism in Darwin's thinking during the voyage of the *Beagle* and its application to the evolution of mind, especially in the few years following the voyage. To say that Darwin's own thinking changed "gradually" is not to imply that the change came easily, without painful struggle. In 1838, in his second notebook[2] on evolution, Darwin wrote:

This multiplication of little means & bringing the mind to grapple with great effect produced is a most laborious & painful effort of the mind (although this may appear an absurd saying) & will never be conquered by anyone (if has any kind of prejudices) who just takes up & lays down the subject without long meditation. (Darwin manuscript, 1837, cited in Gruber & Barrett, 1974, C-notebook, p. 75)

This passage was written only a few months before Darwin decided to keep a separate notebook dealing with psychological issues and mental evolution. The period of the second notebook can be seen as exhibiting complexities and tensions requiring a new branching in Darwin's network of enterprise, which occurred most explicitly when he began the "M notebook," first of two on man, mind, and materialism. Keegan gives a good account of the branchings within the psychology enterprise as it developed further, which we omit here for reasons of space. He also presents a useful picture of Darwin's enterprises as a whole (Figure 10.1). In so doing, he suggests how the thought-form of gradualism permeated the whole of Darwin's thinking.

It is useful to ask what motivated Darwin to keep his earthworm project going for over 40 years from the publication of his first paper on the geological function of worms (Darwin, 1837/1977) to his final book, amplifying the same subject (Darwin, 1881) and combining it with an account of the behavior, even problem-solving behavior, of earthworms. Keegan proposes that the long-term motivating context of the project was twofold: first, Darwin's interest in the thought-form of gradualism; second, the complex assimilation of the project into Darwin's network of enterprises by linking up the geological and the psychological enterprises through the mediation of the worm.

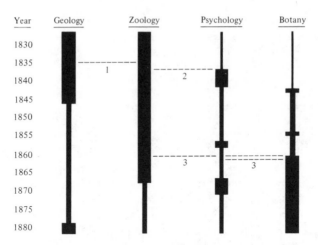

Figure 10.1. Darwin's network of enterprises: 1831–1882. The enterprises are arranged from left to right in the order in which they emerged. The first major connections among enterprises are indicated by dotted horizontal lines. From left to right, the dotted lines stand for (1) the coral reef theory, (2) the M notebook, and (3) the fertilization-of-orchids book. Solid vertical lines indicate the intensity of work during a given period of time. The thickest lines show periods of most active work, moderately thick lines indicate periods of dormancy, and thin lines indicate embryonic periods of the enterprises.

Up to this writing, the network of enterprise has been easier to write about than to diagram perspicuously in all its complexity. Keegan's effort, by painting with a broad brush, gives a useful picture of Darwin's network as a whole. We have yet to find a way of achieving this goal at the same time as we capture the fine structure in its enormous diversity and manifold interconnectedness.

The role of metaphor in creative work[3]

How do metaphors actually function in creative work? Much has been written about the essential nature of structure of metaphor, and sharp lines have been drawn between such ideas as theory-constitutive as opposed to expressive functions of metaphor. In our view, metaphor can serve numerous functions that are not mutually exclusive. The "profile" describing the use of metaphor almost certainly varies from one creative person to another and must also change in different phases of the creative process. This diversity suggests the need for the case study method in order to comprehend the way metaphor actually works in creative processes.

Let us consider some of the possible roles for metaphor. First, metaphor may serve directly as a modality of thought. Just as some thinking goes on directly in visual images and some directly in words, just as Wordsworth seems to have thought directly in iambic pentameter – some thinking can take an immediate metaphoric form. Second, a metaphor may play a synthesizing role, as when it expresses a link between disparate domains. Third, metaphors may play an analytic role, as when a complex idea is broken up into components, each expressed by different metaphors.

Fourth, metaphors may concretize abstract ideas; they may lend palpability to otherwise vague ideas. Fifth, they may illuminate the abstract idea that connects different groups of concrete experiences. Sixth, by highlighting the mismatch between the literal and metaphoric forms of an idea, they may both stimulate the production of new ideas and function as a way of testing a system of beliefs.

Seventh, metaphors may serve a theory-constitutive role, as when they enter directly into the argument being put forth. Eighth, on the other hand, metaphors may play an expressive role, as in cases in which the idea in question has been developed in some other form and is restated metaphorically for purposes of emphasis or communication. Finally, metaphors may play an affective role, as when the evocative power of a metaphor charges an idea with new excitement.

The reader who pauses a moment will have little difficulty extending the foregoing list. It is not intended to be complete, but only to give an initial idea of the complexity and variety of the functions of metaphors in creative work. By now, also, the reader will have recognized that we use the term "metaphor" in a broad sense, much as in *Metaphor and Thought* (Ortony, 1979), where the very distinguished list of authors typically avoided defining the term, or in Leary's ongoing project on metaphors in the history of psychology (D. Leary, personal communication), in which a very catholic idea of the domain of metaphor is made quite explicit.

"Darwin's irregularly branching 'tree of nature' and other images of wide scope" was the title of Gruber's essay in a work on aesthetics in science (Gruber, 1978). A great deal of attention had previously been given to one of Darwin's metaphors: natural selection. We might ask (Young, 1985): Is it a metaphor, properly speaking? In what sense does Nature select? Was Darwin personifying Nature? His other metaphors had been largely neglected.

But Darwin used at least eight major metaphors in developing the theory of evolution through natural selection: tree, tangled bank, wedging, struggle, war, contrivance, and both artificial and natural selection. Overemphasis on the metaphors representing triage in nature – war, struggle, and selection – misrepresents Darwin's thinking. In his theory, it is the interplay between the forces of explosive growth, variation, and enrichment, on one side, and forces of selection, on the other, that produces the evolving panorama of organic nature.

The branching tree diagram appeared in Darwin's thinking in 1837, well before the idea of selection. It evolved into the only diagram in the *Origin of Species* (1859), and it was used to elaborate a number of crucial points in Darwin's complex argument. We do not underline the importance of this one image in order to substitute it for another as Darwin's ruling metaphor. On the contrary, the key point is that Darwin's argument, like any great synthesis, displays a certain organic wholeness, constituted of the assemblage of a number of necessary parts. Among necessary things, one cannot be more necessary than another; so the idea of relative importance loses its meaning.

It might be the case that in a given ensemble of metaphors, one was more original, or another more typical of the author's work, than the others. In Darwin's case, however, the key point is not the reality of his images. His originality lay in the way he assembled them to promote a broad and powerful vision of the evolving natural order.

Darwin's ensemble of metaphors was by no means static. For example, within the family of metaphors representing the diversity of life by branching structures, Darwin tried out a number of different ones as different aspects of his theory became more salient – tree, coral, and seaweed among the more concrete and familiar images – and various more abstract diagrams as well. There is also movement between ideational and imagistic levels, so that each image makes its point, and each point finds its image.

The balance among different images varied from one phase to another of Darwin's life work. His point of departure in biology certainly emphasized the metaphor of "contrivance." This was central to the argument from design propounded by Natural Theologians such as the Reverend William Paley, who had a great influence on the young Darwin. In the *Origin*, the metaphor of contrivance took its place as one in a larger ensemble of metaphors. But in the two decades following publication of the *Origin*, Darwin published his marvelous botanical works, such as *On the Various Contrivances by which British and Foreign Orchids are Fertilized by Insects, and on the Good Effects of Intercrossing* (1862). As the title indicates, neither selection nor branching tree, but rather *contrivance*, moved into the figure role in these works.

Gruber used the term "image of wide scope" where he might just as well have said "important metaphor." An image is " 'wide' when it functions as a schema capable of assimilating to itself a wide range of perceptions, actions, and ideas" (Gruber, 1978). In the present discussion we have used "metaphor" in approximately the same sense. There is probably a place for a special term such as "image of wide scope," distinct from metaphor, to refer to the potential vehicle of a metaphor that has not yet been formulated or to refer to a supple schematization (such as "network") that might enter into a number of metaphors. But in this essay we go no further toward systematizing the variety of figures of thought in creative work.

Ensembles of metaphors in William James's thought

William James both developed and communicated his theories through extended use of metaphors. In his dissertation, Osowski (1986) undertakes a study of the 12-year process (1878–1890) whereby James produced *Principles of Psychology* (1890/1950). He shows the development of James's thought, the questions he was trying to answer, and the role that metaphors played in this process.

Osowski examines the linkages between theoretical ideas and metaphors. He traces the use of metaphors in *Principles* in relation to the emergence of major conceptions in James's theory of mind: continuity, change, unity and identity, selection, and relationships among elements of thought. The development of these concepts was coordinated with the generation of an ensemble of four metaphors: stream of thought, flight and perching of a bird, fringe of felt relations, and herdsman. These major metaphors each embraced subsembles or families, so that several aspects of an idea could be developed through the use of similar but differing images.

The stream-of-thought metaphor was a large and central node around which numerous other metaphors circulated. These satellite images were the following: train, chain, path, current, channel, line, procession, kaleidoscope, and fabric. Through flexible use of these metaphors, James was able to capture concepts of continuity, constant change, direction, connectedness, pace, rhythm, and flow. The stream metaphor allowed James to describe the phenomenology of thought, especially his sense of its fluidity. Complex thoughts could not be built by chaining simple thoughts. James wanted to show that connections in mind are multilinear; the stream, with its branchings and complex flow, could express this idea.

The stream metaphor, however, was not capable of encompassing all of James's ideas. It was necessary to join it with others. In Volume 1 of *Principles*, James linked the stream with both the train and chain metaphors. In Volume 2, another subsemble was more prominent: the stream linked with a path, hydraulic current, and an electric current.

Both the chain and train metaphors helped to clarify the idea of the stream by presenting alternative notions of movement that were antithetical to James's view of fluidity. More positively, they also represented other aspects of mind, such as association and neural functioning, that James wanted to combine with his phenomenological efforts. James also exploited similarities that linked the stream and train: Both move, have their own sources of power, and are able to change pace and direction. He called on the train and chain metaphors to describe a limited linearity in some phases of mental functioning: "There are, then, mechanical conditions on which thought depends, and which, to say the least, determine the order in which is presented the content or material for her comparisons, selections, and decisions" (James, 1890/1950, Vol. 1, p. 553).

Osowski argues that James was unable to find one unifying image to encompass his ideas about both phenomenology and neural functioning. The train, in fact, became two distinct images for James. There was a mechanical or operational train metaphor, used to represent association, and a structural train metaphor, used in contrast to the stream.

Stream, path, and current were used in Volume 2 to explore further the notions of change, continuity, and connection. Both a stream and a path are continuous, but for James what was salient in the path metaphor was its linearity. This helped him deal with the structure of the neurophysiological machinery.

In Volume 1, when James was primarily concerned with phenomenology, the stream metaphor was dominant. In Volume 2, James's concern with neural functioning became more prominent. The path is like the stream in that it remains and may be modified by movement upon or within it. It goes beyond the stream in having a firm structure that can be revisited. This idea of revisitation was important for James because his view of memory and perception entailed reproductive association, and in his neural circuitry model it was necessary to posit a structure that could be modified by repeated use. As James well knew, the Heraclitean flux of the stream conflicts with the requirements of a stable self, and he needed an ensemble of metaphors that could assimilate both.

Current functioned as two distinct metaphors, one denoting the movement of a portion of a larger body of water, the other as the flow of electricity. When the current metaphor was used in the hydraulic sense, James's emphasis was on phenomenology, and he used such terms as "gushing," "swelling," and "bottle up." These water metaphors were particularly evident in the chapters on the will, perception, and emotions – all of which stressed phenomenological over neurophysiological models. For example, in action after deliberation there is a building of tension (as in a dam) and a bursting or flow when the tension becomes too high.

Taken together these metaphors allowed James to expand his explanation of neural mechanisms. The path as an image provided the aspect of a structure that remains after use, yet can be modified through use. The electric current metaphor provided a set of dynamic rules, including notions like excitation and summation. The water current metaphor represented concepts such as tension, blockage, and threshold in both universes of discourse – physiological and phenomenological.

Images of mind in John Locke's thought

Locke's ideas about cognition underwent dramatic change during the course of his work. He began as a nativist, believing that God implants in man necessary knowledge and moral laws. He shifted to sense empiricism, holding that all knowledge arises during the lifetime, from sense perception. He came ultimately to believe in sense experience as a primary and certain way of knowing. In *An Essay Concerning Human Understanding*, begun in 1670 and completed in 1690, he takes the position that men "by the use of their natural faculties, may attain to all the knowledge they have, without the help of any innate impressions" (Locke, 1690/1965).

The development of Locke's theory of cognition was directly influenced by what he perceived to be the causes of men's disregard for one another. As a youth during the English Civil War, he had seen disagreements about the first principles of religious belief and moral conduct shake the foundations of a seemingly stable society. He embarked on an enterprise to search out the foundations of absolute certainty in these things. As he persisted in exploring the problem of certainty and in testing the limits of empirical knowledge, he turned up a wide network of interrelated epistemological and psychological questions. Thus, his transformation from nativist to sense empiricist did not involve only a single change but a slow reorganization of a whole belief system encompassing ideas of cognition, morality, and politics.

Locke relied on a small set of mutually complementary metaphors for knowledge. Some of the more salient ones were as follows: material object, closed space, acquisition, possession, tool or instrument, and wax tablet. This use of metaphor was important because he was able to communicate his ideas in a way that related them to readily recognizable experience. In his writing, Locke made use of his knowledge of commercial, technological, and scientific developments of the time. Was his use of metaphors only communicative, or did they also participate in the actual construction and reconstruction of his thought?

Moore-Russell, in her dissertation, "John Locke on Politics and Cognition: A Case Study of Theoretical Development and Creativity" (1978), asserts that Locke made knowledge objective. In making the idea the object of understanding when the mind thinks, Locke likened knowledge to material objects. The recurrent use of the same metaphorical representations of various aspects of cognition is one of the features of the *Essay* that gives it unity and persuasiveness.

Locke seized on metaphors that occurred to him and examined them for what they could contribute to the problem at hand. For example, the metaphor of the mind as a closed space that contained only its own ideas framed Locke's thinking about the mind and knowledge. It was the metaphor linking ideas and words with objects in motion that permitted him to think about how, given closed minds, apprehension and communication could occur. Each metaphor had a specific role to play in illuminating some aspect of a very broad and complex set of issues. His ensemble of metaphors helped him to think through fundamental questions about human cognition.

Images of gender in Dorothy Richardson's thought

In her dissertation analyzing Richardson's 13-volume novel, *Pilgrimage* (1915–1957/1976), Wallace (1982) shows that Richardson's conceptions of gender were crucial and that they were largely expressed through symbolic language. A group of stable images was used in varying affective climates to express very strong conceptions. Richardson believed that men and women have different natures and that the qualities of their experiences are very different. Her conception of these differences is a major theme in her novel: The image of man centers on the brow (mind) and mouth (body), that of women on a garden. There is a split in men between their minds and bodies; in women there is a different split – between what they really are and what they pretend to be for the sake of men. Women work hard at hiding what they really are; their real selves are secret, beautiful, and connected with nature. Men and women are divided within themselves and from each other. Women are aware of these divisions; men are not. The garden image provides a place where one can experience the joy of existence.

Men are depicted as animals and are seen as dangerous, calculating, secretive, self-important, and deliberately self-segregating. Sentences describing men are full of action verbs like "devour" and "gobble." Through the use of the garden image,

Richardson was able to depict what she considered the live center of women and to demonstrate a basically optimistic view of her inner self.

Wallace examines the complexity of this imagistic structure. Richardson is not always hostile to men. Sometimes she sees them as innocent, unaware, and sad. Although the feelings attributed to men may vary, the structure of the image remains the same. This basic image of men as split between mind and body reappears in different situations.

A reader's use of metaphor

Davis was concerned with how a reader designates and uses symbols in a literary text. Her dissertation centered on one reader's experience in reading two short stories, Bernard Malamud's "The Magic Barrel" (1958) and William Saroyan's "Gaston" (1963). The process of reading could be seen as an interactive, ongoing, reciprocal exchange between text and reader in which the latter actively constructed an interpretation rather than appropriating a preconceived meaning. Metaphors did not exist as such in the text; they became known and designated through the acts of the reader.

Symbols arose for the reader in Davis's study in three different ways. First, certain words and images carried with them direct stimuli to search for their symbolic meanings. The reader described a conscious attempt to generalize from past literary experience. Second, some features of the story gained their symbolic meaning from the textual context supplied by the author, and would not otherwise be seen as symbolic. Third, as she moved through the text, the reader created symbols, often in the form of similes.

Once designated, symbols functioned in different ways in the reader's responses. Some symbols in "The Magic Barrel" were both enduring and stable with regard both to meaning and to symbolic status. These provided a framework against which the reader tested other perceptions and by means of which she organized her ultimate interpretation. They provided an interface between what she read in the text and the ideas with which she approached the text. Other symbols maintained their symbolic status, but their meanings fluctuated. Still other features of the story oscillated between literal and figurative meanings.

Metaphor and the case study method

Our case study work on metaphor brings out certain key ideas. Metaphors do not function in isolation from each other, but in articulated ensembles, each metaphor having its special role in the complex whole constituting the creative work. Each member of an ensemble of metaphors is not so much a sharply defined individual as a family of metaphors, different parts of which become salient at different stages in the development of the work. Members of a family or cluster do approximately the same work, whereas different families play distinct roles in shaping the total configuration of meaning. Both the ensemble of metaphors as a whole and the families of which it is composed evolve through the efforts of the creative person.

It is evident that the development of these ideas about metaphor required the case study method. By using this method, and by focusing on the development of creative works, we have had the advantage of seeing both changes and stability over time and of coordinating the study of metaphor with other developing organizations of knowledge and ideas. What remains to be done is to capture the process of actual generation of metaphors as an individual's thinking progresses.

The interaction between creative person and various worlds

The concept of interaction provides a key to the generation and comprehension of an expressive text. If every literary work has both expressive and communicative elements, how does the manner of expression enter into communication? In analyzing the structures of these works, we can see the ways in which they are organized to communicate the insights and feelings of the writers. How does the reader interact with and transform a text into an understandable form? In the process of creation, the creator necessarily monitors the work as it is being produced, and is necessarily the first audience. Studying the communicative and expressive aspects of creative work together is thus inherent in the evolving-systems approach.

Interaction between reader and text

The Russian filmmaker and theorist Sergei Eisenstein (1947, 1949) discussed artistic communication from the point of view of the creator. He was interested both in the filmmaker's attempt to guide the spectator's response and in the unique contributions of the individual spectator:

In fact, every spectator, in correspondence with his individuality, in his own way and out of his own experience – out of the womb of his fantasy, out of the warp and weft of his associations, all conditioned by the premises of his character, habits and social appurtenances, creates an image in accordance with the representational guidance suggested by the author, leading him to understanding and experience of the author's theme. This is the same image that was planned and created by the author, but this image is at the same time created also by the spectator himself. (1947, p. 33)

The filmmaker, then, organizes the flow of the film in such a way as to present spectators with the content of the film and guide them to recreate the original conception. There is still room for viewers to use their individualities to gain new insights. The work of art can present the viewer with the representations, but it is the viewer who must use them to form an image: A work of art should generate in the spectator the process by which, in life, new images and feelings are built up in human consciousness.

Iser (1974, 1978) discussed the effects on the reader of the basic structural components of a text. For example, the reader's contact with the text extends over time. The reading process, then, involves viewing the text through a perspective continually on the move. One is simultaneously making use of past, present, and future while reading, remembering, and anticipating. Memory requires organizing the material in accordance with the reader's ongoing interpretations. Expectations are generated that are later confirmed, modified, or rejected. The outcome may then have a retroactive effect on what has already been read and interpreted. In addition, the reader is involved in processes of filling gaps and coordinating the different perspectives represented in the text.

Davis devised the "interruption method" to investigate these processes: Texts were divided into sections of several pages. A reader was given each section in turn and asked to read and express all of her responses to the text. Interrupting the reader allowed the experimenter to capture tentative interpretations as they happened rather than retrospectively. The process was repeated in order to examine the effect on the reorganization of the text of having read the whole story and knowing its outcome.

Analysis of the reader's responses gave evidence of a wide range of reactions in which she incorporated diverse ideas into a developing sense of the story. Her responses revealed the breadth of her thinking, how she generated possibilities, and how she coordinated her impressions. Each of the main characters of "The Magic Barrel" was seen in a variety of ways. Statements made by the reader about each of the main characters often contradicted each other. However, the contradictory statements were both developed and, at times, even brought into harmony, so that they embellished each other.

In "Gaston," when the character Gaston, a caterpillar, was introduced, the reader immediately assumed that he would be symbolic and therefore carry more than surface meaning. Thus, while following his part in the flow of events, she was vigilant about any other functions he may have had in the unfolding of the story. He was thus central in her paths toward understanding. He is implicated in the actions of each character, and he also carries major themes and symbolism in the story. This symbolic understanding then serves to enhance a literal construction. Either literal or figurative understandings can serve as the point of departure, and the movement between them nourishes each.

In this way, one can see the spiraling development of meaning. By exploring the possible relationships between Gaston and the other characters, one is symbolically apprised of their situations. By looking at these characters and their responses to Gaston, the reader becomes aware of larger issues and the treatment of helpless beings. Thus, the fluidity extends the meaning.

Life communicated as text

Wallace (1982) studied the development of the writings of Dorothy Richardson, with emphasis on the 13-volume novel *Pilgrimage*. One of the main areas of interest was how the fabric of experience was represented in the texture of the novel. Richardson aimed at writing in a way that life is really experienced – immediately and subjectively. She engaged the reader in the experience, rather than describing it. This she called feminine realism.

The originality of this pioneering example of the stream-of-consciousness genre lay in Richardson's attempt to describe or render the experience from the central character's point of view rather than from an external perspective. This constraint placed certain demands on the writing. For example, it is necessary to depict the passing of time, and with this the developing maturity of the main character. Because the author had chosen not to stand outside her characters' experience, she could not simply tell the reader, from the privileged position of narrator, that time had passed. Instead, she had to convey this through the experience of the main character, Miriam Henderson. Richardson did this in part by her use of sensuous material. She was able to communicate Miriam's increasing maturity by showing that as her experience of the world enlarged, her ways of perceiving and describing it changed.

Because *Pilgrimage* is an autobiographical novel, Wallace could examine the relation between two time frames – that of the novel and that of the real life. Richardson started the novel at the age of 39 and continued it into her seventies. However, the novel covered the ages of 17 to 39 in the life of Miriam. Thus, Richardson had to present states of lesser development from her vantage point of increased maturity. She had to portray a level of thought different from the level she had currently achieved.

Wallace shows how a life itself becomes transformed in the process of turning it into a novel. She describes different levels at which sensuous experience can be viewed: (1) Sense experiences of the external world. The world is full for Miriam because she knows how to ascribe meaning to the things she senses. Sense descriptions are used to convey her responses and impressions. It is important to note that although Richardson is inside Miriam's head in describing the latter's experience, she nevertheless retains authorial control. (2) Sense experience with symbolic implications. Sense experience is symbolized in three different ways: (a) the symbolic meaning is clear to the reader, but not to Miriam; (b) the symbolic meaning is explicitly noted by Miriam and also is clear to the reader; (c) the reasons for the sensations are clear to Miriam, but only gradually become clear to the reader. (3) Sensory experience of fusion with the external world. These are intense occasional experiences in which Miriam reaches another level of awareness and loses her feelings of everyday reality. Richardson was a pioneer in including this kind of experience as a normal occurrence within the framework of the novel. In sum, the complex of sensory experience conveys to the reader much about Miriam: her developing maturity, her sensibility, and her "femaleness."

The process of transforming experience into poetry

Jeffrey (1983), in her study of the writing of the long autobiographical poem *The Prelude* by William Wordsworth, also investigated the transformation of experience into literature. She was interested in the means by which experience is recreated in a text. In a preliminary study, she compared the poem "I wandered lonely as a cloud" (1804) with Dorothy Wordsworth's journal entry describing the precipitating event, and with a poem by Herrick also dealing with the viewing of a field of daffodils. There are two aspects of Wordsworth's poem that distinguish it from these other writings. One is the extended use of poetic phrasing, meter, and tropes or poetic language. The other is the extrapolation of the experience beyond the event – the giving of extended meaning. This involves a pattern of progressive distancing from the raw event. Not only did Wordsworth recount a moving experience, he also showed the mind at work: perceiving, remembering, and imagining. He described the creative mind as imposing its own order and meaning on sensory data.

The growth of the poem about the daffodils illustrates these points. First, there is a series of transformations: from the initial sensuous experience shared by Wordsworth and his sister Dorothy, to her prose recording of the event, and finally to his retransformation into poetic form. Second, the contents of the poem reveal a process of progressive abstraction from the initial sensuous event to a philosophic reflection on imagination and thought.

The Prelude shows Wordsworth's deep interest in psychological questions. Wordsworth described a number of significant memories from childhood, recalling sensory experiences that had special meanings in his mental life.

By reconstructing the order of writing and the pattern and type of revisions in *The Prelude,* Jeffrey concludes that for Wordsworth, writing poetry did not consist of the expression of ideas worked out beforehand, but rather was a process in which new meanings were created and realized. Her findings resemble those of Arnheim (1962, p. 10) in his analysis of Picasso's *Guernica:* "Picasso did not simply deposit in *Guernica* what he had thought about the world; rather did he further his understanding of the world through the making of *Guernica.*"

Jeffrey is particularly concerned with the value and constructive function of repetition (see also Gruber, 1976). She argues that much of the communicative value of the *The Prelude* lies in its repetitive structure. Wordsworth used repetition as a way of deepening and emphasizing the impact of experience. This is essential to the power of the poem. For example, Wordsworth gives 10 examples of nature's formative power over him. This repetition allows the revisiting of a scheme, and represents further investigation, enrichment, and intensification. Through her examination of the poet's worksheets, Jeffrey is able to show how Wordsworth built up this resonating structure of reiteration as the poem evolved over half a century of creative work.

Conclusion: the evolving-systems approach to creative work

Of the many desiderata for a theory of creative work, we have chosen three points for emphasis in this conclusion. First, the distribution of creative work in time; this has clear implications for the motivation and energetics of creative work. Second, the loose coupling of the evolving subsystems of knowledge, purpose, and affect. Third, the need in future efforts to search for and specify nonhomeostatic processes, or "deviation amplifying systems."

Distribution of creative work in time

Perhaps the single most reliable finding in our studies is that creative work takes a long time. With all due apologies to thunderbolts, creative work is not a matter of milliseconds, minutes, or even hours – but of months, years, and decades. The question then arises: What goes on in this time? Why does it take so long?

Once we give up the notion of mysterious gifts disconnected from knowable psychological processes, it seems reasonable that creative work should take a long time. We call it creative because it is difficult and improbable, new and effective. At the same time, we expect the product to receive a favorable reception in at least some quarters. Such a reception, indeed, becomes one of our criteria for judging the work valuable or effective, rather than merely unusual. But in that case, because the creative product met a felt or almost-felt need, it is reasonable to suppose that others were moving in the same direction, and this is what we often find to be so. That is, others are aware, and more than dimly, that some move in that direction is needed. If, in addition, the move or solution were ready at hand, so that any one of a number of qualified workers in the same vineyard might find it, then it would be a general trend, and we would be unlikely to call it "creative." It is this peculiar combination of improbability and fitness that leads people in situations like Huxley's to exclaim, "How stupid not to have thought of that!"

Organization of purpose

The fact that creative work is difficult and therefore spread out over months and years has consequences for the organization of purpose. In order to make grand goals attainable, the creator must invent and pursue subgoals. Delays, tangents, and false starts are almost inevitable. The creative person must therefore have some approach to managing the work so that these inconclusive moves become fruitful and enriching, and at the same time so that a sense of direction is maintained. Without such a sense of direction, the would-be creator may produce a number of fine strokes, but they will not accumulate toward a great work.

Initial sketch

There probably are numerous tools available for helping to maintain such a sense of direction. An important one is the "initial sketch" – the rough draft or early notebook to which the worker can repair from time to time – that serves as a sort of gyroscope for the oeuvre. The notebooks that Darwin kept in 1837–1838 play such a role – also his *Journal of Researches* (1839), the account of the voyage of the *Beagle,* which is full of examples of his style of scientific thought, but withholds any definitive ideas about evolution. Piaget's poem *The Mission of the Idea* (1916/1977) and his novel *Recherche* (1918), both written by the age of 22, before he began work as a psychologist, set out – in a rather romantic form – the major lines he was later to follow persistently throughout his life.

But it is a mistake to identify these early sketches with the later achievement. For Wordsworth there was a series of moves, transforming the brief initial sketch, before he could arrive at his great autobiographical poem *The Prelude.* Although Newton had his annus mirabilis (actually 2 years), it resulted only in initial sketches for achievements that would require the work of the next 15–20 years (Westfall, 1980a, 1980b).

On a different time scale, Arnheim (1962) has shown how Picasso, setting out to make the mural *Guernica,* began with an initial sketch that guided the feverish month of activity that produced the work. But the whole point of Arnheim's analysis is to trace and elucidate the transformations the idea underwent and to understand the artistic and ideological motives that steered these changes.

Closely related to the idea of the initial sketch is Marayuma's (1963) idea of the "initial kick." In a system in the early stages of its formation, and therefore still quite labile, the first few moves can be fateful in determining the pathway that will be followed. The first stroke of the brush transforms the canvas.

Loose coupling of knowledge, purpose, affect, and milieu

In describing the creative person at work, we have found it useful to conceive of the person as a system of three main interacting subsystems: knowledge, purpose, and affect. The fact that they interact is not taken to mean that the state of any one subsystem can be inferred from knowledge of the others. Each has its own independent mode of functioning and its own history. They are only loosely coupled. This provides a prime way for the introduction of some probabilistic aspect into our way of thinking about creative work without being mystified into surrendering the whole to chance. Even if each subsystem were highly deterministic in its mode of operation, which is, of course, not the case, the system as a whole would be nondeterministic because of the partial independence of the subsystems.

To see how these subsystems might work together, let us consider only one hypothetical example. Let us suppose that a creative person at work is baffled by a task, discouraged, and inclined to put it aside. Fortunately, his activity level does not go to zero, because other enterprises are liberated and activated by the very process of stopping work on one project. Fortunately, too, his discouragement and motivational reorganization does not destroy all the knowledge and skill he has acquired relating to the project in question; when his mood shifts or a new opening for further progress on the fallow project presents itself, he does not begin at zero, but takes up more or less where he left off. Serendipitous experiences, such as

Darwin's critical encounter with Malthus's *Essay on Population* (1826), happen to a prepared mind precisely because these organizations of knowledge, purpose, and affect are both enduring and loosely coupled.

All this internal movement takes place within the mind of an individual who is also engaged in rich and complex interactions with his external milieu, both in its social and physical aspects. This milieu is not handed to the person or imposed from without; it is something that the individual plays a part in choosing and constructing. A good example of this is the complex set of relationships among William Wordsworth, Samuel Coleridge, Dorothy Wordsworth, and the world of nature that Wordsworth wrote about so beautifully. William's "I wandered lonely as a cloud" (1804) could not have been written without the celebrated walk in the field of daffodils, or without Dorothy's wonderful notes about the same walk, or without the philosophy of nature that the two poets worked out together – which entailed also Coleridge being steeped in German *Naturphilosophie*.

Nonhomeostatic processes

Let us suppose that creative work is almost invariably organized into a set of tasks and subtasks, with some degree of hierarchical structuring. It is important for the creative person that work be so organized that success along the way does not lead so much to a sense of satisfaction as to a sense of liberation – to do whatever comes next. Westfall (1980b) called his excellent biography of Newton *Never at Rest* to capture just this point. There may be many different configurations of a complex network of enterprise, with its manifold relations with other subsystems in the creative mind, that are capable of generating this consequence that achievement becomes the spur for further achievement. Too much emphasis can be given to the role of extrinsic motivation ("Fame is the spur . . ."). Amabile's book *The Social Psychology of Creativity* (1983) is particularly important in placing the emphasis on intrinsic or task-oriented motivation in creative work. This idea, coupled with attention to the structure of the network of enterprise, is probably what we need in order to understand the seemingly perpetual activity of the creative person.

Besides having an organization of purpose represented by a network of enterprise, there are other conditions that must be satisfied if the creative person is to be kept in goal-directed motion. The most important of these is the perfecting of some heuristics that recognize, preserve, and elaborate embryonic novelties. There probably is an unlimited variety of such "deviation amplifying systems" (Marayuma, 1963) available for the inventing, and any given individual probably can manage only a small number of them – but that may be all that is necessary. This is a subject urgently requiring further research.

One simple example of a deviation amplifying system is the repetition of interesting acts or the revisiting of interesting sites. Variations inevitably occur; the creative person does not suppress them, but builds on them, finds ways of pushing them to their limits. In an earlier study, building on Lewin (1935) and Piaget (1936/1952), who in different ways had written on this subject, Gruber (1976) described "the constructive function of repetition." In the person committed to a line of work, the simple act of constructing a filing system or other mechanism for bringing similar cases together also has the consequence of permitting the deviations to appear and the person to seize on them. When Darwin was having his early love affair with the idea of variation, he came home one day enthralled with the fact that there were, in one London garden, "1,279 varieties of roses!!!"

Notes

1 W. Köhler was Duncker's other mentor. Although his subjects were great apes and not great men, in other respects his methods were similar to those of Duncker and Wertheimer: careful observation and painstaking interpretive reconstruction of pathways taken.
2 Charles Darwin's early notebooks were read in the original manuscript by Howard Gruber in the Cambridge University Library Manuscript Room. They have now been published in various forms, of which the most generally accessible are Gruber (1974/1981) and Gruber and Barrett (1974). In addition, there is a two-volume paperback edition of the same, published by the University of Chicago Press: Barrett (1980) and Gruber (1981).
3 These ideas have also been developed in Gruber (1987), written after the present essay. Jeanne Hersch's essay (1932) on Bergson's imagery studies the relation between Bergson's metaphors and his ideas in a fashion uncannily like our own; we discovered it after the present essay was written. We have searched, without success, for other examples in the psychological literature.

References

Abelson, R. P. (1981). Psychological status of the script concept. *American Psychologist, 36*, 715–729.
Amabile, T. (1983). *The social psychology of creativity.* New York: Springer-Verlag.
Arnheim, R. (1962). *The genesis of a painting: Picasso's Guernica.* Berkeley: University of California Press.
Barrett, P. H. (Ed.). (1980). *Metaphysics, materialism and the evolution of mind: Early writings of Charles Darwin* (with a commentary by H. E. Gruber). University of Chicago Press.
Birch, H. G. (1945). The relation of previous experience to insightful problem-solving. *Journal of Comparative Physiological Psychology, 38*, 367–383.
Burns, C. (1978). *Thinking and the construction of emotion: A case study of the creative thought of Mary Wollstonecraft (1759–1797).* Unpublished dissertation, Rutgers University, Newark, NJ.
Cohen, I. B. (1956). *Franklin and Newton.* Philadelphia: American Philosophical Society.
Darwin, C. (1839). *Journal of researches into the geology and natural history of the various countries visited by H. M. S. Beagle, under the command of Captain FitzRoy R.N. from 1832–1836.* London: Colborn.
Darwin, C. (1859). *On the origin of species.* London: John Murray.
Darwin, C. (1862). *On the various contrivances by which British and foreign orchids are fertilized by insects, and on the good effects of intercrossing.* London: John Murray.
Darwin, C. (1881). *The formation of vegetable mould through the action of worms, with observations on their habits.* London: John Murray.
Darwin, C. (1934). *The Beagle diary* (N. Barlow, Ed.). Cambridge University Press.
Darwin, C. (1977). On the formation of mould. In P. H. Barrett (Ed.), *The collected papers of Charles Darwin* (2 vols.). University of Chicago Press. (Original work published 1837.)
Davis, S. N. (1985). *Constructive acts of a reader: A cognitive case study.* Unpublished dissertation, Rutgers University, Newark, NJ.
Duncker, K. (1945). On problem-solving. *Psychological Monographs, 58*, i–ix, 1–13.

Eisenstein, S. (1947). *Film sense.* New York: Harcourt, Brace & World.

Eisenstein, S. (1949). *Film form.* New York: Harcourt, Brace & World.

Ferrara, N. A. (1984). *Network of enterprise and the individual's organization of purpose.* Unpublished dissertation, Rutgers University, Newark, NJ.

Franklin, B. (1874). *The autobiography of Benjamin Franklin.* (J. Bigelow, Ed.). Oxford University Press.

Gruber, H. E. (1976). Créativité et fonction constructive de la répétition. *Bulletin de psychologie de la Sorbonne: Numéro special pour le 80e anniversaire de Jean Piaget.*

Gruber, H. E. (1978). Darwin's irregularly branching "tree of nature" and other images of wide scope. In J. Wechsler (Ed.), *On aesthetics in science.* Cambridge, MA: MIT Press.

Gruber, H. E. (1981a). *Darwin on man: A psychological study of scientific creativity* (2nd ed.). University of Chicago Press. (Original work published 1974.)

Gruber, H. E. (1981b). On the relation between 'aha experiences' and the construction of ideas. *History of Science, 19,* 41–59.

Gruber, H. E. (1985). From epistemic subject to unique creative person at work. *Archives de Psychologie, 53,* 167–185.

Gruber, H. E. (1987). Ensembles of metaphor in creative scientific thinking. *Cahiers de la Fondation Archives Jean Piaget.*

Gruber, H. E., & Barrett, P. H. (Eds.). (1974). *Darwin's early and unpublished notebooks.* New York: E. P. Dutton. Published in one volume with *Darwin on man;* published separately as *Metaphysics, materialism, and the evolution of mind: Early writings of Charles Darwin,* edited by P. H. Barrett, with commentary by H. E. Gruber (1980), University of Chicago Press.

Gruber, H. E., & Gruber, V. (1962). The eye of reason: Darwin's development during the *Beagle* voyage. *Isis, 53,* 186–200.

Gruber, H. E., & Sehl, I. A. (1984). Transcending relativism: Going beyond the information I am given. In W. Callebaut, S. E. Cozzens, B. P. Lecuyer, A. Rip, and J. B. van Bendegem (Eds.), *George Sarton Centennial.* Ghent, Belgium: Communication and Cognition.

Herrick, R. (1972). "To daffodils." In H. Gardner (Ed.), *Oxford Book of English Verse, 1250–1950.* Oxford University Press.

Hersch, J. (1932). Les images dans l'oeuvre de M. Bergson. *Archives de Psychologie, 23,* 97–130.

Holton, G. (1973). *Thematic origins of modern science. Kepler to Einstein.* Cambridge, MA: Harvard University Press.

Hovey, D. (1962). *Experience and insight: Experiments on problem-solving and a case study of scientific thinking.* Unpublished dissertation, University of Colorado, Boulder.

Huxley, T. H. (1935). *The diary of the voyage of H.M.S. Rattlesnake.* (J. Huxley, Ed.). London: Chatto & Windus.

Iser, W. (1974). *The implied reader.* Baltimore: Johns Hopkins University Press.

Iser, W. (1978). *The act of reading.* Baltimore: Johns Hopkins University Press.

James, W. (1950). *The principles of psychology* (2 vols). New York: Dover. (Original work published 1890.)

Jeffrey, L. (1983). *The thinker as poet: A psychological study of the creative process through an analysis of a poet's worksheets.* Unpublished dissertation, Rutgers University, Newark, NJ.

Keegan, R. T. (1985). *The development of Charles Darwin's thinking on psychology.* Unpublished dissertation, Rutgers University, Newark, NJ.

Kohler, W. (1976). *The mentality of apes* (E. Winter, Trans.). New York: Liveright. (Original work published 1925.)

Labaree, L. W. (Ed.). (1959). *The papers of Benjamin Franklin* (4 vols.). New Haven: Yale University Press.

Lewin, K. (1935). *A dynamic theory of personality.* New York: McGraw-Hill.

Locke, J. (1965). *An essay concerning human understanding* (A. D. Woozley, Ed.). New York: World Publishing. (Original work published 1690.)

Maier, N. R. F. (1940). The behavior mechanisms concerned with problem solving. *Psychological Review, 47,* 43–58.

Malamud, B. (1958). "The magic barrel." In *The magic barrel*. New York: Farrar, Strauss, Cudahy.

Malthus, T. R. (1826). *An essay on the principles of population* (6th ed., 2 vols.). London: John Murray.

Marayuma, M. (1963). The second cybernetics: Deviation-amplifying mutual causal processes. *American Scientist, 51*, 164–179.

Moore-Russell, M. (1978). *John Locke on politics and cognition: A case study of theoretical development and creativity*. Unpublished dissertation, Rutgers University, Newark, NJ.

Ortony, A. (Ed.). (1979). *Metaphor and thought*. Cambridge University Press.

Orville, R. E. (1977). Bolts from the blue. *The Sciences, 86*, 66–73.

Osowski, J. V. (1986). *Metaphor and creativity: A case study of William James*. Unpublished dissertation, Rutgers University, Newark, NJ.

Piaget, J. (1916). *La mission de l'idée*. Lausanne: La Concorde. English translation in H. Gruber and J. J. Voneche (Eds.), *The essential Piaget* (1977). New York: Basic Books.

Piaget, J. (1981). *Recherche*. Lausanne: La Concorde.

Piaget, J. (1952). *The origins of intelligence in children*. New York: Norton. (Original work published 1936.)

Richardson, D. M. (1976). *Pilgrimage* (4 vols.). New York: Popular Library. (Original work published 1915–1957.)

Rothenberg, A. (1979). *The emerging goddess: The creative process in art, science, and other fields*. University of Chicago Press.

Saroyan, W. (1963). "Gaston." In R. Poirier (Ed.), *Prize stories 1963: The O. Henry awards*. New York: Doubleday & Co. (Originally published in *Atlantic Monthly*, February 1962.)

Wallace, D. B. (1982). *The fabric of experience: A psychological study of Dorothy Richardson's "Pilgrimage."* Unpublished dissertation, Rutgers University, Newark, NJ.

Wallace, D. B. (1985). Giftedness and the construction of a creative life. In F. D. Horowitz and M. O'Brien (Eds.), *The gifted and talented: Developmental perspectives* (pp. 361–386). Washington, DC: American Psychological Association.

Wallace, D., & Gruber, H. E. (in press). *Creative people at work*.

Wertheimer, M. (1959). *Productive thinking* (enlarged ed.). New York: Harper & Row. (Original work published 1945.)

Westfall, R. S. (1980a). Newton's marvellous years of discovery and their aftermath: Myth versus manuscript. *Isis, 71*, 109–121.

Westfall, R. S. (1980b). *Never at rest: A biography of Isaac Newton*. Cambridge University Press.

Wordsworth, D. (1974). *Journals of Dorothy Wordsworth* (2nd ed.) (M. Moorman, Ed.). Oxford University Press.

Wordsworth, W. (1979). *The prelude*. In J. Wordsworth, M. H. Abrams, & S. Gill (Eds.), *The prelude, 1799, 1805, 1850*. New York: W. W. Norton & Co.

Young, R. (1985). *Darwin's metaphor. Nature's place in Victorian culture*. Cambridge University Press.

11   Creativity: dreams, insights, and transformations

David Henry Feldman

In February of 1976 I had an experience that was a classic example of insight, with full, blazing impact and dazzling effect. I was even in the shower when it sent me out stark naked to tell the world, or at least a colleague with whom I was then sharing a hotel room. I can still remember that experience in detail, although no doubt it has become somewhat embellished with frequent retelling and reexperiencing. Nonetheless, I would like to use that experience as part of the basis for this essay. With recent emphasis in creativity research on breaking down the process into common elements (Perkins, 1981) or examining it through an information-processing lens (Hofstadter, 1985a, 1985b; Sternberg, 1986), or in terms of persistent lifelong struggles (Gruber, 1981), I think it well to remember that every now and then one of those blinding visions of a new reality actually does occur, and one occurred to me in 1976.

I shall begin by recounting what I saw in the shower, then describe some of the events that led to that moment when things came together so forcefully and dramatically as to nearly knock me off my feet. I shall also summarize what has happened with my insight since it first occurred more than 10 years ago, including a later insight episode. I shall use these personal experiences as a basis for describing certain aspects of creative processes. I make no claim that the way I have gone about it is the only way for creative work to be done, nor do I claim that these particular experiences of insight are of general substantive import. And yes, I am using introspective evidence – that most treacherous source of data. But on the other hand, these are the sources of information about creative processes that I know best, or at least firsthand. Based on my own experience, I am certain that moments of real insight are properly included within the realm of creativity research, even if they are not creativity itself.

I should distinguish at the outset between my own, more holistic work on insight and those efforts to strip insight processes down to their common elements (Perkins,

The support of the Jessie Smith Noyes Foundation, the Andrew W. Mellon Foundation, and the Spencer Foundation is gratefully acknowledged. Also, the members of our research team, the Developmental Science Group, made invaluable contributions: Thanks to Lynn T. Goldsmith, Margaret L. Adams, Martha J. Morelock, and Ronald E. Walton for their help and support.

271

1981; Sternberg, 1986). At least one author, Maria Shrady, has put together a book describing major insight events, appropriately titled *Moments of Insight* (Shrady, 1972), and several others have produced significant works on the subject (e.g., Lonergan, 1957, cited in Shrady, 1972). My own personal favorite is Brewster Ghiselin's inspiring collection of first-person accounts of important aspects of such experiences, including some remarkable insights by notable contributors to the arts, humanities, and sciences (Ghiselin, 1952). Although these volumes may not represent a rigorous scientific literature, they certainly provide grist for the mill and kinship with others who have had moments of deep insight. I can compare my experience with the insights described by others and can look for some patterns that may speak more generally to creative processes; this is what I shall do in the second half of this essay.

An amusement park ride

For at least 3 years before my morning shower in February, I had been having a recurring dream – not every night, but perhaps as often as once a week. The dream consisted simply of an amusement park ride in motion. I was aware after several repetitions of the dream that this image was somehow related to my work, specifically to my efforts to understand development and creativity. I told almost no one about this dream, although I do remember once discussing it with the small group of research assistants I was working with at Yale. It was clear to me that this image was central and intimate and important, and I was embarrassed that I had no idea what it was. Let me try to describe what it looked like. The ride was one of those standard amusement park devices that had a kind of pod in the center, which housed the machinery driving the ride, and a number of struts or spokes emanating from the center to a set of small gondolas that held the riders. The gondolas moved in two planes, both around the central pod and up and down; indeed, the whole thing seemed to be moving and rotating in controlled but complex ways – and because it was a dream, the movements were not always strictly according to the ways in which the parts were connected. I have tried to sketch in Figure 11.1 what the ride looked like.

From time to time the image would change in subtle ways, but the basic parts were always there: central power source, rotating and rising peripheral containers with places for riders in them. Initially, I thought that perhaps the image was a neurophysiological image – something about how the neurons in the brain fire or interconnect – and that I was imaging my own central nervous system working. This left me somewhat dispirited, for I was familiar with enough neurophysiology to know that if this image was indeed neuropsychological, I would be unlikely ever to be able to make sense of it. So I had more or less resigned myself to the presence of this image in my dream life and more or less believed that it probably would be in someone else's lifetime, not mine, that the image would be interpreted.

There was something about this particular image, though, that was different from

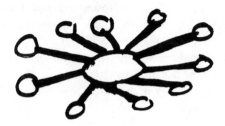

Figure 11.1. The amusement park ride dream image.

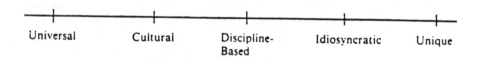

| Universal | Cultural | Discipline-Based | Idiosyncratic | Unique |

Figure 11.2. Developmental regions from universal to unique.

others in my dreams. I came to believe that this image was central to my work and was not about my emotional life, wishes, desires, or what have you – themes that filled many of my other dreams. These other dreams were quite different in how they "felt" to me and in the meaning that I derived from them. I have also had other dreams that were important for other aspects of my work, although none has had the persistent clarity of imagery or the persistent reappearance or has left me with the persistent feeling of importance that the amusement park ride did.

I should mention that my main preoccupation during this period was not with creativity per se. It was definitely on my mind; not long before, I had written a paper on the subject (Feldman, Marrinan, & Hartfeldt, 1972) and also a review (Feldman, 1975), but I did not see creativity research as my central activity. The closest I came to declaring my concern with creativity was shortly before I began having my amusement park dream. I gave a colloquium at Yale in 1973 in which I said that a model of developmental transitions that I was working on would yield some important new insights into creativity (Feldman, 1980). As a matter of fact, about 6 months after making the declaration in public that creativity and developmental transitions were somehow connected (Figure 11.2), I experienced a less dramatic insight than the amusement park ride, an insight that gave me the missing pieces for the "universal-to-unique" model of developmental domains. This model was made possible by my sudden realization (while sitting in a seminar on another topic altogether) that creativity was an extreme version of a stage development shift and could be linked to other such shifts through the conceptual framework for universal and nonuniversal developmental domains that was (I now know) partially completed at the time. By placing creative transformations at one extreme of a continuum and universal transformations at the other end, I was able to construct a

pleasing representation of the range of developmental transitions that I wished to
encompass in my theoretical work.[1] Creativity was thus "discovered" to be a
special case of development in nonuniversal domains. Still, I had no idea that an
image of an amusement park ride would provide me with additional information
about creative processes. The truth of the matter is that 10 years later I am just now
beginning to appreciate that creativity is really what the image was about. But that
gets ahead of the story.

A friendly catalyst

The meaning of the image of the amusement park ride was brought to light through
the catalytic effects of Howard Gruber, who is coincidentally one of the foremost
students of creativity, known particularly for his masterful study of the thinking of
Charles Darwin (Gruber, 1981). Gruber was unaware of the role that he was to play;
in fact, I am not sure to this day that he knows how critical a role he played in this
particular episode of insight. Indeed, there is an irony in the fact that Gruber has
spent much of his career trying to show the relative unimportance of moments of
insight in major works of originality. His research on Darwin, for example, downplays Darwin's so-called Malthusian insight that led to the understanding that natural selection could play a positive as well as a negative role in evolution. Gruber has
shown that this was only one among numerous other insights reported in Darwin's
notebooks and that only in retrospect can it be claimed to be of major importance.
Darwin himself gave no such indication in his notebooks (Gruber, 1981). In my
own case, I know that the particular moment of insight was for me truly momentous
and that it was helped into being by Howard Gruber, a scholar best known as a
skeptic of such moments, an irony appropriate to the topic.

During the fall of 1975, I had been asked to review Gruber's book *Darwin on
Man: A Psychological Study of Scientific Creativity* (Gruber, 1981), and I was so
impressed with it that although I did not know him, I sent him a copy of my review.
Gruber, being the kind of person that he is, called and thanked me for the review
and mentioned that he would be in Boston shortly thereafter to give a lecture. He
invited me to attend the lecture (I had since moved from New Haven to Tufts
University in Medford). I went to his presentation (which was about the imagery
Darwin used in his personal journals), and we met briefly afterward. Because there
was little time to talk, we agreed that it would be worth trying to meet again. As it
happened, Gruber was scheduled to come back to Boston soon.

In the meantime, another colleague and friend, Howard Gardner, was helping the
Social Research Council in New York assemble a committee to review work in the
area of giftedness in children. Gardner wanted both Gruber and me to join him on
that committee. And because the first meeting of the committee was scheduled for
the day after Gruber's next visit to Boston, we made plans to travel together to New
York for the meeting. It was on the air shuttle between Boston and New York that
the critical episode occurred that was to catalyze my insight. It was then that Gruber

described to me his research on "images of wide scope," which had been stimulated by Charles Darwin's "branching tree" diagram – the only illustration in *The Origin of Species* (Gruber, 1981).

Gruber had begun to wonder if this kind of broad metaphorical image was common, particularly among those who had done original work. He was then engaged in an empirical effort to gather as many of these images as he could, and then to study them. He asked me if I was aware of any such images in my own work. For some reason, I felt comfortable enough to tell Gruber that I had been dreaming about the amusement park ride for better than 2 years. I told him also that I knew it somehow had to do with my work, but that I had no idea what its role might be. For the first time, I tried to draw a picture of what the image looked like. Unfortunately, that early drawing was lost. I had no idea that it would be of any particular importance, and I probably threw it away when we left the plane. It was the following morning that I went rushing into his hotel room across the hall and tried to explain what I had just learned in the shower.

The concept of co-incidence

I remember the flash of insight distinctly: What I actually said (out loud, I believe) was, "The ride is not inside, it's outside!" Remember that I had assumed that the carnival contraption was somehow connected with the brain, a neurophysical metaphor. Instead of a mirco model, though, I realized in the shower that it was actually a macro model of the forces that contribute to developmental change. Perhaps I should have known from the outset that my model building would be done at the broadest level, because that is where I am most comfortable theorizing, as my critics well know. But the idea that the image that had preoccupied me for so long would turn out to represent an overarching organizing principle simply did not occur to me. Possibly this was because the ride resembled the way I imagined neuronal activity to occur. In fact, I came to see that there was no physical resemblance between the image and what it actually represents; it is an abstraction representing large-scale dynamic forces and their interrelationships. The image, in short, was one of "wide scope," rather than a reflection of the micro-level processes of the central nervous system.

I later came to label the image and what it represented as the processes of "co-incidence" (Feldman, 1979, 1980, 1986a). I have developed this notion of co-incidence from the original vivid image, and it has come to represent the idea that there are several dimensions of development that must be considered simultaneously if change is to be explained, particularly large-scale or extreme changes (see the chapters by Gardner and Csikszentmihalyi in this volume for complementary views). Development is not solely the result of changes within an individual, catalyzed by transactions with the environment, but is instead the result of a co-inciding of a number of forces – some internal and some external – that set the stage, stimulate, and catalyze change. What I glimpsed in the amusement park ride was a system of great complexity, really a system of systems, that governs the development and expression of human potential. The center, or locus of intersection of the forces, I realized, is the whole individual person, and the surrounding pods represent various other forces contributing to the dynamic developmental calculus.

Co-incidence crystallized for me the idea that people do not master bodies of knowledge solely (or even primarily) because they themselves possess particular abilities, interests, or inclinations. Cognitive development within nonuniversal (and perhaps even universal) developmental domains of knowledge requires the co-inciding and coordinating of a variety of forces and factors that prime, shape, and guide the individual's course of progress. These co-incidence forces include, for instance, the following: the evolving cultural context within the individual; the developmental trajectories of the significant other people who influence the child's development (parents, siblings, relatives, friends, teachers, institutional officials, etc.); the particular set of historical events that bear on that individual; the many disciplines and fields with which the child will come to interact and the developmental histories of these fields; and, finally, long-term evolutionary trends that provide the backdrop for the rest of the process. These trends do not refer simply to the sorting of the genes, but large-scale tendencies in human and other populations and the physical environment. In all, I sensed that there must be hundreds of possible vectors of influence on development, including the centrally important specific physical, emotional, and intellectual qualities of the individual whose development we are trying to comprehend.

When I stepped out of the shower in New York, I understood that the amusement park ride was an image capturing the multiplicity of dynamic forces that influence development and that do not at the same time compromise the integrity or importance of the individual's own contribution to the process. Development does not simply proceed inside the mind of the individual – stages are not inside anyone's head – but as a result of complex, dynamic processes of coordination, change, adjustment, and new coordinations among the individual, the physical environment, the crafted world, and the social milieu. Although this process is extremely complex and ever changing, it is also controlled and lawful.

As with many "new" ideas, there is much about the notion of co-incidence that is not all that new. I am far from the first to point out that development includes more than simply the expression of potential that is carried in the child's genome. A number of other theorists have called attention to the multifold character of the process of development, including most, if not all, of the forces that I discovered when I was able to "read" the image that had been rotating in my head for so long (Cavalli-Sforza, Feldman, Chen, & Dornbusch, 1982). Perhaps the only thing really new was the connecting of the several dimensions of development with an image like a carnival ride, which may or may not actually add anything of importance. For my own part, I can say with certainty that this way of organizing developmental change processes has been greatly illuminating to me, particularly as I have tried to make sense of extreme cases, such as child prodigies. It is more difficult to say whether or not the notion of co-incidence has been of help to others. In fact, it is too soon to say one way or the other, even 10 years later. At this point I am able to say for sure only that the idea of co-incidence has been helpful to me, and also that it was a great relief to have discovered what I was trying to say to myself in my dream. I should also mention that I have not had a dream that included a carnival ride of any description since my rush from the shower. Not once. I take this as evidence that, for better or worse, what I was dreaming was well resolved in the concept of co-incidence that emerged into awareness so suddenly. In contrast to Piaget's idea of "seizing of consciousness" (by which he meant the process of making one's implicit understandings explicit), which became central in his epistemology later in life, I found that the rush to consciousness of this particular concept was not in the least seized. Rather, it seized my consciousness, but through no conscious effort on my part. At least not when it happened.

Co-incidence and child prodigies

When I claim that the insight I now call co-incidence was important to me, I can best illustrate that usefulness with respect to one particular problem I have been working on for more than a decade: how to explain the amazing phenomenon that we call the child prodigy. In fact, I see co-incidence as having been invented, at least partly, so that I might better deal with the matter of the prodigy. Even though I did not begin to study prodigies directly until 1975 (more than 2 years after I began dreaming about the ride with spokes and pods), it was not until I began to prepare to carry out the prodigy research that I made conscious sense of the dream.

That the idea of co-incidence came from a dream image that predated my research with prodigies is not in and of itself a problem for claiming that the concept was invented to explain prodigies. Even before I began a specific research effort, I had thought of the phenomenon of the prodigy as an extreme example of developmental processes that are shared with other individuals of less extreme ability. The amazing reciprocity between child and field that occurs in prodigies is very difficult to explain within traditional theories of development. I knew that I was looking for an alternative perspective to bring to bear on the matter of the prodigy that was part of an effort to bring an alternative perspective to developmental change in general.

It is therefore likely that I was assisted in discovering what my dream image was about by my work on prodigies. It may well have been my focus of attention on the particular and peculiar qualities of prodigies (their extreme precocity, domain-specific abilities, single-mindedness of purpose, seeming wisdom, uncanny maturity, etc.) that moved me toward being able to interpret the carnival ride. It is even possible, I suppose, that co-incidence was one among several interpretations that I might have devised and that it prevailed because of the specific work I was doing on child prodigies. My own belief is that the prodigy work was catalytic, but did not predetermine the final outcome of the construction of the co-incidence idea.

What is it that I was able to say about prodigies after the co-incidence notion that

I was unable to say before? With the co-incidence concept, I think I have been able to present a greater richness of interpretation, a fuller and more articulated explanation (rather than a radically different one) than I had before. I had selected the matter of the prodigy as an interesting topic for research because it seemed to shed light on other aspects of my theorizing (unrelated to the notion of co-incidence), and I had much to say about how prodigies might develop based on those efforts. That theoretical work is summarized elsewhere (Feldman, 1980, 1981, 1983, 1986b), but the basic idea was to try to fill in some of the gaps between universal developmental changes such as Piaget had tried to describe and the remarkable transformations that we associate with the truly unique human contributions. I saw the prodigy concept as a kind of map for some of the territory between these two poles: the universal and the unique (see Figure 11.2).

I did not think that prodigies would necessarily provide examples of the unique end of the spectrum, inasmuch as they do not necessarily transform the fields in which they perform, a critical attribute. Yet there is something about their uncanny mastery, both the speed and depth of it, that suggests a close proximity to creativity. And the frequently cited association between very early mastery and later creativity, although not well documented, seemed plausible to me, especially in music, in which prodigies seem the rule. I labeled the prodigy an example of "idiosyncratic development," along with esoteric specialists and scholars and those who engage in quirky, seemingly useless preoccupations such as collecting thimbles, comic books, or railroad schedules (Feldman, 1980, 1986b). The prodigy seemed to represent an exceptional pretuning to an already existing body of knowledge, one that countless others had spent time and energy developing and refining. It was this remarkable intersection of person and field that was so striking about the prodigy, almost as if the two had been made for each other. I remember wondering what would be the outcome if a child was preorganized to be a chess player but born at a time or in a place where chess was not known. Unhappiness? Frustration? Schizophrenia? Or possibly invention of a proto-chess game? These kinds of thoughts were certainly on my mind as I approached the plane ride with Howard Gruber that was to bring the concept of co-incidence from dream image to interpretive construct.

My assumption, following Piaget, was that developmental changes – major reorganizations of intellectual systems – are brought about by fundamentally similar processes at all places along the continuum of universal-to-unique developmental domains. I thought that because of their rapid movement through levels of mastery in their specific domains, prodigies present an exceptional opportunity to examine transition mechanisms while they are occurring. Instead of interpreting prodigies as anomalous, strange exceptions to the rules of development, I considered them to represent variations in speed and perhaps quality of processing that are not outside the laws of development. Unfortunately, the laws of developmental change still are not well understood; so the assumption that prodigies obey such laws was not a strong claim. It was more of a heuristic, a guiding notion that might allow for extreme examples of human variation in development to be encompassed within a single integrative framework. This has been, more or less, how I have interpreted the matter of the prodigy in my writing (Feldman, 1979, 1980, 1986a).

Once I saw the implications of the co-incidence insight, it seemed as if all development – not just that of the prodigy – could be interpreted as involving the same forces along the same dimensions, with variations in strength and quality of interaction in one or more of these accounting for the differences observed in behavior and abilities. In this account, when a prodigy appears, it is because of a highly improbable but still lawful set of forces that intersect and intertwine over a sufficient period of time. To specify what the forces of such a ''co-incidence calculus'' might be and how to weigh and analyze them seemed a good way to comprehend both the prodigy and other forms of development.

For the prodigy, a number of complementary sets of forces have to be sustained in nearly perfect coordination for early remarkable achievement to occur. In addition to the natural capabilities of the child, a set of responsive and interested parents must be there to recognize and support the early signs of extreme talent. A domain must be introduced early enough and in an appropriate manner to engage the energy, ability, and enthusiasm of the child. Domains themselves evolve and change with time, and the skills and abilities demanded by a domain during one period may not fully duplicate those demanded during another period. When and under what conditions a child comes into contact with a domain may also make a crucial difference. So, too, does the presence of other interests, friends, and practical constraints such as lack of money.

Teachers, schools, guilds, societies, and trades are also critical to the development of the prodigy. A tradition of pedagogy and sufficient structure to move into and through a field must be present for the child and child's parents to chart their way. When dealing with a child 5 or 6 years of age, decisions about who will teach, and how long and in what manner, are vital parts of a co-incidence equation. Cultures and geographic locations vary in their receptiveness to various kinds of talent, to various domains of knowledge and skill. When a climate of receptivity exists for certain fields, such as for the visual arts in fifteenth-century Florence, for scientific fields in Vienna in the 1920s, or for high technology in Silicon Valley in the 1980s, it is because a set of cultural rewards and practices and values crystallizes uniquely in a given place at a given time (Csikszentmihalyi & Robinson, 1986; Feldman, 1986b; Simonton, 1984). Although relatively little is known about just what kinds of things must be present for such an outpouring of creative energy, clearly these aspects of talent expression must be reckoned into any explanation.

Finally, there are longer-term influences that can play vital though sometimes less obvious roles in the appearance and development of extreme early talent. The traditions that run in families are sometimes very explicit and clear, sometimes implicit or even unknown at a conscious level. When known, these traditions can have profound channeling effects, such as in the case of a family of musicians or doctors or artists. For a child born into such a family, the environment is filled with the signs of commitment made by a family and its members, and it seems as natural as any other environment. This is one reason why music prodigies have such an advantage when they come from musical families. Music is all around them from their earliest days, even before birth, and it is played and enjoyed and lived as if it is the most important and central thing that a person can do, and for such families it often is. It should also be noted that strong family traditions can be troublesome for children who have no talent or inclination for the family's preoccupation. This only serves to underline the point that it is the combining and coordinating of all the co-incidence forces that give rise to exceptional early achievement. Remove or mistime any one of these, and the chances are substantially reduced that something really extraordinary will happen with the child.

In families in which there has been a strong tradition, but in which for one reason or another it has been lost or repressed, the effect can still be powerful, but more indirect. In the case of the Menuhin family, for example, a long-standing tradition of producing religious prodigies seems to have been transformed and redirected into preparation of a secular talent: violinist Yehudi Menuhin (Feldman & Goldsmith, 1986). It seems that a centuries-old tradition of producing religious prodigies in this family was suppressed by Menuhin's parents, and the children were unaware of it. Yet, in looking at the pattern of the parents' child-rearing decisions and their organization of resources to bring Yehudi's talent to full flower, the Menuhins repeated many of the same techniques used by their ancestors, even as they re-directed their emphasis into a secular realm.

Another aspect of the prodigy phenomenon that became clearer within the frame-work of co-incidence is the importance of coordination of resources, a task that often falls to families of prodigies. If it is true of development in general that it requires that child, parents, environment, society, and culture be working in harmo-ny, then the prodigy requires a much more precise and carefully timed sequence of appropriate events and experiences. Because the prodigy is unlikely to be capable of making many of the decisions about how to negotiate the early phases of preparation (if for no other reason than extreme youth), others must take on this task. This means that an essential part of prodigy preparation is a finely tuned coordinating function that marshals and deploys just the right kinds of resources and secures optimal early experiences.

Of course, some co-incidence forces simply are not controllable: The child must possess talent, and it must be very powerful; the domain must exist in a form that engages and challenges the child; chance or environmental circumstances that arise must not disrupt the process in any significant way. Only so much of the co-incidence process can be controlled or coordinated by even the most masterful manager. But the things that can be brought into synergistic relationship must be if the co-incidence process is to yield extreme expression of potential.

I am not suggesting that those who have taken responsibility for managing the coordination of co-incidence forces for talented young children are always fully aware of what they are doing. From my experience with several families of pro-digies, it is clear that these parents see their role as simply facilitating and furthering the largely autonomous development of their child's talent. Were they to fully appreciate the magnitude of the problem and the complexity of the task they face, many would no doubt be discouraged from taking it on. The planning, coordination, and execution of a prodigy's preparation is a prodigious task in itself, and only with the full attention and energy of someone very determined is it likely to be successful (Feldman, 1986b).

It is an enormous challenge to raise any child, but at least the target for development is not such a narrow one for most children. Parents of most 6-year-olds want to help their children learn to write and sing, for example, but the children are not specifically driven to write novels or compose symphonies. Although parents often have aspirations for what they would like their offspring to become, uusally it is not obvious what their talents will lead to, so that decisions about how to respond to interests, enrich, and guide have wide margins of error. Parents of prodigies seem to know how crucial their decisions could be for the successful development of their child's talent, particularly in a society like this one, in which the burden for responding to extreme talent falls heavily on the shoulders of parents.

In my research with prodigies, I noticed that most of the families showed signs of stress and were in a continuing (yet, on the whole, successful) struggle against disintegration. The co-incidence notion helped me to see why this would tend to occur in such families. Preparing a prodigy requires vast adjustments in child-rearing, family life, and aspirations, as well as the willingness of at least one parent to devote virtually total attention to the prodigy's development. That these conditions should create stress seems more than reasonable; I began to wonder how the families I observed did as well as they did under the circumstances.

Seeing the development of the prodigy as a process involving several sets of factors that have to be coordinated has helped me to understand why it is important for prodigies also to be blessed with at least a modicum of general organizational/analytic ability, a healthy dose of pragmatism, and a strong sense of inner confidence (Feldman, 1986b). Because so little is explicitly understood about how the various forces of co-incidence intertwine, and even less about how to keep them in effective reciprocal relation to one another, a good deal of the burden for maintaining the trajectory of development falls directly on the prodigy.

Was the insight creative?

I have been trying to describe the episode of insight that was the most dramatic one in my experience. There have been many others, some of which had similar qualities of suddenness and flashing power, most of which did not. I have also elaborated on the meaning of the co-incidence insight itself. Much of what I have said about co-incidence is based on subsequent reflection and analysis of that sudden moment of comprehension. The process of interpretation continued after the insight as it had before, but it was more tightly focused. My insight in the shower transformed a dream image into a tool to work with. Through the process that I have just described, I was able to focus and further my conscious efforts to make better sense of prodigies in particular and the nature of developmental change more generally.

That the co-incidence insight was important for me is, of course, clear. Not only was its arrival marked by fireworks and fanfare, but it has remained an important part of my mental landscape ever since, to be explored over a period of more than 10 years. There is no question, then, that the carnival ride insight was significant for me and, in a real sense, personally creative. I mean that it had the effect of helping transform and reorganize my way of thinking about matters that were and are of vital importance to me. I have found the distillation of the amusement park image into a model of certain aspects of development to be a source of stimulation and satisfaction, and I believe that my thinking is clearer and better organized than it was before. In short, I believe that the experience contributed to my own knowledge and understanding of developmental processes. Of course, it remains to be seen just how much this new knowledge will add to the more formal, distilled body of knowledge we call the field of creativity research or, more broadly, the field of developmental psychology.

How did my personally powerful insight fare in the larger arena of creativity research? I can report one instance in which it seems to have made a difference. My colleague Howard Gardner also studies creativity. He has had a particular interest in co-incidence. His initial reaction to the idea was not enthusiastic. It sounded like overlearning to him, or overdetermined behavior. If the co-incidence concept posits that a large number of forces must conspire to produce prodigious behavior, Gardner reasoned, the outcome is inevitable. Since this first exposure to co-incidence, he has warmed to the idea considerably, as should be evident in his recent writing, including his chapter in this volume. Gardner came to realize, and helped me to realize as well, that it is not enough to invoke a framework that points to the complexity of factors that impinge on and control development, nor even to intone the critical function of qualities like coordination and balance, as I have done. Few would argue that development is not complex, and most would acknowledge that the main vectors of influence identified by the co-incidence model are well chosen. But the manner in which the various forces interact is of critical importance, and this is rarely, if ever, explicitly considered in the co-incidence model.

Asserting that natural talents and personal qualities are not sufficient to account for development, prodigious or not, is of value only if something new about these forces and their manner of interacting is discovered. What patterns of capability, family forces, teachers, peers, institutions, cultural features, and so forth, would lead to one outcome versus another? Is it possible to predict later instances of remarkable behavior from a thorough analysis of the forces that were present during the early years? Given the limited success of psychometric instruments to predict later creativity, might co-incidence offer a way to improve prediction? And what, if anything, does the co-incidence idea have to say about the actual process involved in doing creative work – of carrying out an effort to transform or reorganize a domain?

These well-intentioned challenges led to further reflections about and extensions of the notion of co-incidence. Howard Gardner proposed a possible distinction between a child prodigy and a creative worker. Gardner suggested that co-incidence forces for prodigies tend to work in amazing harmony and coordination, posing few major obstacles or impediments to the fulfillment of their potential, as, for example, was the case with Yehudi Menuhin (Feldman & Goldsmith, 1986). For creativity of a major sort to occur, in contrast, perhaps it is necessary that there be well-timed discordances, failures in coordination, or other instances of less than optimal timing, sequencing, and calibrating of experience. Creativity, then, would depend in part on adversity, on less than optimal circumstances, whereas prodigious achievement would thrive on sustained, amazing coordination among the critical co-incidence forces.

It is true that most child prodigies do not go on to make truly creative contributions, in the sense that they do not bring about significant changes in the structure and organization of a domain. Most prodigies are able to do something very difficult in a very short time, but what they do is not unlike what others do, except that others take more time and perhaps have less natural talent (Feldman, 1986b).

The challenging question, of course, is what combination of qualities and forces, coordinated in what ways, over what period of time, will result in a truly creative contribution to a field of knowledge. At what point will a given combination move in a new direction if it encounters obstacles? Is it true that the old idea of creativity as a response to difficult and frustrating life circumstances has merit after all? Are prodigies an indication of well-being in their own developmental courses and in the domains in which they perform, whereas creative reorganizations and revolutions betoken a malady, plateau, or effort to forestall a dead end in a given field? These seem to be the right sorts of issues to consider when sorting out distinctions between and among different forms of giftedness and talent, and between precociousness and creative accomplishment.

When a domain is stable, it offers a valued place for the canonical performer. It is not likely in such circumstances that a person would find it necessary to transform the field. A case of this sort is provided by the violinist Yehudi Menuhin, whose experience seems to have been one long, happy, highly rewarding road from prodigy to world-class performer. Menuhin's autobiography, written when he was about 60 years old, has an almost smug tone. In the Preface, Steiner (1977) writes:

Luck was there from the beginning: in a brilliantly gifted family, in a childhood guarded but also stretched to fulfillment, in a series of true teachers – Persinger, Enesco, Busch – in an accord between mind and sinew which enabled the very young virtuoso to pass almost unknowing from mechanical display to the inward meaning of a score. International acclaim followed as of itself, in an era, now lost, of transatlantic liners, firelit hotel suites, and a freemasonry of musical culture that admitted no frontiers.

Contrast this with the agonizing of one who has not found that wonderful meshing of talent and domain, who has a need to express himself, but no medium through which to do so. Here are the words of the young Van Gogh, sometime preacher, not yet a painter, who felt himself to be a person with a mission:

Prisoners in an I-don't-know-what-for horrible, horrible utterly horrible cage. . . . Such a man often doesn't know himself what he might do, but he feels instinctively; yet am I good for something, yet am I aware for some reason for existing! I know that I might be a totally different man! How then can I be useful, how can I be of service! Something is alive in me: what can it be! (Ghiselin, 1952, p. 13)

The foregoing examples credibly support Gardner's idea that a major difference between creativity and prodigiousness is the extent to which the forces of co-incidence are in positive alignment. The prodigy takes full advantage of the existing composition of a domain and, through a rapidly accelerated process, masters its expressive potential. Creative work also requires mastery of a domain, but it does not have mastery as an end point; rather, significant extension and transformation of the domain are its goals. Whereas the prodigy experiences an amazing harmony, the creative worker may deliberately attend to misalignments, gaps, and anomalies. In doing so, the creative worker may construct a different perspective on the domain, one that affords perception of its limits and provides glimpses of a fundamental reorganization. For a prodigy, forces must be in nearly optimal and sustained coordination, whereas for significant works of creativity, some misalignments must occur. Precisely which elements must be coordinated or misaligned, for how long, and in what ways, is just the kind of question that I have been exploring (Feldman, 1986b).

The concept of co-incidence, then, may prove useful for thinking about the broad contextual factors that facilitate prodigious behavior or creativity or both. Although this seems to be true, it is also true that creativity will not be adequately explained by a broad framework alone, no matter how appropriate such a framework might be. What we need in order to explain creativity more adequately are models, theories, and frameworks at several levels of specificity. The co-incidence concept provides a general framework, and its usefulness is limited by virtue of this (as is its particular utility defined by it). The more specific qualities and characteristics of each of the major co-incidence forces (individual, society, culture, historical trends, evolutionary patterns, etc.) form more specific processes involved in solving problems and making associations, and they, too, need attention.

Juxtaposing my own experience of a blockbuster insight, for example, and the concept of co-incidence (what that insight turned out to be), it is clear that the latter only loosely and indirectly "explains" the former. That is, the framework of co-incidence is at best a rough guide to the experiences and qualities that may have led me to the moment when reorganization yielded insight. The concept of co-incidence sheds little light on why or how I might have produced such an idea, specifically, or where it might have come from. As a particular component of an overall explanation for creative work and how it is done, co-incidence is of value, but many other components are needed to complement it. In the remaining parts of this chapter I shall briefly discuss some additional possible components, and one in particular that lies at a more fine-grained level of detail.

As it happens, I also came upon this component by way of an insight process, although it was a much more recent one and was more subtle and quiet in announcing itself. I do not believe that the addition of this new component in any sense "completes" the picture of creativity, but it does represent an effort to work at another level and illustrates how efforts at one level of explanation can lead to efforts at another level.

The transformational imperative

Once again there was a series of dreams, and once again there was an insight, but the experience was very different from the co-incidence experience. For the past 2 years or so I have been dreaming in a very particular way, a way different from anything I can remember from earlier dreams. Not a recurring dream, but rather a recurring tendency, it was as if each dream was intended to go a step farther into detail than the last. I do not remember the content of these dreams at all, but I know what my impression was when I would wake and think about them. What was striking about these dreams was the incredible detail that they had generated. The details in these dreams were lovingly displayed, as if my mind were telling me to pay attention and it would show me what it was able to do. Normally I have little interest in details; this certainly tends to be true of my work (as a number of critics have pointed out). I enjoy thinking at broad levels, my theoretical work tends to be about very general phenomena, and I have little memory for specific events. These detail dreams, then, were totally anomalous with respect to both my previous dreams and my normal way of thinking, so far as I am able to determine.

The other thing that was true of these dreams was that the details they produced were of things, people, and places that I had never seen. It was as if each dream was intended to be more amazing than the last in terms of the extent to which the images could not plausibly have come from my direct experience, nor even from my vicarious experience via books, television, hearsay from others, and so forth. The point these dreams seemed to be making was that they could not have come directly from my experience alone. For several months there was a tendency in these dreams to escalate in vividness, specificity, and fineness of detail. It reminded me of the technique of "zooming in" that is used in cinema and video for highlighting the importance of a particular feature of a scene, what is called "lavish" in cinema criticism; indeed, my colleague and friend Gavriel Salomon has used a contrived version of zooming in as a research tool for teaching thinking skills about attention to detail (Salomon, 1979). It felt as though I was teaching myself in my dreams to pay more attention to details – but not just particular details, for almost all details seemed equally important. I also remember something in Stephen Jay Gould's book about intelligence testing to the effect that both God and the devil lie in the details (Gould, 1981). My dreams were telling me that I had been ignoring details for too long, but why were they important?

A clue to why they were important led to the insight that has directed my work on creativity since the fall of 1985. In contrast to the amusement park insight, this one arrived quite without fanfare. It is more than 10 years newer than the co-incidence idea, and already I have all but forgotten when it happened. I simply woke up one morning or sometime during the night and knew what the point of all the details was. As with the previous experience of dreaming described here, I knew for some time that this series of dreams was important for my work, and also that it was of a different character than my usual dream experience. I had been telling my wife Lynn about the detail dreams, but otherwise was not attending to their meaning during consciousness.

For some reason, when I finally realized why the dreams were important, I did not immediately tell Lynn. I sort of let the insight sit for a while, not feeling compelled to run out and tell the world, or even Lynn. Perhaps a week or so later I told Lynn that I knew what the detail dreams were about, but that it would take a while to explain, and so the description in words of the meaning of the detail dreaming process was again delayed. Finally, I began to feel that I might get hit by a truck and not have anyone know about my new perspective on creativity and development; so I managed to find a time to tell Lynn what I thought the dreams were about. As was the case with co-incidence, the effort at explanation did not match the clarity of the feeling of understanding. This lack of ability to articulate what I "knew" did not surprise me this time, and I expect that it will take another 10 years before it becomes clear what the meaning of that set of experiences really is. As best I could articulate it, the important point is that the mind naturally and effortlessly is taking liberties with reality, transforming it.

An additional piece of the puzzle is an extension of something I have been thinking about and saying for several years. I have been involved with efforts to try to demonstrate that major new developmental changes not only occur but also are central features of what it means to be human. This may not sound like much of an issue, because people by and large assume that development of this sort does occur. There are powerful voices, however, that claim otherwise, and these voices have of late been more and more influential in the scholarly field. I am referring to the neonativist views of Noam Chomsky, Jerry Fodor, and others who claim that qualitative changes in thinking not only do not occur but also are in principle impossible (Chomsky, 1980; Fodor, 1983). Their view traces back to Aristotle, who claimed that everything must come from something else and that therefore there is fundamentally nothing new. It also assumes an encoding of reality as its basic process (Campbell & Bickhard, 1986). The argument would apply to creativity, of course, as it does to development in general.

If nothing really new is possible, then development itself is impossible, and it follows that creativity is impossible as well. These sorts of arguments, along with some ideas about genetic determinism, have led to an increasing move in the field in the direction of innatism, even predeterminism, that places the potential for every-thing that a person will ever do as existing at the beginning of life. The argument is clear, it is parsimonious, it is compelling, and it helped Chomsky and his followers shine in the only direct encounter to occur between them and Piaget (Piatelli-Palmarini, 1980).

I have been disturbed by the position taken by neonativists for a number of years and have even written a bit about what form an alternative view might take (Feldman, 1983, 1986a). I also have been encouraged to find that I am not the only one who believes that a radically nativist explanation for change based on encodingism is unacceptable (Bickhard, 1979, 1980; Campbell & Bickhard, 1986). Long before I began dreaming my detail dreams, then, I was consciously working on a solution to the paradox of development, the claim that something new can indeed be constructed even though all the elements of that new thing are not present in the potentials of the physical stuff of the human organism. I even went so far as to assert that there should be a field of inquiry called "developmental science" to balance and contrast with the "cognitive science" that has become such a prominent force in the academic field (Feldman, 1983, 1986a; see Pea & Kurland, 1984, for a complementary view).

As was the case with the co-incidence insight, a series of parallel efforts toward solution of a problem was going on, one set consciously directed toward a solution through direct application, the other set through less conscious, indirectly applied processes that manifested themselves in certain kinds of dreams, of whose purpose I became increasingly aware. At a certain point it seems that the two lines of attack were brought into contact with each other through reflection on a dream or set of dreams, and by my efforts at interpretation of these dreams that I have described as examples of insight.

This experience about how insight works does seem to run counter to David Perkins's recent observations of "loud thinking" by artists, poets, and other workers who reported their thoughts "on line," as it were (Perkins, 1981, 1986). In Perkins's work, insight is seen as relatively mundane and undifferentiated from more typical processing and thinking. For better or worse, however, it is an inescapable conclusion that, in my own case at least, sustained semiconscious and perhaps unconscious processes were applied to problems in parallel with, and eventually in concert with, conscious processes. And the process was not at all mundane or typical. This dual sort of effort took place over a period of years, because in both cases reported here at least a 2-year period elapsed between the earliest dream of a particular type and the insight that, in each case, ended that series. The detail dreams, too, ceased immediately on my realization of what they were trying to "teach" me. And what was that? What was I trying to teach myself?

Essentially, the dreams were showing me that my mind was producing things that I had never seen or heard or been exposed to in any direct way. My mind was quite spontaneously *making new things*. That these new things may have been produced in part out of already existing things does not diminish the fact that by the hundreds and thousands, my mind was showing me that it had the ability to produce a virtual torrent of small transformations and to produce them in coherent, organized ways. I was at times transforming things so rapidly and fluidly that it seemed as if my mind were designed to do nothing else.

I know as well as anyone that in the waking state my mind is not up to these antics. Even daydreaming and preconscious activity touch reality quite actively. But

when I thought about the dreams, the unbelievable dreams of detail, I knew that
their meaning must be to prove that the mind (or at least my mind) works in at least
two complementary ways, one trying to sort, categorize, and otherwise keep things
the same, the other taking the most extravagant liberties with things, sometimes
seemingly just for the hell of it.

Creativity: a three-phase model

There is, of course, nothing really new in the fact that the mind does fantastic
things. Dreams have been subjects of intense investigation for decades and are
known to play a large role in psychological functioning. It is even known that
dreams have sometimes been important for creativity, as in the case of Kekulé's
snake turning on itself as the image for the benzene ring, or Picasso's description of
painting as "successive crystallizations of the dream" (Ghiselin, 1952; Hartmann,
1984). What seems new is to link this large body of evidence to a more general
point of view about mind – that it is capable of producing astoundingly new images,
thoughts, and ideas based only most remotely on anything that came in from
outside, and that these transformations are purposeful and productive. Indeed, they
are part of a larger process of overall coordination and direction in the use of mind.

It seems then that there are at least three essential aspects to creativity. The first I
have just described as a natural tendency of the mind to take liberties with what is
real, mostly in nonconscious ways. These transformations, nonetheless, have the
possibility of being or becoming conscious. Indeed, the manners and kinds of
transformations produced may be directed in some way by the conscious purposes
of the individual, as I had discovered myself through my two series of dream
episodes. The second aspect is the conscious desire to make a positive change in
something real, to, in effect, change the external world to make it conform more
fully to one's wishes. I mean this not necessarily in any lofty or cosmic sense. The
part of the real world that one wishes to change can be modest and mundane; there is
always room for a better mousetrap. The claim here is that it is a natural part of
being human to want to change the world, to experience this wish consciously, and
to set about using whatever resources are available to do so. These resources include
the capability to guide internal transformation and harness its productions to a
conscious goal of change. To do so may not be easy or straightforward (as was the
case with my sets of "harnessed" dreams), but it can be done. This conclusion was
not reached through an insight process, but seemed to follow from the other parts of
the system.

Finally, the third aspect of the process concerns the results of previous efforts by
other individuals labeled at changing the world or their environments. I have labeled
this aspect "the crafted world." The artifacts of creative work are available to the
person who desires to make further changes in the world. These previous efforts, as
represented in a culture's products, models, technologies, and so forth, are of
enormous value to the aspiring creator for at least two reasons: They illustrate that it

is possible to make a difference and have that difference incorporated into the environment, and they make it possible to reduce the "mental distance" one has to go to be able to make a meaningful change. This is at least partially what Newton meant when he exclaimed that he stood on the shoulders of giants.

I shall now try to show how what I have just discussed makes Aristotle's dictum that everything must come from something else true but irrelevant to my point. The Aristotelian tradition, which has seen its fullest expression in Western rationalism, has to do with the part of mind that tries to keep things the same, that gives us something to hang on to, that provides for continuity of experience and a stable sense of reality. The other side of mind aims to continuously change and transform, to show that constructing a stable reality is a device for not going insane, a way to keep the forces of transformation from holding sway. Indeed, conscious versus unconscious thought may have been an evolutionary adaptation for keeping these two functions – transformation and categorization – from destroying each other. This interplay becomes productive and central in the process of making something both new and useful.

Why new ideas really do occur

I have called the presumably universal tendency to produce new things "the trans-formational imperative." I call it this because I want to stress the deep and uniquely human quality that I believe operates when a conscious effort is made to change the world. I think that this tendency is as fundamental a quality of cognition as any. It has even led me to propose that Piaget's two most important change processes are not sufficient to account for new ideas. Piaget proposed that there are two comple-mentary processes, assimilation and accommodation, that account for all change in thought structures. Assimilation refers to the tendency to keep reality just as it is, to take in information and put it into existing ways of organizing experience, even if that information must be distorted in the process. On the other hand, accommo-dation represents the tendency to make adjustments in how reality is interpreted when it becomes impossible to live with the distortions that assimilation demands. The interplay of these two modes of responding to experience accounts for all developmental change, according to Piaget (1971, 1972/1981).

One well-known problem with Piaget's account is that it does not deal well with novelty, with producing really new restructurings of experience. Piaget was well aware of this problem and tried mightily to overcome it (Piaget, 1971, 1972/1981, 1975). Piaget's final attempt to solve the novelty problem was both formal and rational. He claimed that a process called "reflective abstraction" (also sometimes called reflexive abstraction) might be able to explain how genuinely novel ideas could be formed. He was aware that his argument with the nativists hangs on being able to produce a plausible account of novelty (i.e., of changes that represent true advances in thought and that are constructed by the individual mind). Rather than consider the possibility of a nonrational, nonreflective ingredient of the process of novelty production, Piaget persisted in trying to find a conscious, rational, and directed solution to the problem. Of course, there is a conscious, directed aspect to the process, but there is also more. As usual, Piaget was on the right track and laid the groundwork for further progress.

This was not the only difficulty Piaget faced as he worked on the novelty problem (some of the other problems are discussed in Feldman, 1980), but it may have been the most devastating. In order to solve the novelty problem, Piaget would have had to look to an aspect of mind he had self-consciously excluded from his framework for more than 50 years. Little wonder that he was unable to entertain the idea of coordinated efforts between two polar casts of mind in explaining the construction of novelties.

The fact of the matter is that the fruits of the dream or any other transformation process are of little use unless they eventually become connected with the rational, conscious work of the mind aiming to solve a problem or render something more pleasing. As easily as the less conscious mind is able to transform, it seems to have little idea of why it is doing so or how to use its fantastic possibilities. This job is directed by the aspects of mind that are in contact with the world of real things, real people, and real problems. It seems that only when the whole of mind is somehow harnessed to complementary purposes is it likely that something both new and useful will be constructed. And part of what is available is outside the mind altogether. Interestingly, this is more or less what Brewster Ghiselin, a student of creativity, wrote more than 30 years ago:

New life comes always from outside our world, as we commonly conceive our world. This is the reason why, in order to invent, one must yield to the indeterminate within him, or, more precisely to certain ill-defined impulses which seem to be of the very texture of the ungoverned fullness which John Livingston Lowes calls "the surging chaos of the unexpressed." Chaos and disorder are perhaps the wrong terms for that indeterminate fullness and activity of the inner life. For it is organic, dynamic, full of tension and tendency. What is absent from it, except in the decisive act of creation, is determination, fixity, and commitment to one resolution or another of the whole complex of its tensions. (Ghiselin, 1952, p. 13)

Ghiselin had his finger on part of the transformational imperative, but did not extend his description to include use of the external world as well as a critical source of inspiration for creativity. Ironically, some of Piaget's most interesting experiments were with external physical reality of just the sort that I am referring to. He asked children to imagine what a piece of wire would look like when it was bent in various positions, or he asked how a set of two blocks, one on top of the other, would change in appearance if one block was moved a bit off center. What Piaget found was that the ability to mentally represent movement (i.e., physical transformation) was one of the last to be achieved in children. As late as 8 or 9 years, children were unable to carry out even simple mental transformations and make accurate predictions based on an understanding of physical properties in transformation. It was as if the children were locked into the appearance of the object and unable to make it change in state through mental manipulation (Piaget, 1969).

Piaget's ingenious experiments show, I believe, that the conscious rational mind does not deal easily with transformation, but is nonetheless able to learn about it through experience with changed and changing reality. It is as if the conscious mind has been constructed to create a constant world, to behave as if things are not changing, but static, and to go about its business with this purpose as a central goal. Only reluctantly does the conscious mind entertain transformation.

When Piaget's experimental results with physical transformation are compared with dream states, which are suffused with transformations, movements, extrapolations, extrusions, and all manner of wild imaginings, it is a wonder that the conclusion that there are really two quite distinct simultaneously active functions did not occur to Piaget as the key to the novelty problem. As extreme as one way of organizing experience is, the other tends toward the opposite extreme. When both are put in the service of a goal that calls on the best efforts of the full range of waking and dream states, conscious and unconscious processes, conserving and transformational capabilities, a genuinely new idea or work or solution may be constructed. This is a long way from Piaget's idea of reflective abstraction. It is more like reciprocal exchange: on the one hand, an effort to abstract and categorize and organize, to put things in their place; on the other hand, to stir up and change and expand.

Piaget was close to the mark, but he stopped a bit short. He was right to insist that internal novel thoughts are constructed by individuals and that they are achieved through a process of abstraction. Reflection of the sort Piaget described is part of the process, but is limited to conscious effort and directed analysis, necessary but not sufficient for something new to be made. When something new occurs, it is because the fruits of the transformational imperative are made available to the reflective rational mind, and also, in some ways, vice versa. Assimilation and accommodation are useful only if they have the right material to work on, and the transformational imperative helps take care of that. Rather than two invariant functions, assimilation and accommodation, we must propose that there are three: assimilation, accommodation, and transformation. Because the latter, transformation, seems so alien to the rational conscious mind, as Piaget's own experiments showed, Piaget did not see that it is as involved in changes in thinking as the other two functions, but in a different way. The transformational imperative may also be mediated by Vygotsky's "inner speech" (Vygotsky, 1934/1962), as it seems to have qualities of both rational and irrational thought. In any case, the coordinated interplay of the powerful operations that Piaget studied and the fluid productions that I dreamed seems central to the construction of novelty.

Creativity: the construction and appreciation of crafted transformations

Having just proposed to add a third invariant function, transformation, to the broad process of developmental change that Piaget proposed, we may be in range of specifying a mechanism that can account for qualitative change, for novelty. Because the mind is clearly able to construct ideas and images that are not directly part of its experience, it need not be limited to what is represented, copied, perceived, or taught of the world as it exists. In fact, as I have just tried to illustrate, part of the mind seems to do almost nothing but transform. Were it not for the rational, orderly, logical, largely conscious function to balance it, experience would have no stability at all. Yet the transformational imperative is not itself enough to explain development and creativity, to refute the antidevelopmental position of Chomsky and Fodor. It still could be possible that all that is happening in the mind when it "transforms" is to make modifications and combinations based on previous experience, on representation, not really constructing anything new. This would be particularly true if, as the neonativists assert, the basic rules of thought are present, and all that happens is to build even more complex and varied combinations of those rules. This is essentially the argument made by Chomsky for the "creative" feature of language. No two sentences need be quite the same; yet all sentences follow the same deep rules of grammar.

What is needed to complete the mechanism of creativity (or at least to have a sketch of what it might be like) is the additional component I have called the crafted world. It was expressed in nascent form in my work *Beyond Universals in Cognitive Development* (Feldman, 1980) in a chapter with Lynn T. Goldsmith on novelties, where we likened the existence of humanly crafted parts of the environment to Darwin's observations of the unbelievable diversity of living things:

Although we have taken no voyage comparable to Darwin's it occurred to us that the variety of human inventions seems in its own way as overwhelming and inexplicable as the infinite variety of life forms that Darwin saw. (Feldman, 1980, p. 36)

At that time I was not able to say what kind of process might produce human inventions, only to marvel at their variety and pervasiveness. This was true as well of Darwin when he was unable to propose a plausible mechanism for producing variation, a mechanism later identified as genetic recombination (Gruber, 1981).

The full impact of my insight about transformation as an inherent part of human thought – a functional invariant in Piaget's terms – was to come when I combined the two ideas that I have just summarized – the transformational imperative and the existence of innumerable *products* of human invention, perceived and attributed to the efforts of other human beings. I was able at last to glimpse a plausible process that could account for the construction of genuinely new ideas and at the same time refute the antidevelopmental claims of neonativists and other radical, biological determinist types.

The essential point is that thinkers since at least Plato's time have either put the source of creativity outside the individual altogether (coming from the gods or some other unknown place) or put it entirely inside the individual, having no other source of inspiration than the individual's own experience in the use of a developed craft. Piaget went a long way toward breaking this logjam when he claimed that development is not a matter of one source or the other, outside or inside, but must consist of both sorts of forces. Piaget's central epistemological assumption was that knowledge is constructed through the individual's inherent tendencies to know, in confrontation with the inherent properties of the physical world to be known. With this formulation, he had the components needed to show how novelty occurs, except for two: the most internal and the most external aspects of the process. He had the right idea, that it took individuals reflecting on their own experience from transactions with the world of objects and people in order to gain new knowledge (Campbell & Bickhard, 1986). What he missed were the amazing possibilities of the non-conscious, nonrational, expressive side of mind and also the myriad examples of such tendencies expressed in ideas, artifacts, symbol systems, technologies, artforms, and the like, creating an environment that is itself constantly changed through the efforts of purposeful human beings (Gruber, 1981).

To put the matter another way, consider the insight of Aristotle that everything comes from something else. The conclusion that we have incorrectly tended to make from that insight is that nothing new is ever constructed. Aristotle said:

And so, as . . . a thing is not said to be that from which it comes, here the statue is not said to be wood but is said by a verbal change to be wooden, not brass but brazen, not gold but golden, and the house is said to be not bricks but bricken (though we should not say without qualification, if we looked at the matter carefully, even that a statue is produced from wood or a house from bricks, because coming to be implies change in that from which a thing comes to be, and not permanence). (Rothenberg & Hausman, 1976, p. 35)

Aristotle recognized change, but did not seem to notice that the particular *kinds* of changes described, as in this passage, are a consequence of human effort. Or, to be more accurate, he noticed but did not give special status to changes brought about by "thought" or "art." In fact, however, it is a crucial distinction to make between changes that are "natural" and changes that are the result of human effort.

Plato and Aristotle both placed the source of change outside the individual, and in doing so they set the course of Western thought on creativity for more than 2,000 years. Kant put the source of change inside the individual, and only there. It was Piaget who revolutionized thought by placing the source of change in the process itself, a crucial and irreversible change in the history of ideas. Piaget, the quintessential rationalist, ironically opened the door for a dynamic, process-oriented explanation of development that begins to capture the fluid, changing, transformational tendencies of the human mind; in doing so, he made possible an explanation of novelty, the key to creativity.

How, then, is it possible for truly new things to be constructed? It is possible because everything need not come from outside, nor from inside. Things are available in the man-made or crafted environment to provide examples of novel ideas brought to fruition, expressed in real form, by other human beings. They show that it is possible to change the world and make things that are there to be further modified by others. It must, of course, be assumed that something like the transformational imperative exists, that individuals acted on it in the past, and that they externalized their ideas into products. Otherwise, the availability of products of human effort would not necessarily be critical to further change.

The extent to which one might act on a tendency to transform further the crafted world can range from idle "tinkering around" to focused, sustained, systematic, organized, long-term, sophisticated efforts to transform entire fields or bodies of knowledge or cultures. Perhaps the first human to take a stick and make marks in the dirt was exhibiting a playful tendency to bring transformational possibilities to concrete external expression, with eventual profound consequences for all of civilization. Examples of the latter, more deliberate sort include all the great works of Darwin, Freud, Einstein, and Piaget. Transformational tendencies that have taken concrete expression and irreversibly changed the human environment include spiritual, cultural, political, and economic revolutions. And, yes, even the invention of nuclear weapons must be included, for few transformations have had such a profound set of consequences; the context within which every individual uses the transformational imperative has been irreversibly altered by the nuclear threat.

To account for human creativity, then, it is not necessary to assume that something comes from nothing. Something can come in part from the outcomes of innumerable previous efforts at transformation – available, waiting, and also visibly changing the environment. Each one of these products is for a time a survivor of cultural selection pressures somewhat like those of Darwin's "survival of the fittest" (Feldman, 1980). Furthermore, the products of transformational tendencies need not just lie there, waiting for an interested individual to be intrigued with them. Human beings can actively transmit the most important transformations to others, and in doing so they introduce members of the group to the most powerful resources available in their culture. Clearly, such capabilities as speech, writing, reading, counting, and calculating are highly distilled products of many centuries of efforts at expressive transformational possibilities by countless individuals, some of whom were no doubt just tinkering around. These resources provide some of the tools for achieving new products and examples of new products to build on.

Real development, significant internal reorganization that is not preordained, can thus be helped to occur through transactions among individuals who are trying to express their thoughts and ideas and who have done so by changing their cultural world. By being given or taught or confronted with the works of others, the actual material that a person is working with can be added to and enhanced. Therefore, not only is there something new under the sun, there are countless new things being made all the time, each bringing with it the possibility of adding features to the man-made, crafted environment and possibly becoming part of the perceived environment of others.

Development is real even if it is not altogether internally generated. Creativity is therefore also real, a special form of development that yields a product that is new and valuable not only to an individual but also to a field. Spontaneous and directed transformations are the processes that make possible both development and creativity. Plato, Aristotle, Kant, Piaget, and even Chomsky have all contributed to this conclusion, as have countless others. Creativity, therefore, is at once the most individual and the most social developmental process of all, because it depends directly on the efforts of others to provide the material that makes possible a new idea.

Conclusion

In this chapter I have described two insight experiences, one that occurred more than 10 years ago, another much more recent. Each of these experiences has turned out to reflect an aspect of the creative process as well as to provide a source of information about how to form a plausible account of significant acts of creativity. The earlier insight was a blockbuster type, arriving with dazzling suddenness and intensity. The second was the opposite, appearing quietly and with no fanfare. They have been equally important. Each insight was also built over several years, with hints about its meaning in a series of recurring dreams. It was clear long before the meaning of the dreams was discovered that they would shed important light on my work. In the first instance, it was not creativity per se that was the focus of the insight; in the second it was. In both cases, however, the consequences have been profound and continue to be influential.

I have tried to make two points. The first is to show how large-scale insight is a valuable process for studying creativity and for helping to unravel its mysteries. The second is that insight, or, more broadly, illumination, occurs through the loosely directed reciprocal interplay of conscious and less conscious efforts to understand or solve a problem and to produce a work that changes the world, however slightly. The impetus to express a new idea in a form that can be understood and used by others leads to the directed use of both rational and nonrational mental processes for construction of cultural artifacts, which in turn are a unique human environment that may stimulate, nurture, and catalyze efforts at transforming a part of the culture. These new artifacts make the environment different from what it was, an awareness of which is a critical and unique quality of human experience.

Taking the two points together, I have come to the conclusion that genuine, qualitative novel thoughts and ideas do occur. It is possible to make something new under the sun that is not directly a function of the biological potential of the individual. In fact, when one looks around at the results of humanity's efforts to transform the world, it is stunning to reflect on how much of our reality consists of a continuously emerging set of humanly crafted new things. Anyone who argues against development in the sense of true constructed novelty must ignore these manifest fruits of human labor and expression to an amazing degree.

Although I must caution that most of what I have learned is based on my own experience, and is also highly speculative, I know that I did not contrive the typewriter I am using, the chair I am sitting on, or the light that I use to illuminate my office, nor, for that matter, the numerous other things that are being changed in my culture even as I write. To doubt creativity under such circumstances is simply beyond my comprehension.

Note

1 It was somewhat later that I changed the name of creative developmental transitions to "unique" (Figure 11.2).

References

Bickhard, M. H. (1979). On necessary and specific capabilities in evolution and development. *Human Development, 22,* 217–224.

Bickhard, M. H. (1980). A model of developmental and psychological processes. *Genetic Psychology Monographs, 102,* 61–116.

Brandt, R. S. (1986, May). On creativity and thinking skills: A conversation with David Perkins. *Educational Leadership,* pp. 12–18.

Campbell, R. L., & Bickhard, M. H. (1986). *Knowing levels and developmental stages.* Basel: Karger.

Cavalli-Sforza, L. L., Feldman, M. W., Chen, K. H., & Dornbusch, S. M. (1982). Theory and observation in cultural transmission. *Science, 218,* 19–27.

Chomsky, N. (1980). On cognitive structures and their development. In M. Piattelli-Palmarini (Ed.), *Language and learning: The debate between Jean Piaget and Noam Chomsky* (pp. 35–54). Cambridge, MA: Harvard University Press.

Csikszentmihalyi, M., & Robinson, R. E. (1986). Culture, time, and the development of talent. In R. Sternberg & J. E. Davidson (Eds.), *Conceptions of giftedness* (pp. 264–284). Cambridge University Press.

Feldman, D. H. (1974). Universal to unique: A developmental view of creativity and education. In S. Rosner & L. Abt (Eds.), *Essays in creativity* (pp. 45–85). Croton-on-Hudson, NY: North River Press.

Feldman, D. H. (1975). Doing for creativity research what evolution did for biology: A review of Gruber and Barrett's *Darwin on man. Phi Delta Kappan, 57,* 56–57.

Feldman, D. H. (1979). The mysterious case of extreme giftedness. In H. Passow (Ed.), *The gifted and the talented. Yearbook of the National Society for the Study of Education* (pp. 335–351). University of Chicago Press.

Feldman, D. H. (1980). *Beyond universals in cognitive development.* Norwood, NJ: Ablex.

Feldman, D. H. (1981). Beyond universals: Toward a developmental psychology of education. *Educational Researcher, 10,* 21–31.

Feldman, D. H. (1983). Developmental psychology and art education. *Art Education, 36,* 19–21.

Feldman, D. H. (1986a). How development works. In I. Levin (Ed.), *Stage and structure: Reopening the debate* (pp. 284–306). Norwood, NJ: Ablex.

Feldman, D. H. (1986b). *Nature's gambit: Child prodigies and the development of human potential.* New York: Basic Books.

Feldman, D. H., & Goldsmith, L. T. (1986). Transgenerational influences on the development of early prodigious behavior: A case study approach. In W. Fowler (Ed.), *Early experience and competence development* (pp. 67–85). San Francisco: Jossey-Bass.

Feldman, D. H., Marrinan, B. M., & Hartfeldt, S. D. (1972). Transformational power as a possible index of creativity. *Psychological Reports, 30,* 335–338.

Fodor, J. (1983). *The modularity of mind.* Cambridge, MA: MIT Press.

Ghiselin, B. (1952). *The creative process.* New York: Mentor.

Gould, S. J. (1981). *Mismeasure of man.* New York: Norton.

Gruber, H. (1981). *Darwin on man: A psychological study of scientific creativity* (2nd ed.). University of Chicago Press.

Hartmann, E. (1984). *The nightmare: The psychology and biology of terrifying dreams.* New York: Basic Books.

Hofstadter, D. R. (1985a). On the seeming paradox of mechanizing creativity. In D. R. Hofstadter (Ed.), *Metamagical themas* (pp. 526–546). New York: Basic Books.

Hofstadter, D. R. (1985b). Variations on a theme as the crux of creativity. In D. R. Hofstadter (Ed.), *Metamagical themas* (pp. 232–259). New York: Basic Books.

Menuhin, Y. (1967). *Unfinished journey.* New York: Knopf.

Pea, R., & Kurland, D. M. (1984). On the cognitive effects of learning computer programming. *New Ideas in Psychology, 2,* 137–168.

Perkins, D. (1981). *The mind's best work.* Cambridge, MA: Harvard University Press.

Perkins, D. (1986, May). Thinking frames. *Educational Leadership,* pp. 4–10.

Piaget, J. (1969). *The mechanisms of perception*. New York: Basic Books.

Piaget, J. (1971). The theory of stages in cognitive development. In D. R. Green, M. P. Ford, & G. B. Flamer (Eds.), *Measurement and Piaget* (pp. 1–11). New York: McGraw-Hill.

Piaget, J. (1975). *The development of thought: Equilibration of cognitive structures*. New York: Viking Press.

Piaget, J. (1981). Creativity. In J. M. Gallagher & D. K. Reid (Eds.), *The learning theory of Piaget and Inhelder*. Monterey, CA: Brooks-Cole. (Original work published 1972.)

Piattelli-Palmarini, M. (Ed.). (1980). *Language and learning: The debate between Jean Piaget and Noam Chomsky*. Cambridge, MA: Harvard University Press.

Rothenberg, A., & Hausman, C. R. (Eds.). ((1976). *The creativity question*. Durham, NC: Duke University Press.

Salomon, G. (1979). *Interaction of media, cognition, and learning*. San Francisco: Jossey-Bass.

Shrady, M. (1972). *Moments of insight*. New York: Harper & Row.

Simonton, D. K. (1984). *Genius, creativity and leadership: Historiometric inquiries*. Cambridge, MA: Harvard University Press.

Steiner, G. (1977). Foreword. In Y. Menuhin, *Unfinished journey*. New York: Knopf.

Sternberg, R. J. (1986). A triarchic theory of intellectual giftedness. In R. J. Sternberg & J. Davidson (Eds.), *Conceptions of giftedness*. Cambridge University Press.

Vygotsky, L. (1962). *Thought and language*. Cambridge, MA: MIT Press. (Original work published 1934.)

12　Creative lives and creative works: a synthetic scientific approach

Howard Gardner

A visitor to Vienna today finds a lovely Central European capital graced by spacious parks, grand churches and public buildings, intimate cafes and sweet shops, as well as the vigorous Danube flowing along its major boulevards. The population is elegant, and the theatrical and musical stages mount major productions, and yet it is difficult to avoid the feeling that what was once a world-class city is now a living museum.

Less than a century ago, however, Vienna stood at the very center of the world's political and cultural life. Though not as populous as London, nor as historically indispensible as Paris or Rome, Vienna may well have surpassed its competitors in terms of the sheer vitality of its intellectual life. In fin-de-siècle Vienna, living within blocks of one another and hobnobbing at coffeehouses and exchanging views at more formal meetings were such redoubtable figures as members of the Strauss waltz family, composer and conductor Gustav Mahler, playwright Arthur Schnitzler, philosopher Ludwig Wittgenstein, novelist and essayist Robert Musil, painter Gustav Klimt, architect Adolf Loos, satirist Karl Krauss, librettist Hugo von Hofmannsthal, and physicist Heinrich Hertz. Among this illustrious company was an individual fully their equal in creativity, and exerting perhaps an even greater influence on posterity – the neurologist, psychiatrist, and first psychoanalyst, Sigmund Freud.

Whatever one's assessment of the scientific status of Freud's contribution, few would question the fertility of his mind or the creativity of his contributions to an understanding of human nature. Indeed, Freud ranks with such literary giants as Shakespeare and Tolstoy in his capacity to illuminate human nature, and within the ranks of psychology, his contributions surely match those of William James or Jean Piaget or, to choose representatives from a contrasting sphere of psychology, Ivan Pavlov or B. F. Skinner.

In designating these individuals as creative investigators of the human mind and personality, I am making attributions that should be relatively uncontroversial.

Preparation of this chapter was facilitated by support from the John D. and Catherine T. MacArthur Foundation, the Rockefeller Foundation, and the Spencer Foundation. I am grateful to numerous colleagues for their comments on an earlier draft of this chapter: Mihaly Csikszentmihalyi, Yadin Dudai, Howard Gruber, David Perkins, Rick Robinson, Ellen Winner, and Dennie Wolf.

There is little dispute about those few individuals who represent the summit of creativity in a particular field – Mozart or Beethoven, Leonardo da Vinci or Rembrandt, Newton or Einstein. Yet, had I lowered my standards of renown a few notches (Antonio Vivaldi or Jackson Pollock), or singled out an individual work (Mozart's *Magic Flute* or Freud's study of Leonardo da Vinci), I would already have skirted controversy.

There may be an important lesson here. Inasmuch as creativity is difficult to define and challenging to investigate, it is prudent to begin on solid ground – with individuals and with bodies of work that are uncontroversially creative. I shall term this a *holistic* approach, contrasting it with more *atomistic* views of creativity, where the instances or elements studied may appear remote from universally acknowledged instances of creativity. In my view, students of creativity at this point need to develop a framework by which one can adequately conceptualize lifetime achievements of the magnitude of Freud's. We can then determine if it is possible to lower our sights or atomize our instances, still retaining what is integral to the processes of creativity and what is central to persons we deem creative.

Although the adoption of a holistic stance makes a priori sense, particularly in the study of unusual forms of behavior, it may fly in the face of approved scientific practice. Should one approach creativity in the established manner of a cognitive psychologist, a psychometrician, or, for that matter, a geneticist or an anthropologist, there would be certain prescribed disciplinary options to follow. Typically, it would be necessary to study only a very small component of the creative process (e.g., the moment of conscious insight – Koestler, 1964; Wertheimer, 1959) or even to focus on entities that might not be accepted as exemplifying creativity (unusual or "remote" associations – Mednick, 1962). Nor, following the conventional procedure, could insights obtained from a range of disciplinary perspectives be readily combined to illuminate the creative processes in question. By adopting a holistic approach, one encompasses creative phenomena at their full level of complexity – yet at the cost of spurning methods that are more rigorous but less encompassing.

In this chapter, I make a preliminary attempt to develop a framework or model of creativity in the holistic sense described earlier. The framework is multifaceted and complex, as it must be if it is to encompass this mammoth subject. I find it futile to deal with creativity at a single level of explanation, be it the genetic, the psychological, or the historical. I find it equally futile to isolate a single element as the key to creativity, whether that element be a mental process (bi-sociation or fluency), a personality characteristic (doggedness or flexibility), or a cultural ambience (democratic, aristocratic, or irreligious). Indeed, one of the principal reasons why most contemporary psychological accounts of creativity seem so thin (if not irrelevant to creativity writ large) is because they routinely draw on but a single disciplinary lens; creative processes and lives require a combination of disciplines and perspectives.

In my view, creativity is a phenomenon much like prodigiousness: As David Feldman (1986) has argued, a prodigy comes about only when a wide variety of factors all occur at the same "coincident" locus. So, too, creative individuals and creative products come about only when a raft of major facilitating factors are cooperative. It requires several disciplines to bring these disparate factors to the fore, though (unlike the case of prodigiousness) these factors may not always work in synchrony.

When writing about matters creative, one has the option of discussing creative individuals, creative processes, creative works, creative lives, and other cognate entities. Each of these can be defined (and even operationalized) independently. For present purposes, however, it is unnecessary to make a sharp distinction between these entities. Although the focus here will be on creative individuals (with Freud as my chief example), I am comfortable with such a figure exemplifying as well a creative life, exhibiting creative processes, and embodying the more abstract concept of creativity. Should the general framework introduced here seem plausible, there will be opportunity enough to tease apart these different facets of creation.

In what follows, my examples will be restricted to individuals and works that are uncontroversially creative. Both because of his secure status as a creative individual and because the principal facts of his life and work are likely to be familiar to readers of this chapter, I shall focus particularly on the case of Sigmund Freud.

Delineating areas of creativity

My treatment of creativity rests on a key point, one that may be controversial. It is customary to assume (and, indeed, I have assumed it until this point) that creative processes occur in essentially the same way irrespective of the kind of material or subject matter involved. On such an assumption, individuals are creative or not, and, if creative, they ought to be able to manifest their creativity across a range of fields. An eloquent spokesman for this position is Samuel Johnson, who once defined "true genius" as "a mind of large general powers, accidentally determined to some particular direction" (Bate, 1979, p. 252). And even those who concede the existence of specific talents at the highest level are inclined to believe that individuals creative in one area ought to be able to exhibit similar efflorescence in other fields, were they to put their minds to the task.

The thrust of much recent work, however, including my own studies in neuropsychology and developmental psychology, suggests that cognition ought to be decomposed into a number of parts, modules, or factors, with each operating according to its own set of principles (Fodor, 1983; Gardner, 1983). On this contrasting account, cognition consists of such disparate areas as language, logical problem solving, musical competence, spatial skill, and the like. And by a corollary assumption, an individual can achieve a high level of competence, or even the heights of creativity, in a given area of accomplishment without there following any necessary implications about competence in other domains of experience. Should this point of view become accepted, one would no longer speak (except in shorthand) of an individual as creative; instead, one would recognize the possibilities of creativity in specific domains and of individuals who are creative artists, scientists, politicians, or inventors, but who could in no way be substituted for one another.

A first step in studying creativity, then, involves acknowledgment that there are different arenas of potential creativity and that each merits separate investigation. Given provisional acceptance of the idea that cognition and creativity exist in specific spheres of knowledge or competence, it becomes important to discover what those areas are and how the lines between them are best delineated. In earlier work, I proposed a set of seven human intellectual competences or "intelligences" that might serve as an initial list of areas of creativity. However, building on the work of my colleagues David Feldman (1980, 1986) and Mihaly Csikszentmihalyi (Csikszentmihalyi & Robinson, 1986), I have been developing an approach that seems more adequate to the task at hand. We find it useful to distinguish among the following levels of analysis:

1. *The subpersonal.* Any human activity rests ultimately on the biological substrate: the genetic endowment, the structure and functioning of the nervous system, various metabolic and hormonal factors, and the like. Thus far, little has been established for certain about the ways in which these factors contribute to unusual human performances, such as those involved in creative activities over the course of a lifetime. And yet, given the rapid increase in knowledge about the functioning of the nervous system, and the devising of methods whereby neural structures can be studied in vivo and without risk, it appears highly likely that we shall soon be able to pinpoint at least some of the neurobiological facets of human creativity.

2. *The personal.* Consistent with standard psychological taxonomies, it is useful to distinguish two separate perspectives at the level of the person. Adopting the *cognitive approach* mentioned earlier, we can speak of the intellectual competences or intelligences that are manifest by creative individuals. Individuals "at promise" in a particular area as a result of genetic or early environmental factors can advance rapidly in one or more of the seven human intelligences. Ordinarily it is difficult to observe intelligences at work in pure form, but in the case of certain exceptional children, such as those who are autistic, one can peer at an intelligence with little interference. The child artist Nadia, who has very highly developed spatial and bodily kinesthetic skills, exhibits these forms of intelligence with crystalline clarity and insularity (Selfe, 1977). Also, when an individual advances with great rapidity, one has the impression that the faculty or intelligence is again operating with relatively little external molding. Musical prodigies like Mozart, or mathematical prodigies like Gauss, give the impression of an intelligence unfolding or expressing itself in preadapted form. Although creativity involves more than giftedness or precocity, there is little question that a high degree of talent in an intelligence can be an important contributor to a creative life.

In many cases, one can observe a combination of intelligences at work. Thus, Freud seems to have been very gifted in at least three forms of human intelligence – linguistic, logical-mathematical, and intrapersonal – and he combined these talents in his scientific and clinical work. It seem likely that individuals who accomplish a great deal were "at promise" in relevant areas from early in life; and yet it is certainly possible that effective training methods might allow even individuals with relatively modest initial endowments to attain very high levels of accomplishment (Walters & Gardner, 1986).

Complementing the cognitive approach at the personal level is an approach that focuses instead on factors of *personality, motivation,* and *drive.* Even the strongest biological proclivities and the most finely honed set of intelligences are unlikely to yield creative products unless the individual also exhibits certain traits of personality. Indeed, certain degrees of drive, motivation, and energy may even prove more constant concomitants of creativity than any particular pattern of cognitive strengths.

3. *The extrapersonal.* I have in mind here the structure of an area of knowledge or human accomplishment – what I shall hereafter, following David Feldman, call a *domain.* Though initially devised by individuals over the course of years or generations, bodies of knowledge can be examined as extrapersonal phenomena in their own right and analyzed in terms of their principal structures, operations, and so forth. Taken together, these bodies of knowledge constitute what Karl Popper (1976) has termed "World III." Thus, anyone knowledgeable about mathematics can examine the field or a particular subfield (such as calculus or topology), lay out its critical features, distinguish levels of competence within the area, and the like. Often these areas can be instructively examined in terms of their symbolic systems and codes (Gardner, Howard, & Perkins, 1974), as well as the skills needed to master these systems. Such domains may map quite closely onto a single human intelligence – as appears to be the case with music or mathematics. However, they may also draw on amalgams of intelligences. Thus, a domain like chess draws on logical-mathematical and spatial intelligence and may also require a certain degree of interpersonal sensitivity. The practice of psychotherapy stresses linguistic and interpersonal skills, whereas spatial and musical capacities assume little importance in that domain.

A biological potential or intelligence may unfold initially with relatively little influence being exerted by the structure of a particular domain as it happens to be constituted in the individual's milieu. Sooner or later, however, intersection with the relevant domain(s) in the culture becomes an imperative (except in the case of severe pathology). Indeed, one who would engage in creative work must situate oneself in relation to one or more domains. At any particular historical moment, one has a certain level of knowledge or mastery of the domain. Also, the domain itself stands at a certain level of development, with its own problems, questions, unresolved issues, and the like.

The ultimate creativity of an individual is constrained in important respects by the level of development of the body of knowledge when the individual initially confronts it. Thus, Einstein encountered the domain of physics at a time when many fundamental assumptions could no longer be reasonably sustained; his contribution was to reconfigure the domain in ways that proved acceptable for a considerable period of time. Arnold Schoenberg began the study of music at a time when Western diatonic music appeared to be entrenched, but he eventually responded to incipient trends of polytonality and atonality by devising his own system of fully atonal or 12-tone music. Freud was working initially in the relatively well defined domains of neurology and neuroanatomy, but he soon began to pursue issues that did not fall within a recognized scientific domain and that may well have been subsumed in earlier times under the purview of literature, religion, or folk medicine.

Individuals equipped with their own peculiar blend of intelligences must somehow learn about and become engaged with the domains within their culture. This engagement sometimes occurs through "crystallizing experiences" in which a chance (or planned) encounter with some hitherto unfamiliar material or problem has a dramatically motivating effect on the individual (Walters & Gardner, 1986). Subsequently, individuals become involved in one or more projects drawn from the domain. Initially these projects are presented by teachers or drawn from books, but ultimately one devises one's own projects. An individual working on projects that are promising within a given domain has the opportunity to make a creative contribution to that domain.

4. *The multipersonal.* Encompassing both the individual intelligence and the impersonally conceived domain is the social context or *field* in which individuals make (or fail to make) their way. Following Csikszentmihalyi and Robinson (1986), the field may be defined as the social organization of the domain – the pivotal roles that must be filled as well as the behaviors and norms associated with a domain within a particular society. A scientist like Einstein does not simply devise a theory of relativity free of supporting context. He learns about the domain of physics through conversing with physicists, reading books, taking courses, writing papers, exchanging messages and manuscripts with colleagues, attending meetings and presenting papers, and the like. A composer like Arnold Schoenberg does not simply inject 12-tone music into a void or, for that matter, a randomly selected concert hall. Instead, he masters the existing musical literature, begins to compose formally, has his compositions performed and reviewed in respected surroundings, gathers students unto himself, promulgates his new ideas, and is either welcomed or scorned, immediately and in the long run.

Contrary to psychoanalytic mythology, Freud hardly arrived at his contributions in independence of his surroundings. Beneficiary of the greatest teachers of his age, having close confidants on whom he could rely, Freud had ample opportunity to relate his ideas to scientific and medical colleagues. And once it became clear to him – and to others – that he had arrived at an innovative theory of personality and an apparently effective form of treatment, much of the rest of his long life was dedicated to founding and furthering the field of psychoanalysis, into which those interested in his studies would be initiated – not without considerable struggle in many cases.

Just as projects may be viewed as the interface between the individual and the domain, social institutions may be conceptualized as the intermediary between an individual and the field. It is through participation in social institutions – schools, museums, laboratories, journals, meetings, apprenticeship systems – that an individual who aspires to work in a given area of knowledge has the opportunity to become engaged with the relevant persons and platforms.

Creativity: a challenge and an opportunity for "synthetic science"

Cognitive science as synthetic science

In recent years it has become increasingly apparent that issues of the mind transcend the boundaries of any single scientific discipline. This widespread realization gave rise in the last decade to the formation of a new discipline, or supradiscipline, called cognitive science. Inspired in many ways by the advent of the digital computer, and fueled by intriguing convergences in the history of several neighboring disciplines, workers in philosophy, psychology, linguistics, anthropology, neuroscience, and artificial intelligence have banded together in order to tackle major cognitive issues – ranging from the nature of perception to assessment of human rationality (Gardner, 1985).

Cognitive science is still in its earliest phase, and it may be premature to evaluate the achievements of the field, let alone to predict its future. Still, one thing seems clear: If cognitive science is to fulfill its promise, it will have to tackle the most formidable issues concerning the human mind. It is perhaps fitting, therefore, that a self-styled alliance of the disciplines of the mind direct some of its powers to consideration of one of the most difficult – but also most alluring – of cognitive issues: the nature of human creativity.

In truth, few individuals who call themselves cognitive scientists have focused on creativity. The topic seems too large, too elusive, not yet sufficiently defined. It may not be too early, however, to sketch out the form that a cognitive scientific approach to creativity might follow. Such, indeed, is the burden of the remainder of this chapter.

If cognitive science holds promise of illuminating issues of creativity, why speak of "synthetic science" rather than simply of "cognitive science"? The principal reason is that the particular blend of disciplines that seems appropriate today to an investigation of creativity does not map readily onto any current definition of cognitive science. The usual central disciplines of psychology and artificial intelligence are far too narrow to account for creative activities. The broader definition, espoused by the Sloan Foundation and adhered to in my study of cognitive science (Gardner, 1985), includes certain disciplines, such as philosophy, linguistics, and anthropology, that apparently have little to contribute to the present study. Perhaps most important, certain fields, such as the study of personality and motivation, though highly relevant to creativity, clearly fall outside the purview of cognitive science as currently construed. Rather than try to twist the term "cognitive science'' to meet present purposes, it seems preferable to coin the epithet ''synthetic science'' to cover interdisciplinary efforts that seek to illuminate a complex phenomenon like human creativity.

In the remainder of this chapter, I shall in fact suggest some of the features that such an account might exhibit. As noted, my principal example will be the life and work of Sigmund Freud. It should therefore be stressed that I am not a ''Freud scholar'' and that Freud is used here for illustrative purposes. Rather than revolving around the precise facts of Freud's biography, the ensuing discussion is animated by the kinds of questions that his life raises and the suitability of synthetic science for addressing these questions. Like most other amateurs, I rely heavily on Ernest Jones's pioneering biography (1961).

Psychological approaches: the intelligences and the person

Psychology, particularly in its cognitive guise, plays a central role in any cognitive science, and particularly so in the study of a single creative individual. A psychological approach to creativity may begin with an examination of the cognitive strengths or intelligences possessed by the subject. It should also attempt to model the processes exhibited by the subject at work, as well as the ways in which the subject's principal creative products are mentally represented over time.

Creativity extends beyond these cognitive-psychological boundaries. Issues of personality, motivation, and individual style are pertinent to the establishment and maintenance of a creative life. So, too, the social circle in which one spends one's life (in particular, one's friends and family) must be taken into account. Thus, our psychological account must incorporate facets of social and personality psychology and indicate how social, personality, and cognitive factors interact in a given life.

Freud's biographers make it clear that he was an individual who would have been considered highly intelligent by almost any definition – lay or technical. He attended high school a year before the normal age and stood at the head of his class for the last 6 years. His performance was so remarkable that he was hardly ever questioned in class, and he graduated summa cum laude (Jones, 1961, p. 17). Freud's father, himself an intelligent man, once declared that ''my Sigmund's little toe is cleverer than my head'' (Jones, 1961, p. 16).

It is possible to pinpoint Freud's gifts. His memory was astounding. During his youth, photographic recall allowed him to glance at textbooks and then recall the wording exactly (Jones, 1961, p. 38). In later life he remembered many passages he had committed to memory in childhood in a variety of languages (Jones, 1961, p. 161). He invariably lectured without notes and had no need to prepare; in his own words, ''I must leave it to my unconscious'' (Jones, 1961, p. 223).

From a ''multiple-intelligences'' perspective, it appears certain that Freud was extremely gifted in linguistic intelligence. In addition to the evidence for linguistic memory already cited, Freud easily learned English as a child and read voraciously in that language. He was competent in French, quoted comfortably from Latin, and learned Spanish in order to read Cervantes in the original (Gedo, 1983). He was especially gifted as a translator, rendering into German John Stuart Mill from the English and his teachers Charcot and Bernheim from French. According to Jones, "he would read a passage, close the book, and consider how a German writer would have clothed the same thoughts – a method not very common among translators. His translating work was both brilliant and rapid" (Jones, 1961, p. 37). He was able to write with extreme rapidity and with hardly any need for revision.

In 1915, at age 59, he wrote five of his most original and profound essays about metapsychology within a 6-week period. Jones comments, with perhaps a shade of hyperbole, "that they could all have been composed in the space of six weeks seems scarcely credible; yet it happened. Such a factor of activity would be hard to equal in the history of scientific production" (Jones, 1961, p. 344). Then, in the next 6 weeks, he went on to write five more essays. Small surprise that Freud was awarded the coveted Goethe Prize for writing in 1930.

Before entering psychology, Freud had been a major worker in the area of neuroanatomy, where he made a number of important, though not revolutionary, discoveries. It would seem probable, therefore, that Freud possessed logical-mathematical gifts, the kinds of abilities on which scientists characteristically rely. The tightly reasoned quality of many of Freud's writings – in particular the "Project" of 1895 and the metapsychological essays of his mature years – convince me that this was the case. It is therefore revealing to note that Freud himself disagreed. Often in his life he would complain about his lack of intelligence, and it seems clear that he had in mind a deficiency in logic and mathematics that kept him from performing at the very peak of these areas of knowledge. He complained that he had not been given "a better intellectual equipment. . . . I am not really a man of science" (Jones, 1961, p. xi). He once declared "my chief reproach to the Almighty would be that he had not given me a better brain" (Jones, 1961, p. 26). At another time, Freud added, "I have very restricted capacities or talents. None at all for the natural sciences; nothing for mathematics; nothing for anything quantitative. But what I have, of a very restricted nature, was probably very intensive" (Jones, 1961, p. 366).

Lest it be thought that Freud simply held an unjustifiably low opinion of himself, it is instructive to see how he viewed his own powers. Rather than seeing himself as a scientist, or even a scholar, Freud thought of himself as an individual of great curiosity, who felt the need to understand and to speculate (Jones, 1961, p. 23). As a youngster, he had been fascinated by military matters and had strongly identified with the great military leaders of the past (Jones, 1961, p. 19). Although a career in the military was not an option for a Jewish lad growing up in the Hapsburg Empire, Freud persisted in seeing himself as a conqueror or "conquistador." Fiercely ambitious, he cast about for a domain in which he could make a major contribution. Once having decided on a career in medical science, he searched widely for an area of medical science in which he could make a contribution. Having found himself unsuited for many areas, he eventually gravitated toward neuroanatomy, a specialty for which he felt that his configuration of talents was in fact suited (Jones, 1961, p. 29). Within the neural sciences, he soon evinced a preference for examination and observation, rather than experimentation – as Jones puts it, a preference for the eye over the hand. Neuroanatomy remained for Freud a favored area of study, but when he confronted the fact that others were more likely to reach the pinnacle of that field, he began to cast about for an area to which his gifts would be more precisely suited.

Freud attributed his ultimate success less to his intellectual endowment (about which he remained ambivalent) and more to habits of character. As he put it, ''my whole capacity for work probably lies in my character attributes and in the lack of any marked intellectual deficiency. . . . I know that that admixture is very favorable for slowly winning success'' (Jones, 1961, p. 131). Indeed, on the ambitious scale of accomplishment against which Freud measured himself, success did come late – it was only in his late thirties that he entered the areas in which he ultimately became esteemed. This did not surprise Freud, for he saw himself in opposition to very potent forces and knew that he was working in an area that was highly speculative and fraught with scientific traps. It is worth noting that the domain of psychoanalysis is an area in which achievements routinely have come late in life. Indeed, according to John Gedo (1983), analysts almost never make major contributions before the age of 50.

Excellent work habits, a dogged determination, powerful linguistic and adequate logical abilities were enough to ensure that Freud could become a respected scientific worker, but not a world-class creative individual. In Ernest Jones's view, Freud's most irreplaceable gift was his ability to find in an isolated fact the key to a central puzzle: ''When he got a hold of a simple but significant fact he would feel, and know, that it was an example of something general or universal. . . . when Freud found in himself previously unknown attitudes toward his parents, he felt immediately that they were not peculiar to himself and that he had discovered something about human nature in general: Oedipus, Hamlet, and the rest soon flashed across his mind'' (Jones, 1961, p. 68). It is worth remarking that this ability to discover a world view in an isolated fact is often a hallmark of a scientific genius (Lorenz, 1966; Peirce, 1929), but this talent also entails the possibility of jumping prematurely to an erroneous conclusion. In fact, Freud's career is punctuated with just such instances, ranging from his mistaken view of cocaine as a miraculous cure for all manner of illnesses to his belief, which he later rejected, that all hysteria derives from traumatic seduction in early childhood.

Like certain scientific innovators, then, Freud had a peculiar blend of logical-mathematical abilities that was joined to an exceptional linguistic intelligence. There are no signs that Freud stood out in the spatial, musical, or bodily kinesthetic areas; indeed, he may well have been quite poor in one or more of these faculties. On the other hand, there is ample evidence that Freud had unusual personal intelligence: both an interpersonal intelligence that allowed him to grasp the workings of other individuals and an intrapersonal intelligence that revealed many facets (including deep aspects) of his own personality and allowed him to act in light of this penetrating self-knowledge. I would go so far as to say that Freud's genius lay in his virtually unprecedented linking of the intelligences usually associated with science (language and logic) with the personal intelligences that are generally unremarkable in scientific workers, but that in Freud's case gave rise to new areas of knowledge.

Turning from an examination of Freud's profile of intelligences to aspects of his personality, we find that Freud provides eloquent testimony to his belief that the keys to an individual life can be found in one's early experiences. His early life was marked by a series of signs that he was special: He was born in a caul; an old peasant woman asserted soon afterward that an important person had been placed into the world; when he was age 12, a passing poet versified that he would become a cabinet minister (Sulloway, 1983, pp. 476–477). He was the eldest of 7 children and, from all reports, the strong favorite of his mother. As he once declared, "people who know that they are preferred or favored by their mother give evidence in their lives of a peculiar self-reliance and an unshakeable optimism which often seem like heroic attributes and bring actual success to their possessors" (Sulloway, 1983, p. 477). Thus, Freud's formidable talents were reinforced by magical "signs" of his specialness and by unquestioned support on the part of his family.

Although Freud could be very self-critical and underwent definite periods of depression, he was basically a very confident individual – possibly as a consequence of an early life in which he was treated as very important and during which he achieved considerable success. To self-confidence Freud wedded combativeness and tenacity. As he observed to his fiancée in an unguarded moment, "I have often felt as though I had inherited all the defiance and all the passions with which our ancestors defended their Temple and could gladly sacrifice my life for one great moment in history" (Sulloway, 1983, p. 86). And on another occasion, he declared, "I am nothing but by temperament a *conquistador* – an adventurer if you want to translate the word – with the curiosity, the boldness, and the tenacity that belong to that type of being. Such people are apt to be treasured if they succeed, if they have really discovered something; otherwise they are thrown aside" (Jones, 1961, p. 227). And so to talent and magical signs were added a willingness to confront hostility and a strong inclination to persevere.

Whatever Freud's leanings toward conquest, speculation, and optimism, he succeeded early on in uniting these traits with a strong sense of discipline. A telltale marker was his decision to enter medicine, and then the specialty of neuroanatomy, where there was scant opportunity for wild speculative sprees. As he put it, "As a young man I felt a strong attraction toward speculation and ruthlessly checked it" (Jones, 1961, p. 23). In early adulthood he began the practice of working for nearly all of his waking hours and maintained this demanding schedule until near the time of his death (Jones, 1961, pp. 107, 357). Indeed, he would devote up to 12 or 13 hours a day to psychoanalysis, seeing patients until 10 o'clock in the evening, and then writing in the evening from 11 o'clock until 1 or 2 o'clock in the morning (Jones, 1961, p. 358). Even during his infrequent periods of depression, he still continued to be busy and productive. He realized the importance of this dogged dedication when he remarked that there is a vast difference between casual flashes of intuition and taking an idea seriously, working through all of its complexities and winning it universal acceptance (Jones, 1961, p. 162). Moreover, Freud believed in the importance of continuing to work even when ideas were not in abundance; when an idea did not come to him, "now I go half-way to meet it" (Jones, 1961, pp. 224–225).

In one area of his life, Freud differed from nearly all earlier scientists. Whereas most scientists can (and perhaps prefer to) keep their own lives at arm's length, Freud's very scientific being came to rest on the facts and the feelings of his own life. Quite possibly, the most significant and the most daring decision of his professional life was the initiation in 1897 of his self-analysis: the exercise, which he continued until the end of his life, of examining his deepest thoughts for clues about how his mind (particularly its least accessible processes) operated. Moreover, Freud did not simply pursue the self-analysis for his own personal edification; he shared his hopes and fears, his embarrassments and his triumphs, his most profane wishes and most ardent secret hates, with his readers and his live audiences. And even when he may have wished to disguise these experiences, the fact that he was willing to publish his dreams left them as fair game for all succeeding analysts – a challenge that more than few have taken up in the ensuing decades.

As a result of this baring of his soul, we have considerable information about Freud's family life, his friends, and his professional enemies as well. Freud emerges as someone who identified strongly with his roots – with his parents, the rest of his family, his Jewish background – even as he was ultimately quite critical of most of his professional colleagues and of the duplicities and injustices meted out by Viennese society. Freud had a compelling need to form alliances with individuals and an equally strong need to define others as belonging to an out-group. For many years he felt extremely isolated, particularly in view of the skepticism toward his theory expressed by most members of the Viennese scientific and medical establishments. At the same time, however, he had excellent teachers – the neuroanatomist Bruecke and the psychiatrist Charcot – who supported his professional endeavors during the first years of his career, as well as loyal friends, first Josef Breuer and then Wilhelm Fliess, who shared his inchoate ideas and supported him as best they could. Nor were these individuals "fringe characters"; whereas Breuer was more conservative and Fliess yet more radical than Freud, both were highly cultivated and successful physicians whose esteem must have meant a great deal to the struggling Freud.

Once psychoanalysis had been launched, Freud's interactions with others took on a different cast. Instead of being the junior member of a relationship, he became the focal figure, the individual around whom other younger physicians began to gather. In retrospect, it is clear that Freud made mistakes in the way in which he sought to promulgate his views and to organize his followers, and he paid dearly for these errors. And yet it seems apparent that psychoanalysis could not have achieved international success without his considerable gifts of leadership and his ability to mobilize and influence fellow human beings. Freud exploited his formidable talents in both the intrapersonal and the interpersonal domains.

This cursory sketch of Freud's capacities and life experiences as viewed from a psychological perspective reminds us of the multiplicity of factors that interact and contribute to the achievement of a single creative life. In a case study, it is of course impossible to determine which of these factors were truly essential, which could have been dispensed with, which might even have thwarted Freud. The purpose of a psychological investigation of a single creative individual is to come up with the most plausible account of the roles played by various factors and, most especially, to achieve some understanding of how these various cognitive, personality, and social factors interacted at specific points in the individual's life. Only when numerous case studies like this have been carried out does it become plausible to propose models of the creative psychologist, the creative natural scientist, or (should it prove possible) the creative person in general.

The domains of Freud's contributions: cognitive representation and artificial intelligences

Until now, my focus has been on the personal level of analysis – Freud's cognitive profile, his personality traits, his motivation, his relation to important others in his personal and professional circles. It is possible, however, to look at Freud's work – his professional achievement – while factoring Freud's personal contributions out of the picfure. In so doing, in studying Freud's contributions as if they had been achieved by someone else, one focuses on the domain of knowledge.

A study of domains can proceed in one of two directions. On the one hand, there are the particular domains of knowledge in which Freud worked, ranging from neuroanatomy to clinical psychiatry, from literary criticism to sociology. In this case, one views Freud as a contributor to several domains. On the other hand, one can elect to focus instead on Freud's achievement as if it were itself a domain. In this latter case, a domain study amounts to a series of portraits of Freud's own work as it evolved through its various phases. In each case the interest lies not in a summary of what Freud did but rather in the ways in which his life work was original (i.e., made a novel and substantive contribution to an area of knowledge or itself constituted a set of creative products).

To attempt a characterization of the domain(s) of Freud's work would far exceed the scope of this essay – indeed, it is an effort that would require many volumes. My purpose here, far more modest, is to indicate which tools of cognitive science might be brought to bear on this task.

Such a domain analysis begins with a designation of the principal precepts and lines of knowledge that existed prior to Freud's involvement in a given domain of knowledge or practice. Because Freud contributed to approximately a dozen separate areas of science and cultural analysis, this would be a formidable task. (Frank

Sulloway's attempt, 1983, to relate Freud's contributions to the evolutionary biology of his day runs several hundred pages.) Following the opening designation, one would seek in each case to isolate the particular scholarly contributions made by Freud and to determine the ways in which the consequent discipline was affected (or remained unaffected) by his work. Naturally, experts in the history of each domain would need to be recruited for such an endeavor.

In Freud's case, the task becomes yet more formidable, for Freud did not simply contribute to existing areas of knowledge. In some cases, such as the psychology of personality, he radically reshaped the domain. In others, such as the treatment of neurosis, it might equally well be said that he created an entirely new domain.

So far, the study of domains of knowledge has been approached principally from the point of view of the historian of science. However, the same task can and should be approached as well by the scientist interested in cognitive representations. Here the task entails an effort to describe Freud's "mental models" as they existed, and as they changed at crucial times during his scientific evolution (Gentner & Stevens, 1983; Johnson-Laird, 1983). Such an endeavor would include microscopic examinations of particularly crucial intervals: for example, the frequent changes in Freud's conceptualizations during his work on the "Project for a Scientific Psychology" of 1895 (Pribram & Gill, 1976). It would also include more macroscopic examinations: for instance, a tracing of the evolving conceptions of the ego, or of anxiety, over several years. In addition, such an enterprise would involve consideration of which aspects of Freud's scientific development exploited knowledge obtained far earlier in his career and which aspects were genuinely dependent on new findings or insights obtained from recent reading or clinical experience.

The observer will legitimately ask if the nascent discipline of cognitive science possesses special tools for such efforts. The answer, in truth, must be tentative, for as I have noted, few cognitive scientists have directed their attention to creative products of any scope. In Howard Gruber's pioneering investigation (1981) of the notebooks of Charles Darwin, however, we encounter a useful model of how such a cognitive analysis might work. What is needed, at one extreme, is the most fine-grained analysis of the degree of knowledge possessed, and the way it is organized, during every step of a creative scientific breakthrough. (This is what Gruber achieved in his examination of the notebooks kept by Darwin during a crucial period of his thinking.) On the other extreme, equally necessary, are more general concepts: for example, images of wide scope that will guide an inquiry, a network of enterprise that will incorporate the various kinds of questions on which engaged scientists find themselves working at any one time, and so on (Gruber, 1982).

Although none of these tools is the exclusive possession of contemporary cognitive scientists, our understanding of mental representations (schemas) and transformations should facilitate a more systematic and testable analysis than was hitherto possible (Gentner & Stevens, 1983; Johnson-Laird, 1983; Perkins, 1981). Moreover, it is so complex a task to keep track of the various schemata of knowledge possessed by any individual, let alone the creative scientist, that only powerful computers have the potential to handle this task. Even casual consideration of the many different enterprises in which Freud worked over 70 years, the hundreds of projects in which he became engaged and brought to fruition, should underscore the need for powerful computational aids in any comprehensive analysis of the domain we might term FREUD.

Here lies the opportunity for artificial intelligence. A principal goal of this new field is to devise clear models of cognitive processes and to determine if these models are viable (e.g., whether or not they exhibit psychological plausibility). We are still some distance from being able to model the understanding of an expert in a given field, let alone the contributions of a genius caught in the process of founding a new field. And yet, in principle, it should be possible to model the changing thought processes of an active scientist and to ascertain whether or not that model is in fact viable. If one can seek to model the mind of a paranoid (PARRY) or the processes of induction used in arriving at a scientific principle (BACON) (Boden, 1976), why not attempt to model the mind of a creative scientist? Furthermore, if the modeling of a mind of a creative artist or scientist still has a science-fiction flavor to it, that is not the case for the modeling of individuals who are in the process of gaining knowledge about a new area. Individuals training to be psycho-analysts (or psychological theorists) pass through a sequence that can be well described as a novice-to-expert transition; the modeling of such a passage is cer-tainly within the purview of artificial intelligence.

An approach via artificial intelligence exhibits another advantage. In considering the contributions of an individual like Freud, who was in many ways an authentic hero, one is prone to become enwrapped in the mythology of psychoanalysis and to attribute more originality to his discoveries than may actually be warranted. Com-putational models allow one to examine the sources and the transformations of ideas without any interference from knowledge of the personal circumstances surrounding the creation. If Frank Sulloway is correct, nearly all of Freud's major discoveries had been anticipated – in some cases by well-known predecessors like Darwin or Krafft-Ebing, in other cases by his own intimates whom he did not adequately acknowledge, such as Wilhelm Fliess or Alfred Adler. Doubtless one result of the domain study espoused here would be to document the extent to which Freud stood on the shoulders of giants and peers. One trusts that his contribution is sufficiently singular that it would survive such dissection.

A final question concerns the limits of domain study. Where does humanistic scholarship stop and cognitive science commence? The beginnings of an answer lie in the search for general patterns and for replicability. Whereas a study of creative lives and products should, in my view, begin with a sophisticated understanding of particular instances, it need not end there. The cognitive scientist is on the lookout for principles and laws that will pertain to groups of individuals, if not to all instances of creativity. The humanistic scholar does not have such generalizations as a major goal and indeed may be more interested in particularities, peculiarities, and exceptions than in universals. Thus, in considering the foregoing sketch of

Freud, the cognitive scientist is not interested primarily in the particular set of intelligences or social factors that produced Freud, but rather in the ways in which intelligences or social factors coalesce, more generally, in order to produce multiple exemplars of creativity. And by the same token, construction of models is intended not merely to account for the contributions of one individual – no matter how outstanding – but rather to understand altogether the nature of creative enterprises.

This statement of the potential contributions of artificial intelligence also points to a possible test of the effectiveness of a model. Individuals of high creativity are generally able, when confronted with new information or arguments, to formulate responses or solutions that grow out of their schemas of knowledge. If a model of an individual's capacities and skills is truly comprehensive, it ought to be able to simulate the kinds of conclusions to which an individual would come if presented with new data of this sort. Successful performance at this simulation could serve as a confirmation that the model has appropriate information embedded within it. As Csikszentmihalyi (personal communication) has pointed out, however, it is far more challenging to find new problems, or to determine which data are relevant to a problem one is attempting to solve.

The field of Freud: the historical-cultural context

The "genetic" Freud could have lived anywhere on the planet, but the "historical" Freud spent most of his life in Vienna. Around the turn of the century, Vienna was in many ways unique, and it is appropriate to assume that this cultural "field" exerted an important, if not decisive, impact on Freud's lines of development (see Janik & Toulmin, 1973, and Schorske, 1981, for detailed descriptions of fin-de-siècle Vienna).

On the surface, Vienna seemed the stable and powerful capital of the spacious and long-lived Austro-Hungarian Empire. Ruled by Emperor Franz Josef from 1848 to 1916, it seemed to represent solid Catholic values that were shared by aristocrats and leading members of the bourgeoisie. As a place of learning, Vienna had few peers, and as a medical center, it was arguably the best in the world. There was a liberal minority whose members occasionally occupied positions of influence, but in general the community embraced reactionary positions and spurned novel political ideas. Curiously, however, there was a guarded tolerance rather than repression of innovative ideas in the arts and sciences.

In this peculiar tension between political and social conservatism, on the one hand, and tacit support for the exploration of new ideas in arts and sciences, on the other, lay the special genius of fin-de-siècle Vienna. Those involved in these speculative areas formed a small but influential group that was essentially cosmopolitan and supranational rather than narrowly Viennese or Austro-Hungarian. In a way difficult for us to appreciate, disciplinary specialization was scarcely known. Whatever their major professional identifications, Viennese citizens were exposed to a wide range of ideas, and most leading intellectual figures were familiar with the currents in disparate areas. Moreover, these individuals frequently invaded one another's life spaces. To take just a few examples, composer Anton Bruckner taught piano to physicist Ludwig Boltzmann; Gustav Mahler brought his psychological problems to Freud; Breuer was the physician to philosopher Franz Brentano; the home of philosopher Ludwig Wittgenstein was a center of discussion in areas ranging from music to psychology (Janik & Toulmin, 1973, p. 92).

Finding themselves at the cutting edge in their respective fields, yet in touch with the range of disciplines, living in a seat of power, but within a community that was somewhat marginal, wrestling with the tension between conservatism and tolerance, brilliant young Viennese were in a privileged position to rethink the basic assumptions of their chosen domains. And that is what they did, in domain after domain, in the period from 1880 to 1920. Cherished ideals such as belief in progress, reason, and order; entrenched assumptions such as the need for disciplined conformity; aesthetic norms such as musical tonality, visual realism, and literary restraint; articles of faith such as the Kantian conceptions of space and time – all of these and many more were challenged by the best minds of the time. There was a widespread desire to cut oneself off from historical precedents, to open oneself to hitherto mysterious psychic states, to cast an ironic glance at entrenched values, to locate or found key conceptions that could set the tone for the unknown century ahead.

Sigmund Freud was as sensitive to, and as much an instrument of, these features as any of his contemporaries. Indeed, trained in the sciences, but working in areas abutting the humanities, he was especially alert to the collapsing of norms and the undermining of shibboleths everywhere. He was politically liberal in a conservative epoch, a Jew in an environment in which anti-Semitism was rife (if not always overt), a champion of sexual issues in an environment that suppressed explicit mention of erotic themes. Freud felt the tensions acutely. Freud often spoke critically of the Viennese surroundings, and as a practical matter he avoided ''high society'' of any sort and remained within his small and almost entirely Jewish circle. And yet it can be argued that Freud had a symbiotically productive relationship with his home territory; living elsewhere, he might not have had the opportunity to make many of the observations that were key to his theory. Nor would he have felt that intense struggle between the expression of human instincts and the dictates of a repressive society that ultimately animated his theoretical edifice.

One cannot perform the crucial experiment and move Freud to another location, any more than one can exchange Ludwig Wittgenstein with Jean-Paul Sartre, Arnold Schoenberg with Charles Ives, or Gustav Klimt with Aubrey Beardsley. Yet the incredible flowering of talent in Vienna during a relatively brief period of time is powerful evidence that the particular atmosphere was conducive to creativity – even as Florence in the Renaissance and China during the T'ang dynasty were similarly catalytic. Perhaps the best evidence for this massive ''field effect'' lies in the poignant fate of Vienna in the latter period of Freud's life. Franz Josef died in 1916, the Hapsburg house did not survive the end of World War I, and Vienna as a major intellectual community did not outlast Hitler's regime. Indeed, it could be argued that there has not been a single figure in the post–World War II era in Vienna who can match the dozens of luminaries who frequented the coffeehouses in Freud's time. President Kurt Waldheim epitomizes the current gray era.

Cultural-historical studies connect human cognition to the environment or field in which it is nourished or where it is redirected or thwarted. No matter when or where one lives, an individual confronts a domain of knowledge within particular fields, ranging from the intimate family circles where education begins to the larger institutions of society in which one ultimately traffics. Placing Freud at the center, one can draw circles of various radii extending outward and including his early family and school environments, the university and medical schools, his post-university training in France as well as Vienna, the laboratories and clinics where his crucial observations were made, the lecture halls and journals where his ideas were first tried out publicly, the columns of newspapers in Vienna in which they were sometimes ridiculed, his first group of intimate followers who met Wednesday evenings in his home, and, eventually, his ever expanding circle of students, peers, friends, admirers, and detractors all over the world, beginning in the 1910s and extending even until today.

Again, these issues routinely have been considered the realm of biographers and historians. The anthropologist or historian of science with a cognitive scientific slant will adopt a comparative approach: a contrast of Vienna with other cities, of Freud's circle with other circles, of progress in a field like psychology with comparable progress in physics, poetry, or pottery. Of special interest here will be those rare communities, institutions, or situations in which creativity seems to flower – which may range from a period of several generations in Florence to the ambit of a particular high school in Budapest or the Bronx. And by the same token, it will be of interest to carry out studies of communities or schools in which high creativity might have been anticipated, but where, for reasons as yet undetermined, there were few, if any, creative individuals or creative products.

For those of a psychological persuasion, the field may seem a simple backdrop against which individual human talents and creativities exhibit themselves. It is possible – and salutary – to shift this emphasis and to view the field as the "prime mover." On such an analysis, it is the particular era and institutions that are in need of a breakthrough of one or another sort – and a particular individual is simply a vessel through which these needs can be satisfied. If Freud had not existed, perhaps he would have had to be invented? Or perhaps his role would have been taken instead by Pierre Janet of Paris, Carl Jung of Zurich, or William James in the United States. In all probability, the extent of contribution of individual genius will depend on the particular area of knowledge at issue and the particular contribution that has been made. In other words, individuals will differ in terms of indispensability.

In at least one respect, however, the field proves indispensable. Without the criteria and standards imposed by the field, it is simply impossible to determine which individuals have made genuinely important contributions (e.g., Freud) and which are better regarded as "false positives" (e.g., Fliess). For this reason it is impossible to demonstrate that an individual is both creative and obscure. The very act of determining that an individual is genuinely creative rather than fraudulent necessitates imposing some communal standards. One might even speak here of an indeterminacy principle at work in the case of the proverbial "hermit creator": In the absence of imposed standards, it is impossible to determine whether or not the hermit is indeed creative. Once standards are imposed, the hermit has been reintroduced into society.

Biological foundations of creativity

Even as cultural studies of the "field" define the upper bound for a study of creativity, the biological and neurological disciplines delineate a lower bound (analyses at the level of atomic particles are simply irrelevant). Logically, in fact, a synthetic scientific account of creativity ought to begin with consideration of these biological factors, for they are antecedent to any behavior whatsoever.

I have deliberately postponed consideration of these factors, however, for two related reasons: (1) so little is known at this time about biological facets of creativity; (2) the impulse to analyze the biological basis of creativity and giftedness has been a controversial issue, partly for good reasons.

Let me consider the controversy first. For many years, psychologists preferred to adopt a "black-box" approach to mental phenomena. The drive to avoid biology (to which Freud subscribed) reflected the need to establish autonomy for the field, lest it remain forever in the shadow of the "wet" sciences (Gardner, 1985). Added to this disciplinary chauvinism has been a second factor. In many eyes, the search for a biological basis for, say, intelligence or talent has been coterminous with a desire to establish that these factors are innate or predetermined – and hence with a justification of the status quo (Block & Dworkin, 1976). And, indeed, among biological workers of many stripes who have at one time or another directed their attention to such psychological issues, there has been a tendency to minimize environmental contributions to unusual promise or unusual performance.

Neither of these reasons, however, suffices to preclude a genetic or neurobiological approach to issues of creativity. First of all, cognitive studies have established the legitimacy of an analysis on the level of mental representation. The likelihood that a cognitive approach will ever be engulfed by a reductionist approach seems remote (see Gardner, 1985, for extensive discussion of this point). As for the sometime equation of biological with predeterminist or nativist analyses, this may well be a contingent fact, but it is certainly not a necessary conclusion. For that very reason, individuals pursuing a neurobiological analysis of creativity or giftedness ought to be especially vigilant that their findings not be uncritically absorbed into such a framework.

I believe that tools and insights that have been developed in the biological sciences ought to be brought to bear on important facets of human thought and behavior – including the area of creativity. Indeed, just because of the many path-opening findings in biology in the past decades, it is high time to reopen the issue of the biological bases of creative behavior. In this spirit, my colleagues and I have recently convened a conference on the topic of the biology of giftedness (Gardner & Dudai, 1985), and 1 have also explored dimensions of this subject in occasional writings (Gardner, 1975, 1982a, 1982b).

At the present time, it is probably fair to say that biological approaches are more immediately relevant to issues of giftedness than to issues of creativity. That is, it is easier to speculate about the biological bases of unusual precocity or exceptional adult performance than to make analogous inferences about heightened creativity. Indeed, Yadin Dudai has hypothesized (personal communication) that structural differences in the nervous system are more likely to be associated with giftedness, whereas creativity is more likely to be a characteristic of the mode of functioning of an otherwise unremarkable nervous system. Animal models of unusual precocity are also easier to envision than animal models of creative behaviors, especially because the whole realm of creativity – with its heavy "field component" – may be a peculiarly human arena.

Despite these caveats, it is not a difficult matter to list areas of biology that might be relevant to a study of creativity. Any such accounting would certainly include the following: studies of the genetics of unusual abilities and unusual performances; the relevance of animal models and experiments to exceptional human performance; the development of the nervous system in early life and the way in which it comes to be organized in normal and exceptional individuals; the relationships among patterns of cerebral lateralization, neuroanatomic structures, and exceptional capacities (Geschwind & Galaburda, 1986); the processes of cerebral blood flow in unusual individuals as they are engaged in solving problems or creating products; patterns of precocity and aging in individuals with different cognitive profiles: measures of the hormonal and neurochemical patterns of individuals engaged in highly creative activity; studies of energy, drive, and sleep cycles in creative individuals; and dozens of other equally pertinent indices.

What is much more difficult, however, is to institute such lines of research and to determine the ways in which they might genuinely illuminate creative individuals and behaviors. Our own survey has indicated that neurobiological and genetic studies have advanced most rapidly when dealing with systems that are relatively simple and that unfold over a brief span of time. Creativity, however, involves systems of great complexity that unfold over extensive periods of time. Neurobiology is as ill-prepared as cognitive psychology for dealing with these macroscopic phenomena; we do not know how to model events or processes that unfold over many years.

An equally enormous problem involves the issue of individual differences. Until now, studies of individual differences have assumed little import in the neurobiological sciences; universal or species-specific behaviors have (understandably) been at a premium. Indeed, most studies of the aforementioned topics have focused on the species as a whole, or on the grossest individual differences, such as gender or handedness. Yet, as stressed throughout this chapter, creativity must be studied in the *individual* who is creative. Ultimately, then, neurobiologists will need to consider the ways in which particular individuals, and individuals in particular situations, may differ from their peers. Because we do not know if they will differ – let alone in which ways they may differ – the stakes are high in these scientific gambles. Even if we were to have Einstein's or Freud's brain completely at our disposal, it is not clear where we should look or what we should count.

Still, I have little doubt that the speculative leap is worth taking. Just as the mind in its many facets stands as the major "general" target for current neurobiological work, creative efforts are among the most important "specifics" in need of elucidation. Numerous electrophysiological and neuroradiological tools now make feasible studies of individual differences. And there exists within the biological sciences ample precedent for dealing with processes that take place over long periods of time – whether it be studies across the life span or investigations spanning millions of years. What is needed, as in any new scientific pursuit, is a few pioneering researchers who will investigate particular creative persons or processes in a way that is appropriate to the phenomena and that can be transported to other laboratories.

One other point worth stressing is that neurobiologists can now expect to receive aid from researchers working at the other side of the cognitive-scientific interface. Many psychologists and artificial intelligence researchers working at the level of "domain" or "intelligence" are now probing cognitive processes in great detail; an account in terms of underlying neurophysiological or neurochemical processes is no longer remote. And when it comes to the study of particular human faculties, ranging from language to vision, there is again a cadre of workers prepared to see their work analyzed in terms of underlying biological systems. Such common interest is no guarantee of success, of course, but it makes initial collaborative efforts more tenable.

Concluding remarks

Rather than reporting the results of a particular research program, this chapter peers toward a possible scientific future. We know very little about creative individuals or creative works; and, as I have indicated, much of what passes for knowledge is not readily linked to an understanding of unambiguous instances of human creativity. My faith, which I have articulated here, is that a cooperative synthetic scientific effort to illuminate creativity has become a possibility. One can begin by examining the four levels of description – the subpersonal, the personal, the extrapersonal, and the multipersonal – from the perspective of several appropriate disciplines. In my view, few challenges should be more attractive to a unified cognitive or synthetic science than a fresh attack on the problem of human creativity.

I want to touch on the moral aspects of creativity. There is a tendency to equate creativity with positive contributions, and yet a moment's reflection reveals that there is nothing inherently moral or positive about a creative individual or product: Adolf Hitler wandered the same city streets as Sigmund Freud, admired some of the same buildings, musical works, and individuals as did Freud's contemporaries, and began to hatch some of his diabolical plans during his years in Vienna.

Risk is entailed in associating issues of creativity with issues of morality, particularly because so many creative individuals have apparently been unconcerned with issues of morality, and many others have led lives and espoused values that few would admire today. Still, I believe that a study of creativity ought to have a moral dimension. First, I think it is important to consider the moral stances taken by creative individuals – or, in selected cases, to consider why moral issues were *not* considered part of an individual's personal or professional agenda. One wonders, for instance, why Einstein (who worked in an area remote from human affairs) was drawn deeply into the politics of his era, whereas Freud (deeply immersed in human investigations) generally spurned topical debates. Second, and more controversially, I believe that those of us who elect to study creative processes assume a special burden with respect to the knowledge that we acquire. Just because creative individuals are likely to have a disproportionate impact on the circle in which they live – be it limited to their friends or extending to the larger society – it is important to understand how these effects are wrought and how they might be channeled to the advantage of society and human societies in general.

In arguing that students of creativity ought to ponder the moral implications of their findings, I am under no illusion that we bring any special insights to bear on this matter. Indeed, it may well be questioned whether any individual has special insight in this area (Gruber, 1985). But just because these individuals and these issues are so important for human survival and for human thriving, I think it is important for us to make public our findings and to discuss what the moral implications of our findings *might* be. No doubt, subsequent discussion will reveal which ideas or implications (if any) are worth pursuing.

I return in conclusion to the realm of science and in particular to the scientific status of the framework proposed here. It should be evident that my remarks here are in no sense a scientific theory: There are no laws or principles that lend themselves to empirical test, nor even a set of propositions that can be evaluated on the plane of logic. What I have put forth is more properly considered a framework for organizing and synthesizing information so as to illuminate important, but as yet largely elusive, phenomena.

At the same time, I would be disheartened were the ideas presented here disregarded as irrelevant to scientific practice. I hope, first of all, to have made the case for attending to certain large-scale phenomena that prove easy to bypass in the pursuit of "normal science." I hope as well to have suggested, through some remarks about one creative individual, how the framework might someday illuminate diverse instances of creativity and perhaps even lead to laws that have some scientific permanence.

Moreover, and perhaps of greater scientific importance, there are many lines of ongoing work in the cognitive sciences today that could readily and appropriately be redirected so that they would pertain more directly to creative phenomena. The list would range from studies of brain-wave activity in children with various talents to investigations of friendship patterns among creative persons with different cognitive profiles. One assignment for the student of creativity is to aid in this process of reorientation. A second assignment is to direct particular attention to the ways in which findings at the intersection of two or more disciplines may relate to and inform one another and, ultimately, to attempt to piece together findings from disparate sciences that may jointly help to illuminate creativity.

When the ultimate story of creativity comes to be written, it may well turn out that creative individuals benefit from the confluence of a great many disparate factors whose coming together allows them to carry out their work. In my own view, however, the ultimate story may turn out quite different. Having reviewed the facts of the lives of many creative individuals, I have been struck by the lack of synchrony – indeed, frequently the *asynchrony* – among the various factors and levels of analysis introduced here. Creative individuals often are marked by an anomalous pattern of intelligences, by a tension between intellectual and personality styles, and by a striking lack of fit between personality and domain, intelligence and field, and biological constitution and choice of career. Indeed, it sometimes appears as if the very lack of fit served as a primary motivation for the individual to strike out in a new direction and, ultimately, to fashion a creative product. Should this impression be confirmed by more systematic study, it would bolster our opening speculation that creativity is a phenomenon radically different from giftedness.

To test such propositions, we shall require analytic frameworks and synthesizing procedures of great scope and subtlety. Most scientists are uncomfortable at undertaking such a mission of analysis and integration, though it is a mission at which some great scientists (like Darwin and Freud) have excelled. Perhaps it is fitting that a trait that has characterized the most creative individuals is also at a particular premium in contemporary efforts to offer a holistic account of creativity.

References

Arieti, S. (1976). *Creativity*. New York: Basic Books.

Bate, W. J. (1979). *Samuel Johnson*. New York: Harcourt, Brace, Jovanovich.

Block, N., & Dworkin, G. (1976). *The IQ controversy*. New York: Pantheon.

Boden, M. (1976). *Artificial intelligence and natural man*. New York: Basic Books.

Csikszentmihalyi, M., & Robinson, R. (1986). Culture, time and the development of talent. In R. Sternberg & J. Davidson (Eds.), *Conceptions of giftedness* (pp. 264–284). Cambridge University Press.

Ellenberger, H. (1970). *The discovery of the unconscious*. New York: Basic Books.

Feldman, D. (1980). *Beyond universals in cognitive development*. Norwood, NJ: Ablex.

Feldman, D. (1986). *Nature's gambit*. New York: Basic Books.

Fodor, J. (1983). *The modularity of mind*. Cambridge, MA: MIT Press.

Gardner, H. (1975). *The shattered mind*. New York: Knopf.

Gardner, H. (1982a). Giftedness: Speculations from a biological perspective. *New Directions for Child Development, 17*, 47–60.

Gardner, H. (1982b). *Art, mind, and brain*. New York: Basic Books.

Gardner, H. (1983). *Frames of mind*. New York: Basic Books.

Gardner, H. (1985). *The mind's new science*. New York: Basic Books.

Gardner, H., & Dudai, Y. (1985). Biology and giftedness. *Items, 35*, 1–6.

Gardner, H., Howard, V., & Perkins, D. (1974). Symbol systems: A philosophical, psychological and educational investigation. In D. Olson (Ed.), *Media and symbols* (pp. 27–55). University of Chicago Press.

Gedo, J. (1983). *Portraits of the artist*. New York: Guilford.

Gentner, D., & Stevens, A. (1983). *Mental models*. Hillsdale, NJ: Lawrence Erlbaum.

Geschwind, N., & Galaburda, A. (1986). *Cerebral lateralization*. Cambridge, MA: MIT Press.

Gruber, H. (1981). *Darwin on man*. University of Chicago Press.

Gruber, H. (1982). On the hypothesized relation between giftedness and creativity. *New Directions for Child Development, 17*, 7–30.

Gruber, H. (1985). Giftedness and moral responsibility: Creative thinking and human survival. In F. D. Horowitz & M. O'Brien (Eds.), *The gifted and talented: Developmental perspectives* (pp. 301–330). Washington, DC: American Psychological Association.

Janik, A., & Toulmin, S. (1973). *Wittgenstein's Vienna*. New York: Simon & Schuster.

Johnson-Laird, P. N. (1983). *Mental models*. Cambridge, MA: Harvard University Press.

Jones, E. (1961). *The life and work of Sigmund Freud*. New York: Basic Books.

Koestler, A. (1964). *The act of creation*. London: Hutchinson.

Lorenz, K. (1966). The role of gestalt perception in animal and human behavior. In L. L. Whyte (Ed.), *Aspects of form* (pp. 157–178). Bloomington, IN: Midland Books.

Mednick, S. (1962). The associative basis of the creative process. *Psychological Review, 69*, 220–232.

Newell, A., & Simon, H. (1972). *Human problem-solving*. Englewood Cliffs, NJ: Prentice-Hall.

Peirce, C. S. (1929). Guessing. *The Hound and Horn, 2*, 267–282.

Perkins, D. (1981). *The mind's best work*. Cambridge, MA: Harvard University Press.

Popper, K. (1976). *Unending quest*. London: Fontana.

Pribram, K., & Gill, M. (1976). *Freud's project reassessed*. New York: Basic Books.

Rothenberg, A. (1976). *The emerging goddess*. University of Chicago Press.

Rothenberg, A., & Hausman, C. (Eds.) (1976). *The creativity question*. Durham, NC: Duke University Press.

Schorske, C. (1981). *Fin-de-siècle Vienna*. New York: Vintage Books.

Selfe, L. (1977). *Nadia*. London: Academic Press.

Sternberg, R. (Ed.) (1984). *Mechanisms of cognitive development*. San Francisco: Freeman.

Sulloway, F. (1983). *Freud: Biologist of the mind*. New York: Basic Books.

Torrance, E. P. (1965). *Rewarding creative behavior*. Englewood Cliffs, NJ: Prentice-Hall.

Vernon, P. E. (Ed.). (1970). *Creativity*. London: Penguin Books.

Walters, J., & Gardner, H. (1986). The crystallizing experience. In R. Sternberg & J. Davidson (Eds.), *Conceptions of giftedness* (pp. 306–331). Cambridge University Press.

Wertheimer, M. (1959). *Productive thinking*. New York: Harper & Row.

Winner, E. (1982). *Invented worlds*. Cambridge, MA: Harvard University Press.

The study of creative systems

13   Society, culture, and person: a systems view of creativity

Mihaly Csikszentmihalyi

The constitution of creativity

It is customary to date the renewal of interest in creativity among psychologists to Guilford's presidential address to the APA more than 30 years ago (Guilford, 1950). Ever since that date, an increasing tide of publications on the subject has been appearing in our journals. Many of these books and articles have tried to answer what has been thought to be the most fundamental question: *What* is creativity? But no one has raised the simple question that should precede attempts at defining, measuring, or enhancing, namely: *Where* is creativity?

On hearing this question, most people would answer "Why, in the creative person's head, of course." Others might demur at such a subjective location and say that creativity is in the thought, object, or action produced by the person. At any rate, all of the definitions of creativity of which I am aware assume that the phenomenon exists, as a concrete process open to investigation, either inside the person or in the works produced.

After studying creativity on and off for almost a quarter of a century, I have come to the reluctant conclusion that this is not the case. We cannot study creativity by isolating individuals and their works from the social and historical milieu in which their actions are carried out. This is because what we call creative is never the result of individual action alone; it is the product of three main shaping forces: a set of social institutions, or *field,* that selects from the variations produced by individuals those that are worth preserving; a stable cultural *domain* that will preserve and transmit the selected new ideas or forms to the following generations; and finally the *individual,* who brings about some change in the domain, a change that the field will consider to be creative.

So the question "Where is creativity?" cannot be answered solely with reference

---

Three colleagues from three different generations have been especially helpful in developing the ideas in this chapter. J. W. Getzels, who inspired me to the study of creativity, has always been a source of fresh insights and strong values. Howard Gardner, as stimulating and generous a colleague as one might wish for, sharpened the thoughts in this chapter through the numerous conversations we have had over the years. And so did Rick Robinson, who is starting out now on the long journey of scholarship.

to the person and the person's work. Creativity is a phenomenon that results from interaction between these three systems. Without a culturally defined domain of action in which innovation is possible, the person cannot even get started. And without a group of peers to evaluate and confirm the adaptiveness of the innovation, it is impossible to differentiate what is creative from what is simply statistically improbable or bizarre.

The importance of this distinction is shown by the muddle that people who ignore it are prone to get into. For instance, Herbert Simon (1985), in his 1985 address to the APA, made the claim that his computer program BACON could replicate the solutions of some of the most creative problems in science – such as the derivation of Kepler's and Newton's laws – and therefore it should be considered to have the attribute of "creativity" (Csikszentmihalyi, in press). His conclusion would follow if one were to accept the premise, clearly articulated by Simon, that if an object or idea A is undistinguishable from another object or idea B, and if we agree that B is creative, then it follows that A must be creative too. This argument might work in the domain of logic, but it does not apply in the empirical world, where creativity exists only in specific social and historical contexts.

To see the weakness in Simon's argument, we need only to consider the case of a forger who can exactly reproduce some painting that we have agreed to recognize as creative – one originally painted by, let us say, Rembrandt. The two canvases, the original and the forgery, are completely indistinguishable. Does it follow from this identity between the two products that Rembrandt and the forger are equally creative, or that the two paintings are equally creative? If we say yes, then there is no more point in talking about creativity.

My argument, of course, is that the two paintings may be of equal technical skill, of the same aesthetic value, but they cannot be considered to be equal in creativity. Rembrandt's work is creative because he introduced some variations in the domain of painting at a certain point in history, when those variations were novel, and when they were instrumental in revising and enlarging the symbolic domain of the visual arts. The very same variations a few years later were no longer creative, because then they simply reproduced existing forms. The same argument applies to BACON and to any other procedure that replicates a creative achievement.

It is impossible to tell whether or not an object or idea is creative by simply looking at it. Without a historical context, one lacks the reference points necessary to determine if the product is in fact an adaptive innovation. An unusual African mask might seem the product of creative genius, until we realize that the same mask has been carved exactly the same way for centuries. A complex mathematical equation that purports to explain teleportation might impress the layman, but be recognized as pure gibberish by the mathematically trained.

I realized only recently, after writing for over two decades about creativity, that I had never "seen" it. Of course, like most people, I have been exposed to many objects and ideas that we call creative. Some of these might have been arresting, or interesting, or impressive, but I cannot say that I ever thought of them as "creative." Their creativity is something that I came to accept later, if at all, after comparing the object or idea with others of its kind, but mostly because I had been told by experts that these things were creative.

When I was a young child, we lived for a while in Venice, a few steps from St. Mark's Square, in a spot where the density of original works of art is one of the highest in the world. Later we moved to Florence, and every morning I walked past Brunelleschi's elegant Foundling Hospital with its priceless round Della Robbia ceramics. As a teenager I lived on the Gianicolo Hill in Rome, overlooking Michelangelo's great dome. During this time, my father, a redoubtable amateur art historian, made sure to point out to me the flowering of Renaissance creativity that surrounded us. I believed him, but I must confess that those masterpieces by and large made no impression on me. Some of them did produce an uncanny sense of serenity; others conveyed a great sense of power, or an undefinable excitement. But creativity? The great breakthroughs of Western art all looked equally old and decrepit to me; to think of them as innovations seemed a silly convention. I am afraid that in those years I would have gladly exchanged Giotto's frescoes in the Scrovegni Chapel for some Donald Duck comics illustrated by Walt Disney.

One might ask what this proves – only that I was ignorant and that it requires a certain amount of sophistication to recognize genuine creativity. I grant my ignorance, but I beg to raise what I think is an important point: Where does the information that gives us the ability to make sophisticated judgments come from? The information does not seem to be in the object itself. If we think about it, the reason we believe that Leonardo or Einstein was creative is that we have read that that is the case, we have been told it is true; our opinions about who is creative and why ultimately are based on faith. We have faith in the domains of art and science, and we trust the judgment of the field, that is, of the artistic and scientific establishments.

There is nothing wrong with this, because it is an inevitable situation. But by recognizing it, we must also accept some of its consequences, namely, that any attribution of creativity must be relative, grounded only in social agreement. And from this it also follows that social agreement is one of the constitutive aspects of creativity, without which the phenomenon would not exist.

It is easiest to see this process in art, where the selection criteria of the field change rather erratically. Kermode (1985) tells how Botticelli was for centuries considered to be a coarse painter, and the women he painted "sickly" and "clumsy." Only in the mid-nineteenth century did some critics begin to reevaluate his work and see in it creative anticipations of modern sensibility. To what extent was creativity contained in Botticelli's canvases, and to what extent did it emerge from the interpretive efforts of critics like Ruskin? One might argue that Botticelli's creativity was constituted by Ruskin's interpretations, that without the latter the former would not exist, and hence that Ruskin and the other critics and viewers who have since looked closely at Botticelli's work are just as indispensable to Botticelli's creativity as was the painter himself.

Similar situations abound in the history of art. In his lifetime, Rembrandt was thought to be a less important painter than Jan Lievens, who was also working at the same time in Amsterdam. How many people know of Lievens now? The powerful canvases of Francisco de Zurbaran were eagerly sought after in the royal court of Madrid until around 1645, when Murillo began to show his more graceful and lively paintings; after a few years Zurbaran was forgotten, and later died in poverty (Borghero, 1986). To understand creativity, it seems necessary to know how the attributions of creativity are made. By what process does Rembrandt emerge as more creative than Lievens?

The notoriously fickle realm of the arts is by no means the only one in which social processes determine what is and what is not to be considered creative. As Kuhn (1970, 1974) has noted, the same forces are at work in the hard sciences. In the domains of physics and chemistry, in the domain of mathematics, originality is attributed by social processes that are relative and fallible and that sometimes are reversed by posterity.

Augustine Brannigan (1981) has reviewed several instances of scientific discoveries in which retrospective reinterpretation was at least as important as the original contribution had been. For example, he makes an interesting case to the effect that our view of Mendel's contribution to genetics is generally quite wrong. The impression we have is that Mendel made a series of epochal experiments in the genetic transmission of traits in the 1860s, but that his creativity was not recognized by the scientific community until about 40 years later. This view, according to Brannigan, is radically mistaken in a subtle but essential respect. He argues that Mendel's experiments were not and could not have been contributions to genetics at the time they were made. Their implications for the theory of variation and natural selection were discovered only in 1900 by William Bateson and other evolutionists looking for a mechanism that explained discontinuous inheritance. Within their theoretical framework, Mendel's work suddenly acquired an importance that it had lacked before, even in the mind of Mendel himself. So where was Mendel's creativity? In his mind, in his experiments, or in the use his results were put to by later scientists? The answer, it seems to me, must be that it is to be found in all three. Just as the interpretations of Ruskin and other critics are inseparable from Botticelli's creativity, so the interpretations of Bateson and his fellows are constitutive parts of Mendel's creativity.

Brannigan forces us to see how even ostensibly simple facts, such as what is or is not a "discovery," are really the results of social processes of negotiation and legitimation. Most people would agree, for instance, that Columbus discovered America. But what does "discovery" mean in this context? Certainly it does not mean that he was the first man to set foot on the shores of the Western Hemisphere. Nor does it mean that Columbus knew that he had found a new continent previously unknown to Europeans; until the end he was convinced he had landed in Asia.

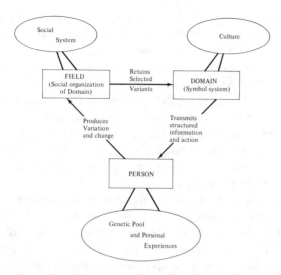

Figure 13.1. The locus of creativity. This "map" shows the interrelations of the three systems that jointly determine the occurrence of a creative idea, object, or action. The individual takes some information provided by the culture and transforms it, and if the change is deemed valuable by society, it will be included in the domain, thus providing a new starting point for the next generation of persons. The actions of all three systems are necessary for creativity to occur.

It means, as Brannigan shows, that he was the man for whom the field that could legitimize such things (which in his case included the Spanish crown, its royal commission, and various scholars and cartographers) was willing to make a claim of discovery. Not until Vespucci recognized that the so-called West Indies were part of an entirely different continent did Columbus's almost superhuman efforts get retrospectively revised as a "discovery." And if in the fullness of time it turns out that it was Erik the Red who really discovered America, that "discovery" will be as much a result of scholarship and politics as a result of Erik's travels.

A dynamic model of the creative process

One way to represent the set of relationships that constitutes creativity is through the "map" provided in Figure 13.1. It is important to realize that the relationships shown in the figure are dynamic links of circular causality. In other words, each of the three main systems – person, field, and domain – affects the others and is affected by them in turn. One might say that the three systems represent three "moments" of the same creative process.

The starting point on this map is purely arbitrary. One might start from the "person," because we are used to thinking in these terms – that the idea begins, like the lighted bulb in the cartoon, within the head of the creative individual. But, of course, the information that will go into the idea existed long before the creative person arrived on the scene. It had been stored in the symbol system of the culture, in the customary practices, the language, the specific notation of the "domain." A person who has no access to this information will not be able to make a creative contribution, no matter how able or skilled the person otherwise is. One needs to know music to write a creative symphony. It is difficult to become recognized as a creative Mandarin chef without knowing quite a bit about Chinese cooking.

A corollary of this relationship is that depending on the structure of the domain, it might be either relatively easy or more difficult for a person to innovate. The more precise the notation system, the easier it is to detect change and hence to evaluate whether or not the person has made an original contribution. Other things being equal, it should be easier to establish creativity in mathematics, music, or physics than, say, philosophy, the visual arts, or biology.

But returning to the system "person," we see that its contribution to the creative process is to produce some variation in the information inherited from the culture. The source of the variation might be an inherited or learned cognitive flexibility, a more dogged motivation, or some rare event in the life of the person. Of course, this is the aspect of the process that almost all psychologists interested in creativity have been studying – unfortunately, this usually is the only aspect studied. And by itself, the process of generating variation will not reveal what creativity is about. The reason is that focusing on the individual out of context does not allow the observer to evaluate the variation produced. It has been said that 99% of all new ideas are garbage, regardless of the domain or the status of the thinker. To sift out the good ideas from the bad, another system is needed.

It is the task of the "field" to select promising variations and to incorporate them into the domain. The easiest way to define a field is to say that it includes all those persons who can affect the structure of a domain. Thus, the field of art includes the following: art teachers and art historians, because they pass on the specialized symbolic information to the next generation; art critics, who help establish the reputation of individual artists; collectors, who make it possible for artists and works of art to survive; gallery owners and museum curators, who preserve and act as midwives to the production of art; and, finally, the peer group of artists whose interaction defines styles and revolutions of taste.

Thus, the field of art, like any other field, is made up of a network of interlocking roles. Some of them have a better chance than others of incorporating a selected variation into the domain. The people who fill these privileged roles act as "gate-keepers" to the domain. For instance, in a field like nuclear physics, the conviction of a thousand high school physics teachers that a new idea is pure genius probably would not be enough to get the new idea into the journals and textbooks that define the domain, whereas the same conviction held by half a dozen Nobel Prize winners might do it. During the Renaissance, the attention of a pope, or his mistress, was enough to select out the work of a young artist and slate it for preservation; once preserved, the work becomes part of the canon and will filter through, as one item of information in the domain, so that following generations of artists can be inspired to imitate it or reject it.

It goes without saying that fields will differ in the stringency of their selective mechanisms, the sensitivity of their gatekeepers, and the dynamics of their inner organization. The fields of botany and genetics in the USSR had only one gate-keeper for almost a generation, and his criteria of selection were based more on ideology than biology (Lecourt, 1977; Medvedev, 1971). Critics complain that the fate of American art is decided by only ten thousand inhabitants of Manhattan, but compared with most of the past stages of Western civilization, during which a few princes and bishops held the keys of artistic survival, this is a huge field.

It also follows that a field with fuzzy selection criteria, or one with gatekeepers who are not highly respected, will have great difficulty in establishing the creativity of a new idea. Similarly, but for opposite reasons, a new idea will face difficulties in being recognized as creative if the field is defensive, rigid, or embedded in a social system that discourages novelty. For instance, the aridity of Soviet genetics in the thirties was not, strictly speaking, a fault of the scientists who made up the field, but of the peculiar agenda of the broader social system of which the field was a part.

Every field is embedded in a specific social system. The resources of the larger society help to support the recognition of new ideas. The flowering of new ideas in Athens in the fifth century BC, or in fifteenth-century Florence, nineteenth-century Paris, or twentieth-century Vienna and New York, was due in large part to the fact that these centers at those times were in the position to pay attention to an unusually great number of new ideas. What does it take for a community to be able to do so? To a certain extent the materialist explanation applies: Disposable wealth is one of the conditions that makes the selection of novelty possible. In addition, it takes disposable attention – people who in addition to being wealthy have the time to take an interest in the domain (Csikszentmihalyi, 1978, 1979). A hundred years ago, every aspiring artist in Europe dreamed of being in Paris, where the field of art had the greatest financial clout, as well as being numerically the largest and most sophisticated. It is sobering to remember that even the great Leonardo, that most protean of all known creators, timed his moves to the tides of his patrons' fortunes. As soon as Sforza started spending lavishly, he left Florence for the ducal court in Milan; when the pope became more solvent than the duke, he moved to Rome; he went back and forth between the two Italian courts, but when the finances of King Francis I began to outshine those of both, he packed up for France.

Occasionally, great creative reformulations appear to take place outside of all constituted fields. Gardner (1986) makes this case for Freud: Essentially, he invented psychoanalysis, and at the time he did so there was no social organization specifically qualified to support or supress his ideas. In a certain sense, the founders of all great systems are in the same position: Galileo may be said to have started the field of experimental physics, and at the time of the Wright brothers there was no field of aeronautics. What happens in such cases is that a subset of people from related fields recognize the validity of the new variation and become identified with the emerging field. In the case of Galileo, it was mathematicians, astronomers, and philosophers who were attracted to his ideas; in the case of the Wright brothers, it was automobile and bicycle mechanics; Freud's first followers were other medical men.

But the model suggests that without people in neighboring fields who become attracted to the new idea, the creative process will be aborted. If no qualified persons are willing to invest their energy in preserving the variation, it will not become one of the "memes" that future generations will know about. In a setting with not enough mechanics interested in flying, the Wrights' efforts would eventually have been forgotten, and aeronautics would not have developed.

The element of time in the constitution of creativity

In looking again at the complex dynamics represented in Figure 13.1, it should be clear that time plays an important role in the creative process. It is here that the folk view of the creative idea as a bolt of lightning is least realistic. First of all, an important breakthrough usually follows a long period of gestation in the domain. The atomic theory of matter existed, in embryonic form, 25 centuries before it was given its first satisfactory shape. Medical advances, engineering triumphs, and artistic revolutions typically exist for a long time as unclearly formulated possibilities. During this period of gestation, new converts to the field become imbued by its "problematics." Occasionally there seems to be a discovery that truly comes from nowhere: Roentgen's discovery of radiation and Fleming's discovery of penicillin usually are held to be accidental. But they appear to be accidents only if we abstract the creative person from the context. The behavior of electric current in a cathode tube and the effects of various substances on bacterial cultures were problems that existed in Roentgen's and Fleming's respective domains; we might perhaps even say that they provided an implicit tension, a demand for resolution that exerted an invisible pull on workers in the field. If Roentgen and Fleming had not been sensitive to these potentialities in their work, no number of lucky accidents would have produced a discovery.

It is not only in the transition from the domain to the person but also in the move from the person to the field, and from the field back to the domain, that time is involved. The only way to establish whether or not something is creative is through comparison, evaluation, and interpretation. Sometimes, as we have seen, the field reverses its judgment: Botticelli moves to the forefront, and Lievens fades into the background; Mendel is hailed a genius, and Lysenko is revealed a fake.

And once the field makes up its collective mind – at least temporarily – it takes a while for the new idea to be included into the canon of the domain. Given current technology and the highly rationalized organization of most fields, this time lag is shorter than at some times in the past. But it has been estimated that it still takes an average of 7 years for a bona fide new discovery to make its first appearance in the textbooks of most domains. This process is faster or slower depending on the structure of the domain and of the field.

I know a particle physicist of great renown who likes to tell a story about an advanced seminar he has taught in Munich, where one of the students once interrupted his blackboard demonstration and jotted down a formulation of the equation different from the formulation he had been developing. The student's version appeared to be more elegant and suggestive than the professor's had been. The story goes that in a matter of weeks, every theoretical physicist in Germany knew of the event, and within a month, physicists on the West Coast of the United States were toying with the new equation. Eventually the student got himself a Nobel Prize.

Such a denouement would be impossible in most other disciplines. It could never happen, for instance, in psychology. Imagine a student, even if he had the most brilliant mind in the world, being able to impress his peers, his teachers, and the community of psychologists by something he said in a seminar! Not even the best-known psychologist could achieve such a result. Perhaps in very limited, very specialized subfields it is possible to earn instant recognition for a creative idea, but the lack of common conceptual commitment, the fragmentation of the domain, guarantees that the recognition will remain for a long time parochial.

There is another sense in which time is implicated in the systems model developed in Figure 13.1. The arrows pointing from person to field to domain actually describe an ascending spiral, because every new bit of information added to the domain will become the input for the next generation of persons. Thus, the model represents a cycle in the process of cultural evolution. As the terms suggest, *variation, selection,* and *transmission* are the three main phases of the cycle, and these are also the main phases of every evolutionary sequence (Campbell, 1965, 1976). We might conclude that creativity is one of the aspects of evolution. But contrary to biological evolution, in which information relevant to phenotypic behavior is changed chemically in the genes, cultural evolution involves changes in information coded extrasomatically. Dawkins (1976) coined the term "meme" to refer to a "unit of imitation" that was transmitted from one generation to the next. A meme could be a tool like a stone ax, a formula for smelting copper, the Pythagorean theorem, the first bar of Beethoven's Fifth Symphony, the concept of democracy, the smile of the Mona Lisa – in short, any structured information that could be remembered and that was worth passing on through time. Using Dawkins's term, we would say that a domain is a system of related memes that change through time, and what changes them is the process of creativity (Csikszentmihalyi & Massimini, 1985).

The generative force of the field

In Figure 13.1, the arrows go in a clockwise direction from domain to person to field, and then again to the domain – at a later point in time. This sequence, although it accurately represents the main trends, does not exhaust all the possibilities. A field – or the society that harbors it – may stimulate directly the emergence of new ideas in people who otherwise would never have taken up work in a particular domain.

The case of Brunelleschi is a good example. He was clearly one of the most creative individuals of the Renaissance, whose impact on the future of architecture is indisputable. Yet by all accounts he never would have became an artist and architect if he had been born a generation earlier, when the community of Florence was less interested in sponsoring art. Brunelleschi was the son of an upper-class professional, a notary with good political connections, and he went through the best educational training the city had to offer. Everyone expected him to follow a career in the liberal professions. Yet at the age of 23, in 1398, Brunelleschi joined the goldsmiths' guild and started practicing the plastic arts. It was a startling choice for a scion of the oligarchy (Heydenreich, 1974, p. 31), but as the demand for good artists became more intense, more of his peers followed Brunelleschi's example.

Florence in the first 25 years of the fifteenth century illustrates well how the field can stimulate the emergence of creativity. There is general agreement that during those few years some of the most enduringly original works of art were produced in what was a relatively small community. An approach to creativity that focused on the person would have to explain what happened in Florence by postulating a sudden and temporary increase in the originality of individual artists, presumably based on genetic drift or some environmental change that increased originality. But the more likely explanation is that individual potentialities remained constant, and the changes that produced the Renaissance took place in the social system, the field of art, and, to a lesser extent, the culture and the domain.

By the dawn of the fifteenth century, Florence had been the foremost financial center of Europe for almost two centuries, and one of its main manufacturing centers. By judiciously lending money to various kings and princes in England, Germany, and France, at least a dozen families in Florence (the Mozzi, Peruzzi, Bardi, Spini, Scali, Pulci, Abbati, Falconeri, Alfani, Alberti, Chiarenti, Cerchi, Buonsignori, Franceni, Rimberti, not to mention the latecomers Strozzi and Medici) had become the leading capitalists in the Western world. There were several dozen wealthy merchant families, and hundreds profited from the making of wool and silken textiles and from working metals. In the words of one historian, "the other great requirement of art, patronage, sprang from the same financial source" (Cheyney, 1936, p. 273).

The social situation was not one that would appeal to our democratic sensibilities. According to one sociologist, the Florentine worker was "completely deprived of all civil rights . . . capital [ruled] more ruthlessly and less troubled by moral scruples than ever before or after in the history of Western Europe" (Hauser, 1951, p. 20). Nor were foreign affairs in better shape; during those years, Florence was engaged in constant life-and-death struggles against Milan and Naples (Hartt, 1979). Yet rising production led to increased home consumption, and by a fortuitous chain of events, such as the discovery of long-buried Roman buildings and sculpture, and the influence of new ideas from the Middle East, the consumption of the wealthy Florentines was channeled into the patronage of works of art.

It might help to understand the genesis of creativity if we review briefly the events of those crucial 25 years of Florence. Most art historians agree on what were the greatest accomplishments of that period. Any list would include, at the very least, the following: the making of the north doors of the Baptistery by Ghiberti (1402–1424); the statues of St. Mark (1411) and St. George (1415) that Donatello placed in the chapel of Orsanmichele; the statue of St. Philip (1414) by Nanni di Banco in the same location; Brunelleschi's start on the Foundling Hospital (1419), the cathedral cupola (1420), and the Sacristy of San Lorenzo (1421); the frescoes of the Adoration of the Magi by Gentile da Fabriano (1420–1423); and those Masaccio painted in the Brancacci Chapel (1424–1427). These three works of architecture, three sculptures, and two sets of paintings are generally held to be the most notable achievements of the early Renaissance in Florence (Hartt, 1979; Heydenreich, 1974).

Now, in each of these eight cases, the impetus for doing the work came either from a rich individual who wanted to celebrate the name of his family (the works of Masaccio and Gentile da Fabriano and Brunelleschi's sacristy were commissioned, respectively, by the bankers Brancacci, Strozzi, and Medici for their churches) or from one of the political or guild unions (Ghiberti's doors were commissioned by the merchants' guild; the Signoria asked for and paid for the statues of Donatello and Nanni; the silk weavers' guild got the Foundling Hospital built; and the wool guild supervised the building of the dome).

The building of this famous dome gives a glimpse of how the community directed artistic production. The executive power was in the hands of a 12-man committee, the Operai del Duomo, who were selected from various corporations, with a preponderance of wool merchants and manufacturers. The function of this committee was to organize competitions, select the best entries, commission the winning artists, supervise the work in progress, and pay for the finished product. In the case of the cupola, general plans had been drawn up as far back as 1367, but despite several competitions, no architect had been able to satisfy the stringent requirements of the Operai. It is well known that during this period a large proportion of the populace took part in the selection process: suggestions, letters, and criticism flowed steadily from citizens to the Operai, expressing their ideas of how the dome of the cathedral should be built. Finally, more than 70 years after the first plans, Brunelleschi and Ghiberti were entrusted with the great task.

The "Gates of Paradise" that Ghiberti finally built for the Baptistery went through a similar close scrutiny. The Calimala, or merchants' guild, appointed a jury of 34 experts to review the entries. Before the contest, the jury consulted some of the leading scholars of Italy about what the subject matter of each of the 28 panels of the doors should be. Of the several dozen artists who prepared sketches for the commission, six were chosen for the final list. They were given 1 year to prepare a bronze relief that would serve as the test entry, and during this period their production costs and living expenses were covered by the Calimala (Hauser, 1951, p. 39). The test consisted in making a panel illustrating the sacrifice of Isaac. After the year had passed, Ghiberti, who in 1402 was only 23 years old and almost unknown, was judged to have done best. For the next 50 years he worked first on the north, then on the east doors, with the continuing financial and critical backing of the guild (Heydenreich, 1974, p. 129).

It was this tremendous involvement of the entire community in the creative process that made the Renaissance possible. And it was not a random event, but a calculated, conscious policy on the part of those who had wealth and power. The goal of the Florentines was to make their city into a new Athens (Hauser, 1951, p. 23). In terms of our model, an unusually large proportion of the social system became part of the art "field," ready to recognize, and indeed to stimulate, new ideas.

"In this environment," wrote Heydenreich (1974, p. 13), "the patron begins to assume a very important role: in practice, artistic productions arise in large measure from his collaboration." Hauser's position is even more extreme: "[In] the art of the early Renaissance . . . the starting point of production is to be found mostly not in the creative urge, the subjective self-expression and spontaneous inspiration of the artist, but in the task set by the customer" (Hauser, 1951, p. 41).

Implications of the model

At this point, some readers used to the person-centered perspective on creativity might begin to feel that the argument I am developing is a betrayal of psychology in favor of historical or sociological approaches. This is surely not my intention. It seems to me that an understanding of the complex context in which people operate must eventually enrich our understanding of who the individual is and what the individual does. But to do so we need to abandon the Ptolemaic view of creativity, in which the person is at the center of everything, for a more Copernican model in which the person is part of a system of mutual influences and information.

The domain level

A long agenda of questions can be generated from this approach, questions that usually are ignored in creativity research yet might hold the key to many important findings.

In terms of the domain, the basic question is "What are the various ways in which information can be stored and transmitted, and how does the structuring of information affect creativity?" We need to develop concepts and measures to evaluate the structuring of information, so as to discover which symbol systems are better able to store creative ideas, and to transmit them over time. The work of Feldman (1980) was a pioneering attempt in this direction, and so is the direction of research pursued by Project Zero at Harvard (Perkins, 1981). The newly emerging fields of cognitive science and artificial ingelligence (Gardner, 1985) also will have much to contribute to answering such questions.

We also need to understand better how access to information is differentially open to various categories of individuals. Basically, this amounts to the question

"How can we make past creativity available to the most people, so as to facilitate future creativity?"

The other side of the coin is the question "How can we motivate people to become involved in a particular domain?" The issue here is not how to provide extrinsic motivation like money and recognition, which more properly belong to the concerns of the field, but rather how to ensure intrinsic motivation, which hinges on the inherent attractiveness with which the information is presented. For no matter how original one might be, if one is bored by the domain, it will be difficult to become interested enough in it to make a creative contribution. The ability to attract and sustain interest rests in part on how well the domain is internally organized. How motivation and personality more generally are implicated in creativity has been extensively studied (Amabile, 1983; Csikszentmihalyi, 1986; Csikszentmihalyi & Getzels, 1973; Roe, 1946), but we still know very little about the specific motivational values of different ways of patterning information.

The person

Because most studies of creativity focus on individual processes, this is the phase of the creative cycle that needs the least attention, being the best known. The main conceptual question here is "How do some individuals get to produce a greater amount of variation in the domain than others?" The answer to this question is going to involve motivational and affective variables as well as cognitive ones. It is likely that some children are born with more sensitivity to certain ranges of stimulation – to light as opposed to movement, or to sound – and therefore might be more advantaged in dealing with the memes to which they are more sensitive (Gardner, 1983). The ways in which various information-processing strategies are used by creative children are being actively investigated (Bamberger, 1986; Siegler & Shrager, 1984; Sternberg, 1984). It is also likely that early experiences (Walters & Gardner, 1986) and demographic variables such as sibling position, social class, or religious upbringing will have their effects. The importance of "problem finding" as an approach to creative tasks has been documented longitudinally with artists (Csikszentmihalyi & Getzels, 1971; in press).

Careful studies of truly creative individuals that take into account all the facets of the complex interactions among person, field, and domain are especially needed and in scarce supply. Some examples of attempts in this direction are Gruber's study (1981) of Darwin, Getzels and Csikszentmihalyi's longitudinal study (1976) of young artists, and Feldman's continuing investigations (1986) of prodigiously gifted children.

The field

It is probably true that less is known about the effects of the social system on creativity than about the other two phases of the cycle. The theoretical issue here is

"What forms of organization facilitate the selection of new variants and their inclusion in the domain?" Bloom (1985) has documented the extensive support system, including devoted parents and committed teachers, that gifted children need in order to master the skills required by a domain. Getzels and Csikszentmihalyi (1968) and Csikszentmihalyi, Getzels, and Kahn (1984) have shown how social roles interact with artists' personalities to determine success in the field. Simonton (1978, 1984) has conducted extensive studies of the relationship between features of the social system and the frequency of creative behavior.

A start in the right direction has certainly been made. Psychologists studying creativity have begun to realize the relevance of related approaches. The history of science, the history of ideas, cognitive science, artificial intelligence, and organizational sociology are no longer out of bounds for those who wish to get a strong grip on the issues. But all these promising studies – and the many others there was no room to mention – are thus far unrelated to each other, as if these distinct aspects of the creative process could be understood in isolation from each other. Perhaps even more than new research, what we need now is an effort to synthesize the various approaches of the past into an integrated theory. Of course, all this poaching in neighboring territory places an added burden of scholarship on the psychologist. The systems approach demands that we become versed in the skills of more than one discipline. The returns in knowledge, however, are well worth the effort.

References

Amabile, T. (1983). *The social psychology of creativity*. New York: Springer-Verlag.

Bamberger, J. (1986). Cognitive issues in the development of musically gifted children. In R. J. Sternberg & J. E. Davidson (Eds.), *Conceptions of giftedness* (pp. 388–416). Cambridge University Press.

Bloom, B. (1985). *Developing talent in young children*. New York: Ballantine.

Borghero, G. (1986). *Thyssen-Bornemisza Collection. Catalogue Raisonné*. Milano: Edizioni Electa.

Brannigan, A. (1981). *The social basis of scientific discoveries*. Cambridge University Press.

Campbell, D. T. (1965). Variation and selective retention in socio-cultural evolution. In H. R. Barringer, G. I. Blankston, & R. W. Monk (Eds.), *Social change in developing areas* (pp. 19–42). Cambridge, MA: Schenkman.

Campbell, D. T. (1976). Evolutionary epistemology. In P. A. Schlipp (Ed.), *The library of living philosophers* (pp. 413–463). La Salle, IL: Open Court.

Cheyney, E. P. (1936). *The dawn of a new era: 1250–1453*. New York: Harper & Bros.

Csikszentmihalyi, M. (1978). Attention and the holistic approach to behavior. In K. S. Pope & J. L. Singer (Eds.), *The stream of consciousness* (pp. 335–358). New York: Plenum.

Csikszentmihalyi, M. (1979). *Art and problem finding*. Paper presented at the 87th annual convention of the APA, New York.

Csikszentmihalyi, M. (in press). Motivation and creativity: Towards a synthesis of structural and energistic approaches to cognition. *New Ideas in Psychology* (in press).

Csikszentmihalyi, M., & Getzels, J. W. (1971). Discovery-oriented behavior and the originality of creative products. *Journal of Personality and Social Psychology, 19*(1), 47–52.

Csikszentmihalyi, M., & Getzels, J. W. (1973). The personality of young artists: An empirical and theoretical exploration. *British Journal of Psychology, 64*(1), 91–104.

Csikszentmihalyi, M., & Getzels, J. W. (in press). Creativity and problem finding in art. In F. H. Farley & R. W. Neperud (Eds.), *The foundations of aesthetics, art, and art education*. New York: Praeger.

Csikszentmihalyi, M., Getzels, J. W., & Kahn, S. (1984). *Talent and achievement: A longitudinal study with artists.* Unpublished manuscript, University of Chicago.

Csikszentmihalyi, M., & Massimini, F. (1985). On the psychological selection of bio-cultural information. *New Ideas in Psychology, 3*(2), 115–138.

Csikszentmihalyi, M., & Robinson, R. (1986). Culture, time, and the development of talent. In R. J. Sternberg & J. E. Davidson (Eds.), *Conceptions of giftedness* (pp. 264–284). Cambridge University Press.

Dawkins, R. (1976). *The selfish gene.* New York: Oxford University Press.

Feldman, D. (1980). *Beyond universals in cognitive development.* Norwood, NJ: Ablex.

Feldman, D. (1986). *Nature's gambit.* New York: Basic Books.

Gardner, H. (1983). *Frames of mind.* New York: Basic Books.

Gardner, H. (1985). *The mind's new science.* New York: Basic Books.

Gardner, H. (1986). Freud in three frames. *Daedalus,* 105–134.

Getzels, J. W., & Csikszentmihalyi, M. (1968). On the roles, values, and performance of future artists: A conceptual and empirical exploration. *Sociological Quarterly, 9,* 516–530.

Getzels, J. W., & Csikszentmihalyi, M. (1976). *The creative vision.* New York: Wiley.

Gruber, H. (1981). *Darwin on man.* University of Chicago Press.

Guilford, J. P. (1950). Creativity. *American Psychologist, 5*(9), 444–454.

Hartt, F. (1979). *History of Italian Renaissance art.* Englewood Cliffs, NJ: Prentice-Hall.

Hauser, A. (1951). *The social history of art* (Vol. 2). New York: Vintage.

Heydenreich, L. H. (1974). *Il primo Rinascimento.* Milano: Rizzoli.

Kermode, F. (1985). *Forms of attention.* University of Chicago Press.

Kuhn, T. S. (1970). *The structure of scientific revolutions* (2nd ed.). University of Chicago Press.

Kuhn, T. S. (1974). Second thoughts on paradigms. In F. Suppe (Ed.), *The structure of scientific theories.* Urbana: University of Illinois Press.

Lecourt, D. (1977). *Proletarian science.* London: New Left Books.

Medvedev, Z. (1971). *The rise and fall of Dr. Lysenko.* Garden City, NY: Doubleday.

Perkins, D. (1981). *The mind's best work.* Cambridge, MA: Harvard University Press.

Roe, A. (1946). The personality of artists. *Educational and Personality Measurement, 6,* 401–408.

Siegler, R. S., & Shrager, J. (1984). A model of strategic choice. In C. Sophian (Ed.), *Origins of cognitive skills.* Hillsdale, NJ: Lawrence Erlbaum.

Simon, H. A. (1985). *Psychology of scientific discovery.* Paper presented at the 93rd annual APA meeting, Los Angeles, CA.

Simonton, D. K. (1978). History and the eminent person. *Gifted Child Quarterly, 22,* 187–195.

Simonton, D. K. (1984). *Genius, creativity, and leadership.* Cambridge, MA: Harvard University Press.

Sternberg, R. J. (1984). Toward a triarchic theory of human intelligence. *Behavioral and Brain Sciences, 7*(2), 269–316.

Walters, J., & Gardner, H. (1986). The crystallizing experience. In R. Sternberg & J. Davidson (Eds.), *Conceptions of giftedness* (pp. 306–331). Cambridge University Press.

Herbert J. Walberg

Since 1975, educational psychologists have synthesized several thousand studies on how learning can be enhanced (Walberg, 1984b). The syntheses show that the amount and quality of instruction and the degree of psychological stimulation in classrooms, homes, peer groups, and mass media have consistent and powerful effects on learning. This work has implications for talent and creativity for two reasons: The studies include learning outcomes ranging from basic knowledge and skill acquisition to creativity and the "higher mental processes." Creativity, moreover, nearly always requires general knowledge as well as disciplined mastery of the basic elements of special fields. Achieving general knowledge and specialized mastery quickly and efficiently not only enables creativity but also allows additional time for its development.

From the perspective of an educational psychologist, this chapter addresses the following topics: definitions of creativity, "human-capital theory," exceptional performance and talent, educational productivity, childhood environments of eminent adults of history, and the family and school environments of talented contemporary adolescents. My interests are in child-rearing, education, and national welfare, and my profession is called on to recommend policies and practices. This chapter, accordingly, emphasizes an understanding of what should be done as much as what seems known and what else deserves investigation.

Toward a definition of creativity

What is creativity? More than 30 years ago, Morgan (1953) culled from the psychological literature 25 definitions. They had only one common element – the development of something unique. But should uniqueness be the ruling criterion? Does creativity have to be unique in the experience of the individual, the individual's culture, or the world? How should we count simultaneous and multiple discoveries? Rediscoveries?

Is it the creative person, the product, or the process that is held unique? Are people who are unusual in some way – bohemians, or those with high IQs – creative? Uniqueness, strictly speaking, implies a qualitative distinction – one of a kind. But creative fields usually have several first-rate talents contending for the

340

highest place; they differ more in degree than in kind, and no clear line separates them from others. Yet, what must we think about the accomplishment of a unique first, such as a new world time for the 100-meter dash, or a virtuoso violin performance – each perhaps a quantitative increment in highly competitive fields, but not a qualitative breakthrough that some have in mind in speaking of creativity?

Does the act, or the process, or the outcome of creativity have to be socially significant, competitively won, useful, or in some way satisfying? Can it be recognized by creative individuals themselves, or must it be certified by qualified judges? Does significant application or implementation count for as much as merely unusual ideas and discoveries? Can contemporary society really judge those in its midst who will be recorded in history? Reasonable people of good will answer these questions in different ways; they illustrate the difficulty of a definition that will satisfy everyone.

Cognitive psychology

Newell, Shaw, and Simon (1963) set forth several useful criteria of creative thinking:

1. The product of thought has novelty and value for the thinker or for the culture.
2. The thinking is unconventional in modifying or rejecting previous ideas.
3. The thinking requires high motivation reflected in persistence and intensity.
4. The problem solved was initially vague and ill-defined, so as to require reformulation.

A more recent and comprehensive approach that links creativity to general mental abilities is Sternberg's triarchic theory of human intelligence, which posits:

1) internal, mental mechanisms responsible for intelligent behavior; 2) the external contextual setting which defines what will be labeled as intelligent within a given societal milieu; and 3) the level of experience an individual has with a given task or situation intended to measure intelligence. According to Sternberg, individuals may be gifted in cognitive functioning of the kinds measured by conventional tests; contextual fitting that requires adaptation to, selection of, or shaping of environments; and the ability to deal with novelty or to automatize information processing effectively. (Sternberg & Davidson, 1985, p. 42)

As applied to giftedness, Sternberg isolates three basic kinds of elementary information processes:

metacomponents, which are high order control processes that are used in executive planning and decision making in problem solving; performance components, which are lower order processes used in executing a problem-solving strategy; and knowledge-acquisition components, which are lower order processes used in acquiring, retaining and transferring new information. (Sternberg & Davidson, 1985, p. 51)

Both views are comprehensive and insightful with respect to ideation. Psychology's rediscovery of thinking, indeed, is all to the good; behaviorism and motivational theories by themselves have been too narrow. But the "new cognitive psychology" also presents the danger of undue emphasis on thinking over behaving and feeling in psychology's ancient triumvirate. A balance must be sought, especially with respect to creativity that derives partly from the affective or behavioral domains, such as musical, visual, and written composition and dramatic, musical, and rhetorical performance.

Talent and creativity

Just as surely, creativity must depend on talent – constitutional or acquired. "A talented or gifted child is one who shows consistently remarkable performance in any worth-while line of endeavor" (Havighurst, 1958, p. 19). Yet practice helps make talent perfect, and persistence can overcome initial deficits, handicaps, and inabilities. Is the essence of creativity external stimulation, or internal motivation to persevere in the face of inevitable difficulties?

It is perhaps premature to set forth a definition and typology of creativity in the hope of agreement from various investigators. But many of the elements referred to earlier can help to discriminate between lower and higher degrees of creativity, even though none seems a perfect indicator. With more of the elements present, the person, process, and product can be said to be more creative. Creativity may be thought of as a constellation of attributes, such as the family resemblance of faces with more or less common but not universally distinguishing features. "Human-capital theory" offers a useful organizing framework for thinking about such elements of creativity and learning.

Human capital theory

"Capital" can be defined as an asset that gives rise to income, or, more broadly, utility that includes nonpecuniary or "psychic income" such as tranquillity and honor. Although money, land, buildings, and machines come to mind as financial and physical capital for production and income, it is useful to consider humans as capital investments or assets to themselves and society. The MacArthur Foundation, for example, following the Japanese recognition of "living human treasures," established no-strings grants to its fellows to enhance the nation's human assets in the arts, science, and practical affairs.

"Human capital" refers not to mere hours of labor but to the quality of work or the motivation, skills, and creativity of the worker. It was Adam Smith's original theory that the wealth of nations depends on the ability of people, but such economists as Becker (1976) and Mincer (1979) have recently enlarged greatly the scope of such human-capital theory.

Perhaps because human capital is largely acquired in nonmarket activities, particularly child-rearing and education, it seems novel if not provocative to speak of people as capital assets to themselves and others. If people's time is valuable, however, it is all the more reason to allocate it efficiently to attain human purposes. Society, especially through parents and educators, can be viewed as developing an individual's portfolio of knowledge, skills, and talents. In addition, the young and old themselves face choices between working and various investments in enhancing their capital, and between investment and consumption of their time and talent – all of which involves risky short- and long-term opportunities, costs, and benefits.

To economize or allocate scarce resources such as human time to competing purposes in this way, standard microeconomic theories and empirical techniques need not be reformed, but merely extended to valuable but nonmarket or unpriced activities that produce valuable changes in people (Becker, 1976; Mincer, 1979). To understand the production of talent, it is possible but often unnecessary to impute costs and benefits: Child-rearing costs, for example, may be estimated as forgone earnings of parents; benefits may be measured as added earnings and psychological satisfaction.

Of course, technical and substantive problems of measurement, analysis, uncertainty, and subjective value abound and are far from solution, and the great significance of human capital for human welfare has been incompletely recognized. Nor has it been scientifically exploited sufficiently and practically tested. Despite the immense value of human capital, we have less scientific and practical knowledge of its production, price, and value than we do about such things as automobiles and corn.

National welfare

From a national standpoint, the growth of human capital is both a condition and consequence of economic growth and other aspects of well-being (Mincer, 1979). Its promotion is more than the transmission of knowledge and its embodiment in people; it refers also to the new knowledge and techniques that yield worldwide economic growth.

In an era of convenient travel, quick global communication, and streamlined technology transfer, the benefits of original discoveries and new knowledge are unlikely to be restricted to countries of original discoveries (Walberg, 1983). It seems possible, indeed, for countries to overvalue and overinvest in original creative discoveries; rights to patented and copyrighted material, for example, are cheap compared with implementation costs and difficulties.

Because a great array of new discoveries and possibilities for exploitation confront individuals and nations, the most valuable kinds of creativity may be acquisition, selection, and implementation (Walberg, 1983). For example, in contrast to England and the United States, with their many Nobel laureates, Japan exemplifies mass social creativity in the acquisition and implementation of ideas; its use of the creative minds and hearts as well as the hands of workers is well known. It seems possible to allocate too much of a nation's finite amount of total human capital to elite and original discovery at the expense of less prestigious creativity more vital to a nation's future welfare (Walberg, 1984c). The quality of child-rearing and elementary and secondary education may be more important than universities and graduate schools for national prosperity and welfare.

Individual welfare

Investments in education, learning, talent, and creativity are like other investments that produce utility – both financial and nonfinancial returns (Mincer, 1979). Employers hire and pay higher wages to talented workers because presumably they are more skilled and productive; outstanding artists may be compensated by their value in the marketplace. Utility also includes nonfinancial rewards – psychic income, altruistic satisfaction, prestige, expected heavenly compensation in afterlife, or the inner feeling of artistic virtue despite society's indifference – all vital but subjective determinants of human nature.

Despite the value of human-capital investment, it entails risks. For example, increases in the supply of workers trained for specific jobs without corresponding increases in demand can reduce the value of the investment, at least with respect to earnings. Some occupations and professions, of course, fare much better than others: Generally, the higher the investments, the higher the utilities; arduous medical training, for example, has yielded high income and prestige. In creative performance, something essentially beyond the ordinary, the costs, rewards, and risks may be correspondingly greater. How many artists ever receive the compensation and fame of Picasso, or even make a living at painting?

Human-capital theory alerts us to the value of early investment and initial advantage. Cumulative advantages or "Matthew effects" (Walberg & Tsai, 1984) characterize human-capital investments over the life course (Mincer, 1979). The amount invested in a person in a given period is statistically proportional to that already invested; "To him that hath," according to Matthew, in the Bible, "shall be given, and he shall have abundance"; precociousness attracts parental encouragement and superior teaching.

The amount of specific human capital added over time is likely to be proportional to the child's personal stock, because incentives and opportunities tend to remain stable over the life course (Mincer, 1979). Psychological environments, too, are correlated over time and place (Walberg & Tsai, 1984). Parents, for example, may transfer wealth as well as genetic and environmental advantages to their children; piano-playing parents, for example, may transfer ability, provide models, and enrich the child's musical environment. Children with greater endowments and acquired advantages and skills can afford, and have greater opportunity, to acquire still greater advantages over the life course; they may, indeed, be able to acquire further advantages more efficiently than others even from the same environments and opportunities (Walberg & Tsai, 1984).

Human capital may be general or specialized. General knowledge and skills acquired in early life, and mastery of the liberal arts and sciences in high school and college, are surely valuable for many expected and unexpected purposes; they lay the foundation for safe occupations and other common pursuits. Relatively good amateur performance, moreover, can be attained in a specialty by means of 1 or 2 hr of daily practice for a few years; think of chess, painting, or *ikebana*. But the highest accomplishments, eminence or adjudicated creativity, demand great costs and sacrifice – nearly full concentration of one's life on a specialty for one or more decades. Even among those who make such an effort (e.g., violinists, writers, and ballet dancers striving to be world-class), many will remain unrecognized and obscure.

Investment in a portfolio of stocks or a manufacturing plant involves imperfect knowledge; it is risky. So it is with societies and individuals who invest their time and talents. In view of vast uncertainties, decisions can be said to be good or bad only in retrospect, if at all. Rather, most decisions must balance trade-offs between poorly estimated costs and benefits in view of possible vicissitudes. Prediction is difficult, especially if it involves the future.

Yet, in uncertainty lies hope; pursuit may be worth more than accomplishment. Mediocrity may be fun, and certainly is better than poor performance. What is worth doing may be worth doing poorly. Learning to dance at age 55, like Socrates, and making a joyful noise may be counted as time well spent.

Exceptional performance

Creativity may involve rare rather than unique accomplishments, and it may be useful to think of it as being on one end of a continuum of performance or learning that is attainable by nearly anyone with sufficient instruction and perseverance. Learning Japanese may appear daunting, but Japanese children have done so and are able to make creative use of it. Learning a language, though one of the most difficult human tasks, is accomplished by children learning their native languages the world over. Even though vocabulary constitutes the most common test of intelligence, children's native abilities in their native languages dwarf the abilities of adults exposed to a new language. Linguistic and other environments, especially if they are enduring and powerful, strongly shape accomplishments; societies and individuals, moreover, can choose or determine their environments.

Contrary to the notion of instant creativity that was popular in the 1960s, distinguished accomplishment seems partly a matter of continuous and concentrated effort over a decade or more. When Newton was asked how he managed to surpass the discoveries of his predecessors, in both quality and quantity, he replied, "By always thinking about them." Gauss said, "If others would but reflect on mathematical truths as deeply and continuously as I have, they would make my discoveries." Discovery may occur in an instant, but it usually requires decades of preparation in the special field.

Intense perseverance, however, seems necessary but insufficient: Getzels and Csikszentmihalyi (1976), for example, found that those who turned out to be eminent visual artists could find appropriate problems on which to work; problem finding, aesthetic ability, and originality – more than mere craftsmanship and mastery of basics – seemed the keys to later success. Psychological studies of the lives of eminent painters, writers, musicians, philosophers, religious leaders, and scientists of previous centuries, as well as prize-winning adolescents today, have revealed early, intense concentration on previous work in their fields, often to the near exclusion of other activities. It appears, though, that science and mathematics, because of their specialized and abstract symbolism, may require the greatest concentration and perseverance.

The same fundamental thought processes, moreover, appear to be required in both elementary learning and advanced discovery, as Simon (1981), Sternberg, and others have shown. Acquisition of knowledge and problem solving for beginners differ in degree rather than in kind from the mental activities of experts. The scarce resources are opportunity and concentration rather than the amount of information available or the processing capacity of the mind, both of which, for practical purposes, are unlimited.

The major constraints on the acquisition and processing of knowledge, according to Simon, are the few items of information, perhaps two to seven, that can be held in immediate, conscious memory, and the time required (5–10 s) to store an item in long-term memory. Experts differ from novices in science, chess, and other fields that have been studied not only in having more information in permanent memory but also, and more significantly, in being able to process it efficiently. Among experts, for example, items of information are more thoroughly indexed and thus can be rapidly brought to conscious memory. The items, moreover, are elaborately associated or linked with one another. Two consequences of these associations – the ability to recover information by alternative links, even when parts of the direct indexing are lost, and the capacity for extensive means–ends or trial-and-error searches – are the essential steps called into play in problem solving from the most elementary to the most advanced.

Talent and expertise

For my purposes, creative talent is a rich and complex association of cognitive elements (perhaps also involving affective and psychomotor connections). Achievement is the acquisition of such elements from the environment and their recall to conscious memory or recognition in the environment. Creativity (including problem finding and solving) is the trial-and-error search for novel and useful solutions by combinations of stored and externally found elements. As Sternberg and Davidson (1985, p. 44) concluded, "Precocious children form connections at a much more rapid rate than do ordinary children, and exceptional adults have formed exceptionally large numbers of variegated stimulus-response connections."

Following Aristotle, Herbart, and Simon, this parsimonious account calls attention to the time for acquisition and association of elements, the importance of the richness of the environment, and the natural continuity and linkage of creativity with achievement. Because the account also emphasizes mental constraints, it can help to explain why creativity has appeared mysterious: If creative problem solving consumes the time and exhausts mental resources, it leaves no capacity to observe and understand the detailed mechanisms and processes.

Increased understanding of such cognitive mechanisms and processes is likely to result in greater efficiencies in memory and thought and in teaching and learning. Ericsson, Chase, and Faloon (1980), for example, showed that an undergraduate of average intelligence given 230 hr of instruction and practice based on such notions raised his memory for numbers from 7 to 79 digits – nine times larger than the value taken by psychologists as indicative of superior intelligence, and as large as the capacity of stage mnemonicists. It will be difficult, of course, to produce such results for higher cognitive processes, such as analysis and synthesis, and to use their implications in educational practice. Thus, human time and concentration are likely to remain essential for learning and creativity in the foreseeable future.

The greatest advantage of the expert and difficulty for the novice is "chunking," the representation of abstract groups of items as linked clusters that can be efficiently processed. Such chunks may underlie mental processes ranging from childhood learning to scientific discoveries. Simon estimates that 50,000 chunks, about the same magnitude as the recognition vocabulary of college-educated readers, may be required for expert mastery of a special field. The highest achievements in various disciplines, however, may require a memory store of 1 million chunks, which may take even the talented about 70 hr of concentrated effort per week for a decade to acquire, although 7–9-year exceptions such as Mozart and Bobbie Fisher occasionally occur.

The prospect of such prodigious and sustained concentration should impress – if not defeat – the novice. Yet only a small fraction of the total is required for basic mastery. An extra 1 to 2 hr per day, perhaps taken from the usual 4 to 5 hr that American schoolchildren typically spend watching television, might enable them to attain levels of achievement and creativity far beyond the ordinary in many fields.

The performance distribution

By definition, creative or exceptional performance may be unique, rare, or unusual. But what does the shape of the human-performance distribution actually look like? Psychologists' first inclination is to assume normality revealed in a bell-shaped Gaussian curve, but the actual plots of distributions and other evidence suggest that human performance is highly skewed to the right (Walberg, Strykowski, Rovai, & Hung, 1984). Most people exhibit null or mediocre performances on most concrete tasks, but any person is likely to be exceptional on a few tasks.

Most people tend to produce the lowest possible performances on nearly all specific human tasks, even though they could, in principle, work to achieve very high performances, given the time, instruction, and environment. Few people, for example, can speak more than one or two of the world's thousands of languages. Few can play the many games that have been invented in the course of human history. Few can name 10 streets in Kyoto, state the rules governing national collegiate debates, play a tune on a violin, run a 4-min mile, or write a Shakespearean sonnet.

In the real world, however, some exceed average performance by several orders of magnitude. Such distributions, in which most people are at or near zero, but a few are far above average, are known as high-positive-skew or J curves, following the laws of Pareto, Allport, or Zipf (Walberg et al., 1984). These laws describe the extreme asymmetric distributions common to many fields and one of the most common phenomena of human behavior (although less well known because research measurements often are artificially constrained to normality). For example, 20% of salespeople may account for 75% of sales, 15% of scientists may account for 85% of scientific publications and citations, 10% of the books in a library may account for 60% of the circulation, and 15% of the opera and rock singers receive 65% of the income in their fields.

Competence and productivity

These laws have led to great efficiencies in special fields. Star performers, for instance, may be recruited for teams and institutions, or they may be studied, and their productive traits may be emulated by, or developed in, others.

One critical ingredient in exceptional performance is attention to costs, which often are neglected in much casual behavior and in academic writing on achievement, performance, and creativity. Oddly, sports and industrial training show what systematic approaches to cost control can accomplish. Several quotations from Gilbert's *Human Performance* (1978) illustrate: "Roughly speaking, competent people are those who can create valuable results without using excessively costly behavior" (p. 17). "Knowledge, motivation, and work, when used competently, are to be husbanded and spent wisely" (p. 18).

A system that rewards people for their behavior encourages incompetence. And a system that rewards people only for their accomplishments, and not for the net worth of their performance, is an incomplete system that fails to appreciate human competence. When such a system is used by managers in the world of work, and teachers in the world of school, it invites them to squander other people's energies. (p. 19)

To optimize achievement and creativity, measurement of results and careful allocation of scarce human resources are required. Gilbert shows how rigorous programs can improve outcomes by multiples if not magnitudes. His "potential for improving performance" (PIP) is the ratio of exemplary performance to typical (median or mean) performance.

PIP ratios tabulated by Gilbert show small values of 2.0 or less in national and world-class athletic competition, which indicates that precise ratio measurement and optimal training regimens have nearly maximized performances. The highest number of runs scored in a baseball season, for example, was Babe Ruth's 177 in 1921, which yields a PIP of 2.02, or twice the average of 87.5 runs. Recent world-class competitors, however, such as Mark Spitz and Jim Ryun, despite superb performances in swimming and track, attained PIPs of less than 1.5, indicating that there was highly intense competition and that their competitors were close behind them.

By comparison, PIPs in education, business, and manufacturing are large, indicating great potential for improvement. Gilbert's figures show that outstanding workers outperform the average by as many multiples as 30. Gilbert shows that careful study of outstanding performance and rigorous implementation of its causes can greatly increase human performance. This usually entails setting forth a few well-defined objectives, studying the most efficient ways to meet them, and paying careful attention to detail and monitoring.

Studies of consultant-induced work changes have also revealed that moderate to large gains in productivity can be expected in newly industrializing countries. Leibenstein (1976) has pointed out that the use of management consultants can repay companies as much as 20 times their fees. Kilby's analyses (1962) of international consulting missions, for example, showed that labor productivity can be increased dramatically. These missions were able to induce productivity gains of 500% in textile mills in India, 200% in Burmese manufacturing assembly, and 45% to 91% in diamond cutting and orange picking in Israel.

Motivation and innovation

Kilby (1962) reported that when members of productivity missions returned to firms they had helped improve, they often found reversion to previous methods and productivities. Leibenstein (1976) offers a theory of "X-efficiency" to explain such suboptimal performance: First, tight, calculated decision making, especially concerning the use of one's own time, to achieve maximal performance is disliked outside the "circles of economists, accountants, and engineers" (p. 73). Second, other components of rationality, such as objective assessment of reality, independence of mind, prolonged reflection, deferral of short-term gratification, and learning from experience, are costly and rare. Third, maintaining old ways avoids the costs of "rate busting," search for and selection of new ways, breaking old social relations, and forming new ones (pp. 82–89).

Sustained organizational productivity and individual innovation may have little to do with simple recognition and installation of apparently superior procedures. Strong motivations and traditions may curb what seem to be rational improvements in techniques. What seems irrational, however, is simply the analyst's ignorance of the complete pecuniary and psychological costs and rewards of people's opportunities and choices as they view them. Exceptional performance may have to do with long-term motivations and habits that grow over a lifetime and may be somewhat independent of immediate perceptions and ideas.

Matthew effects

Current learning and behavior are strongly determined by the past; a good start enhances later opportunities and environments. Considerable evidence, compiled by Walberg and Tsai (1984) in the areas of communications, early childhood, cognitive psychology, and education, shows that early advantages confer future advantages.

Such evidence corroborates Merton's theory (1968) of "the rich getting richer" (from the Gospel of Matthew in the Bible). With respect to scientific creativity, he argued that initial advantages of university study, work with eminent scientists, early publication, job placement, and citation and other recognitions combine multiplicatively over time to confer tastes, skills, habits, rewards, and further opportunities that accumulate to produce highly skewed productivity in scientific work. Similarly, outstanding science departments attract distinguished or potentially distinguished faculty and students, grants, facilities, intellectual contacts, and other factors over time that lead to probable continuing distinction.

The effects are dynamic in that they affect one another over time. The theory, however, is parsimonious and highly generalizable in another sense: It may be said that environments affect growth, and growth affects subsequent environments. The specifics of development and creativity in science are merely instances of the general and pervasive phenomenon.

What such Matthew effects accomplish, in essence, may even be simpler: sustained and concentrated effort necessary for distinction. Such effort is well exemplified by Simon (1954) in the "Berlitz model" of learning a foreign language – one of the more difficult adult tasks that requires perhaps as much effort and time as do the lower levels of creativity. Simon assumes that an individual can choose the amount of practice, that practice makes the language activity easier, that ease increases the pleasantness of the activity, and that pleasantness increases practice. He hypothesizes that excessive difficulty slows practice because it is unpleasant, but if practice persists through temporary difficulty, it will become pleasant and can persist through to mastery.

With respect to creativity, something more than mastery, it can be imagined that early encouragement, specific goals, clear attainments, continued effort, and appropriately high standards are required. Such things lead to further effort, attract the attention of outstanding teachers and coaches, and result in the usual positive-skew distribution of achievement and performance, creativity and eminence.

It seems parsimonious and useful to view the acquisition of knowledge and skill in schools and in societies as similar to, and continuous with, the attainment of creativity and eminence. The differences are not matters of kind, but of degrees of difference with respect to natural and contrived social environments, stimulation and encouragement, and concentration and effort.

Families, schools, and universities are the chief agencies for acquisition, and they can also foster creativity. To the extent that they are more efficient, they can accomplish more of both; and they can foster more creativity not merely in elites but in masses of students. In child-rearing and education for the first two decades of life, moreover, greater productivity can enhance creativity in individuals and society. Cultural literacy and a general education, acquired more fully and quickly, leave more time for advanced acquisition and creativity.

Generally, the scarce resources are educational expertise and human time – the time of parents, educators, coaches, and of learners or creators themselves. To the extent that educational institutions can make early acquisition more efficient, however, they allow more youth more time to go farther in attaining creativity. Because we now have a reasonably good understanding of educational productivity, the problem of increasing acquisition and creativity, in large part, lies in putting efficient procedures into place and finding time to make use of them.

Educational productivity

A compilation of quantitative effects measured in nearly 3,000 studies of learning in homes and schools shows that education can be made far more productive. Nine factors require optimization to increase learning; potent, consistent, and widely generalizable, these nine factors fall into three groups:

A. Aptitude includes:
   1. Ability or prior achievement, as measured on the usual standardized tests
   2. Development, as indexed by age or stage of development
   3. Motivation or self-concept, as indexed by personality tests or willingness to persevere on learning tasks
B. Instruction includes:
   4. The amount of time students engage in classroom learning
   5. The quality of the instructional experience, including both its psychological and curricular aspects
C. The aspects of the psychological environment that bear on learning are:
   6. The curriculum or academic environment of the home
   7. The social climate of the classroom group
   8. The peer group outside school
   9. Exposure to mass media, notably television.

The categorization of these factors is somewhat arbitrary, but it reflects the disparate traditions of research that bear upon learning in natural settings. The more specific aspects of the factors and the magnitudes of their effects on learning are specified elsewhere (Walberg, 1984b).

The specific educational techniques and aspects of environments that enhance one aspect of learning also tend to enhance others. Important aspects of talent and creativity, nonetheless, are poorly measured, and we cannot be certain that they trade off against one another and achievement. For example, we cannot be sure that achievement, as measured on the usual standardized tests, enhances or detracts from creativity.

Generally, what makes a difference in the home and school are stimulation and encouragement. The curriculum of the home, for example, refers to informed parent–child conversations about school and everyday events, encouragement and discussion of leisure reading, monitoring and joint critical analysis of television and peer activities, deferral of immediate gratifications in order to accomplish long-term human-capital goals, expressions of affection and interest in the child's academic and other progress as a person, and, perhaps, among such serious, unremitting efforts, smiles, laughter, caprice, and serendipity.

Specific methods of teaching and certain new programs in schools are much more effective than others. These include mastery learning, cooperative learning, and adaptive education. These and other methods and their comparative effects on learning are described elsewhere (Walberg, 1984b). Most of these methods are well researched insofar as acquisition is concerned. Here it seems useful to describe a nearly forgotten method of education that may be particularly useful in fostering creativity.

Open education

"Open education" has been dismissed by many educators, but surveys of research findings have now illuminated its beneficial effects. From the start, "open" educators tried to encourage educational outcomes that would reflect the goals of teacher, parent, student, and school board, such as cooperation, critical thinking, self-reliance, constructive attitudes, lifelong learning, and other objectives that technically oriented psychometrists seldom measure. A summary (Raven, 1981) of surveys in Western countries, including England and the United States, shows that when given a choice, educators, parents, and students rank these goals above standardized test scores and school marks.

Moreover, studies of the relationships between grades and adult success have shown their slight association (Samson, Grave, Weinstein, & Walberg, 1984). Thirty-three post-1949 studies of the college and professional-school grades of physicians, engineers, civil servants, teachers, and other groups showed an average correlation of .155 for these educational outcomes with life-success indicators such as income, self-rated happiness, work performance and output indices, and self, peer, and supervisor ratings of occupational effectiveness.

These results should challenge educators and researchers to seek a balance and to seek connections between continuing autonomy, motivation, responsibility, and skills to learn new tasks as an individual or group member, on the one hand, and memorization of teacher-chosen textbook knowledge that may soon be obsolete or forgotten, on the other. Perhaps since Socrates, however, these views have remained so polarized that educators find it difficult to stand firmly on the high middle ground of balanced or cooperative teacher–student determination of the goals, means, and evaluation of learning.

Although open education, like its precursors, faded from view, it was massively researched by dozens of investigators whose work has been little noted. Perhaps a study of this research may be useful to educators who want to base practice on research rather than on fads, or those who will evaluate future descendants of open education.

Hedges, Giaconia, and Gage (1981) surveyed 153 studies of open education, including 90 dissertations. The average effect was near zero for achievement, locus of control, self-concept, and anxiety (which suggests no difference between open and control classes on these criteria), about .2 for adjustment, attitude toward schools and teachers, curiosity, and general mental ability, and about .3 for cooperativeness, creativity, and independence. Thus, students in open classes do no worse in standardized achievement and perform slightly to moderately better on several outcomes that educators, parents, and students hold to be of great value.

Unfortunately, the negative conclusion reported in Bennett's single study (1976) – introduced by a prominent psychologist, published by Harvard University Press, publicized by the *New York Times* and by experts who take the press as their source – trumpeted the failure of open education, even though the conclusion of the study was later retracted (Aitkin, Bennett, & Hesketh, 1981) because of obvious statistical flaws in the original analysis (Aitkin, Anderson, & Hinde, 1981).

Giaconia and Hedges (1983) took another recent and constructive step in the synthesis of open-education research. From their prior survey they identified the studies with the largest positive and negative effects on several outcomes to differentiate more and less effective program features. They found that programs that were more effective in producing the nonachievement outcomes – attitude, creativity, and self-concept – sacrificed academic achievement on standardized measures.

These programs were characterized by emphasis on the role of the child in learning, use of diagnostic rather than norm-referenced evaluation, individualized instruction, and manipulative materials, but not three other components sometimes thought essential to open programs – multiage grouping, open space, and team teaching. Giaconia and Hedges speculated that children in the most extreme open programs may do somewhat less well on conventional achievement tests because they have little experience with them. At any rate, it appears from the two most comprehensive surveys of effects that open classes, on average, enhance creativity, independence, and other nonstandard outcomes without detracting from academic achievement unless they are radically extreme.

University research

Research in higher education and graduate education seems to corroborate such findings. Chambers (1973), for example, asked several hundred creative psychologists and chemists to describe the teachers who had had the greatest facilitating and inhibiting influences on their creative development. The most facilitative had the following characteristics (in order of importance): treated students as individuals; encouraged students to be independent; served as a model; spent considerable amount of time with students outside of class; indicated that excellence was expected and could be achieved; enthusiastic; accepted students as equals; directly rewarded students' creative behavior or work; interesting, dynamic lecturer; excellent on one-to-one basis. Inhibiting teachers, on the other hand, had the following characteristics: discouraged students' ideas and creativity; insecure; hypercritical;

sarcastic; unenthusiastic; emphasized rote learning; dogmatic and rigid; did not keep up with field; generally incompetent; had narrow interests; unavailable outside the classroom.

These results seem plausible and reasonable even though the research basis was far smaller and less rigorous than that supporting conclusions on knowledge and skill acquisition. Other research on eminent or highly creative people supports the notion of the special importance of encouragement and stimulation in fostering creativity.

Childhoods of highly eminent adults

Involving 76 other scholars, our research reveals common psychological traits, as well as family, educational, and cultural conditions, for more than 200 highly eminent men born between the fourteenth and twentieth centuries, such as Mozart, Newton, and Lincoln (Walberg, 1982). Ratings of their childhood characteristics and environments made on the basis of respected biographies show their distinctive intellectual competence and motivation, social and communication skills, general psychological wholesomeness, and versatility and concentrated perseverance during childhood. Most were stimulated by the availability of cultural stimuli and materials related to their fields of eminence and by teachers, parents, and other adults. Although most had clear parental expectations for their conduct, they also had the opportunity for exploration on their own (Cox, 1926; McCurdy, 1957; see Simonton in this volume).

The sample of persons for our research traces back to the turn-of-the-century work of James McKean Cattell, founder of the biographical volumes *American Men of Science* (now called *American Men and Women of Science*). In 1903, Cattell listed, in order of imputed eminence, the 1,000 most eminent people according to the number of words that had been written about each in American, English, French, and German biographical dictionaries.

Soon after Cattell's publication, Catherine Cox and Frederick Terman (the developer of the Stanford-Binet Intelligence Test) began a fascinating psychological study of part of Cattell's sample (Cox, 1926). They eliminated the least eminent half of the sample, persons who had apparently been included only because of aristocratic or noble birth, and those born before 1450. Cox and several associates combed more than 3,000 sources, including encyclopedias, biographies, and collections of letters in the Stanford and Harvard libraries, for information on the mental development of each of the remaining 282 persons (including 3 women). From this information, Cox and two associates independently estimated the IQ for each person. Cox's analysis and our own reanalysis of Cox's data show that the reliability of these careful estimates compares reasonably with that for group IQ tests now given to children in school classes.

For additional estimates of eminence, we counted the numbers of words in the primary biographical articles on each of the 282 persons in the 1935 *New International Encyclopedia* and the 1974 *Encyclopaedia Britannica*. The indices of eminence are in substantial agreement from one period to the next, but there are some interesting changes. For example, philosophers lost and musicians and artists gained in estimated eminence from 1903 to 1974. Individuals also shifted in estimated eminence. (For example, starting with the most eminent, the top 10 in the 1903 estimates were Napoleon, Voltaire, Bacon, Goethe, Luther, Burke, Newton, Milton, Pitt, and Washington. In the 1935 word counts, the top 10 in order were Samual Johnson, Luther, Rembrandt, Da Vinci, Napoleon, Washington, Lincoln, Goethe, Beethoven, and Dickens. In the 1974 citations, the top 10 were Descartes, Napoleon, Newton, Leibnitz, Luther, Hegel, Kant, Darwin, Galileo, and Da Vinci.

Confirming Cox's analysis, we found that persons with the highest averages on the four indices of eminence had slightly higher estimated IQs (the correlation is +.33) than others in the sample. There is no doubt that IQ and eminence are linked, but the linkage is by no means tight; the brightest, by measured IQ, are not necessarily the best. Research on recent samples of writers, scientists, and adolescents who have won awards and prizes suggests that outstanding performances in various fields require minimal levels of intelligence. Intelligence higher than these levels, however, seems less important than the presence of other psychological traits and conditions (Walberg, 1969a, 1971).

Minimal levels of intelligence, however, seem required. The most distinctive of all the childhood traits was rated intelligence; 97% of the sampled men and women were rated intelligent, which confirms the Cox-Terman IQ estimates. Other, more wide-ranging cognitive traits were also highly characteristic of the sample. The group as a whole exhibited convergent and divergent abilities ranging from concentration and perseverance to versatility and fluidity.

The majority of the sample also showed a large number of distinctive affective traits that collectively suggested psychological wholesomeness: The majority were rated as ethical, sensitive, solid, magnetic, optimistic, and popular. About a quarter to a third of the sample, however, showed introversion, neuroses, and physical sickliness. Only 38% were rated tall, but the majority were handsome and possessed vitality.

Large percentages of the sample were exposed to stimulating family, educational, and cultural conditions during childhood. Only slightly more than half were encouraged by parents, but a solid majority were encouraged by teachers and other adults and were exposed to many adults at an early age. Significantly more than half (60%) were exposed to eminent persons during childhood.

About 80% were successful in school; the majority liked school, and less than a quarter had school problems. Seventy percent had clear parental expectations for their conduct; but nearly 90% were permitted to explore their environments on their own – obviously a delicate, important balance in child-rearing and teaching.

"The childhood shows the man, as morning shows the day," wrote John Milton in 1667. Our research on childhood traits of highly eminent people confirms the poet's wisdom. Outstanding traits and conditions of childhood can be identified that foreshadow the degree and kind of eminence that history records.

But as rainy afternoons sometime follow sunny mornings, the identified childhood traits and conditions are possible clues or indications of adult eminence rather than certain predictors. The remnants of the records of eminent men are likely to be biased; contemporary ratings of their traits and conditions by biographers and psychologists are no doubt subject to further bias.

Still, the criterion of eminence – how much is written about one in encyclopedic history a century or two later – is more certain, at least more certain than recognition of creativity among our contemporaries is likely to be. These findings appear to be corroborated in my studies of contemporary youth.

Artists and scientists

From a national sample of 771 high school students, I identified three groups: those winning competitive awards in science, those winning awards in the arts, and those not winning awards (Walberg, 1969a). Then I compared them on 300 biographical items on a long, self-administered questionnaire.

In social relations, both creative groups tended more often than did the others to describe themselves as friendly, outgoing, and self-confident. Yet they were also more likely to find books more interesting than people. Both groups had earlier and stronger interests in mechanical and scientific objects, as well as the arts; they more often enjoyed professional and technical books, visited libraries for nonschool reading, and had greater numbers of books at home. They were more interested in work with fine detail, more persistent in carrying things through, and had less time to relax. They liked school and applied themselves to their studies. They also did their work faster than their classmates.

The creative groups felt more creative, imaginative, curious, and expressive and tended to make more original suggestions to childhood playmates and to feel that it is important to be creative. In contrast to some previous formulations and findings in empirical work, they had no greater propensity to suggest "wild" ideas, although they did find satisfaction in expressing ideas in new and original ways. They indicated that they were brighter than their friends and quicker to understand. Larger proportions of the creative groups expected to earn graduate degrees and higher salaries after graduation. They also attached greater importance to money and thought that responsibility is a relatively desirable job attribute. However, in choosing the best characteristics to develop in life, they selected "creativity" more often and "wealth and power" less often. In short, these young creative artists and scientists were more friendly, outgoing, curious, attentive to detail, interested in and self-confident of their own creativity and intelligence, and ambitious for their own education, salary, and, most important, creativity.

In contrast to the artists, the winners of science awards indicated that people had more difficulty in talking to them about personal problems and that they had more difficulty making friends after changing schools. The young scientists more often did not date or dated different girls, rather than dating only one at a time. They were less bothered by humiliating experiences and took less interest in other people's interests. They read biography, but generally were more bookish and were interested, as one would expect, in books about science and mechanics rather than the arts, music, and writing. The scientists were also more interested in finely detailed work and were more apt to bring work to completion in the face of difficulty and distraction. They were less involved in organized school activities and more inclined academically, as expected, to mathematics and science than to music and the arts. There were significant tendencies for the scientists to value and express more confidence in their own intelligence, whereas the young artists felt this way about their creativity. The scientists had higher educational aspirations, were more definitely decided about their future occupations, and tended to make carefully detailed plans rather than let fate take its course. In contrast to the artists, the scientists tended to favor ''security'' as the best characteristic of a job.

In short, the scientists seemed preoccupied with things and ideas rather than people and feelings. They avoided intense emotional closeness to others, persisted in the face of difficulty, were attracted to academic work and detail, and were actively task-oriented. Obviously, mastery is crucial in the arts, and subconscious feelings play an important role in science. But the differences found here imply that communicated inner feeling is the essential preoccupation of the artist (Beauty), whereas single-minded conceptual grappling with external realities is the sine qua non of science (Truth).

In contrast to the responses of those winning no awards, both the artists' and scientists' responses were wholesome and indicative of high aspirations for social status. Comparisons of the award-winning groups suggests that social communication of inner feeling was the preoccupation of the artists, whereas scientists were more intent on single-minded conceptualization of external reality.

Varieties of adolescent creativity

I was able to follow up this original survey with another national sample of nearly 3,000 high school physics students, many of whom had taken an IQ test. In no case was measured intelligence correlated with membership in prize-winning creative groups. This lack of relationship confirms prior studies of creativity and intelligence that have shown weak associations.

Chambers (1969), after reviewing research in this area, hypothesized that a minimal level of intellectual ability is essential for creative productivity, but beyond a given ''floor,'' which varies in different fields, there is no relationship between measured intelligence and creativity. A fairly typical result is that of MacKinnon (1961). He found that a sample of creative architects scored higher on intelligence tests than did undergraduate students. However, when the architects were ordered according to their peer-rated creativity, the correlation between intelligence and creativity was found to be nonsignificant ($-.08$).

Based on his own research on creative writers and on the work of others, Barron (1961) concluded that there are correlations around $+.4$ between the two variables over the total range of intelligence, but that beyond an IQ level of 120, intelligence is a negligible factor in creativity. The mean IQs for boys and girls in my sample were 117 and 119. The group that elected to take physics in high school was generally higher in measured intelligence than the rest of the high school population. Moreover, the criteria for creativity employed in the study were not as stringent as those used by Barron and MacKinnon for creative architects and writers who had won national recognition. Nevertheless, a large part of the total sample in the study may be beyond the minimal levels of mental ability required for winning awards and prizes in adolescent competition – thus explaining the lack of relationship between intelligence and creativity.

Creative groups among the sample of boys were different from students who did not achieve distinction. In contrast to other students, the creative groups more often reported themselves as more creative and imaginative and as having more creative opportunities. They more often liked school, got high marks, and questioned their teachers. Also, they more often thought that it is important to be intelligent, had at least two cases of books in the home, studied and read outside school, and talked to adults about future occupations. Lastly, they more often followed through with work despite difficulties and distractions.

These relationships confirm several findings from prior research and suggest that the creative groups in different fields resemble one another more than they resemble students who have not won distinction. The data from this research and two prior studies (Schaefer & Anastasi, 1968; Walberg, 1969a) and several hypotheses from a multidimensional theory of creativity (Chambers, 1969) converge on several general factors associated with creativity in adolescence. As identified by teacher nominations, creativity test scores, and self-reports, creativity is associated with (a) the stimulating qualities of the home, (b) a wide range and high level of involvement in both school and outside activities, (c) persistence and single-mindedness in following through activities despite difficulties, and (d) strong intellectual motivation, although not necessarily extremely high levels of ability.

However, several differences are worth noting. Artists characteristically had more diversified, less concentrated interests and opportunities than scientists. Performers and musicians tended to do more studying outside of school, to have more creative opportunities, to think less of the importance of intelligence, and to be less persistent. Creative leaders and scientists, however, seemed to concentrate their energies more in school; they were more likely to question teachers, to be persistent, and to think it important to be intelligent. Thus, although all creative groups shared a high degree of involvement in all activities, as compared with other students, after these differences are considered, scientists and leaders tended to be more involved in academic life than did performers and musicians.

Specialized performance and creativity

It is not philosophically unpleasant to contemplate positive skew of exceptional performance and creativity as long as a variety of skills are valued. To make everyone alike, as some educators wish to do, is impossibly difficult, as collectivist and totalitarian societies have demonstrated. Biologists celebrate diversity, and agricultural experience warns of the danger of uniformly optimizing crop characteristics for only one condition or against a single threat of disease.

Modern portfolio theory suggests that risks are lower if several stocks are held, rather than only one, because they are unlikely to decline in value all at the same time. The law of comparative advantage in economics suggests, by analogy, that people with different skills may raise each other's welfare more than can those who are similar. And it has been known for two centuries, since the time of Adam Smith, that division of labor can enhance individual and national welfare.

Should educators allow more specialization? A synthesis of 35 post-1950 studies showed that grades in college and professional schools, such as business, education, engineering, and medicine, account, on average, for 2.4% of the variance in later indications of career success, such as income, effectiveness ratings, and happiness (Samson et al., 1984). The results suggest that it may not be critical for educators and students to cover all topics and subjects equally well, as they often try to do. Because human energy and time are finite, trying to master a little of everything (or what other people know, or what can be looked up) may hamper efforts to get to the bottom of a question, to pursue a skill to one's personal limit, to acquire exceptional expertise, to encourage and recognize skill in others, and to appreciate groups that combine diverse, specialized skills. Considerable research in a variety of academic, artistic, athletic, scientific, and other fields suggests that world-class performance demands intensely specialized efforts for as much as 70 hr per week for a decade (Walberg, 1983).

It may be well to allow and encourage students, even young students, more often to pursue various topics and skills, perhaps of their own choice, to the low or even high end of exceptionality. Such exceptionality may be brought about not only by acceleration programs and extramural study but also by more individualization and student choice in ordinary school classrooms. Skimming off "the best and the brightest," however, may isolate them from "normal" students to the disadvantage of both groups. The disadvantage is especially risky if only conventional measures of academic verbal ability are employed.

Life is a series of such trade-offs, and educators, parents, and students themselves will have their own preferences regarding the decision to strive for exceptional performance in one field or opt for some degree of balance among fields. Whatever one's views on these matters, however, neither "all-roundedness" nor exceptional performance is likely to be increased dramatically until more comprehensive and explicit theories of educational productivity are formulated, better measures of causes and effects are developed, and more comprehensive studies of productivity are completed.

References

Aitkin, M., Anderson, D., & Hinde, J. (1981). Modeling of data on teaching styles (with discussion). *Journal of the Royal Statistical Society, Series A, 144,* 419–461.

Aitkin, M., Bennett, S. N., & Hesketh, J. (1981). Teaching styles and pupil progress: A re-analysis. *British Journal of Educational Psychology, 51,* 170–180.

Barron, F. (1961). Creative vision and expression in writing and painting. In D. W. MacKinnon (Ed.), *The creative person* (pp. 237–251). Berkeley: Institute of Personality Assessment Research, University of California.

Becker, G. S. (1976). *The economic approach to human behavior.* University of Chicago Press.

Benbow, C. P., & Stanley, J. C. (1983). *Academic precocity.* Baltimore: Johns Hopkins University Press.

Bennett, S. N. (1976). *Teaching styles and pupil progress.* London: Open Books.

Bloom, B. S., & Sosniak, L. A. (1981). Talent development vs. schooling. *Educational Leadership, 39*(2), 510–522.

Cattell, J. M. (1903, February). A statistical study of eminent men. *Popular Science Monthly, 359–377.*

Chambers, J. (1969). A multidimensional theory of creativity. *Psychological Reports, 25,* 779–799.

Chambers, J. A. (1973). College teachers: Their effect on creativity of students. *Journal of Educational Psychology, 65,* 326–334.

Cox, C. M. (1926). *The early mental traits of three hundred geniuses.* Stanford, CA: Stanford University Press.

Ericsson, K. A., Chase, W. G., & Faloon, S. (1980). Acquisition of a memory skill, *Science, 208,* 1181–1182.

Getzels, J. W., & Csikszentmihalyi, M. (1976). *The creative vision.* New York: Wiley.

Getzels, J. W., & Jackson, P. W. (1962). *Creativity and intelligence.* New York: Wiley.

Giaconia, R. M., and Hedges, L. V. (1983). Identifying features of open education. Stanford, CA: Stanford Center for Educational Research.

Gilbert, T. F. (1978). *Human performance.* New York: McGraw-Hill.

Havighurst, R. J. (1958). The importance of education for the gifted. In N. B. Henry (Ed.), *Fifty-seventh Yearbook of the National Society for the Study of Education* (pp. 14–33). University of Chicago Press.

Hedges, L. V., Giaconia, R. M., & Gage, N. L. (1981). *Meta-analysis of the effects of open and traditional instruction.* Stanford, CA: Stanford University Program on Teaching Effectiveness.

Kilby, P. (1962). Organization and productivity in backward economies. *Quarterly Journal of Economics, 76,* 306–316.

Leibenstein, H. (1976). *Beyond economic man.* Cambridge, MA: Harvard University Press.

McCurdy, H. G. (1957). The childhood pattern of genius. *Journal of Elisha Mitchell Science Society, 73,* 448–462.

MacKinnon, D. W. (1961). Creativity in architects. In D. W. MacKinnon (Ed.), *The creative person* (pp. 291–320). Berkeley: Institute of Personality Assessment Research, University of California.

Merton, R. K. (1968). The Matthew effect in science. *Science, 159,* 56–63.

Mincer, J. (1979). Human capital and earnings. In D. Windham (Ed.), *Economic dimensions of education* (pp. 1–21). New York: National Academy of Education.

Mincer, J. (1981). *Human capital and economic growth* (Working Paper No. 803). Cambridge, MA: National Bureau of Economic Research.

Morgan, D. N. (1953). Creativity today. *Journal of Aesthetics, 12,* 1–24.

Newell, A., Shaw, J. C., & Simon, H. A. (1963). The process of creative thinking. In H. E. Gruber (Ed.), *Contemporary approaches to creative thinking* (pp. 43–62). New York: Atherton.

Orczyk, C., & Walberg, H. J. (1983). Psychological traits and conditions of eminent artists. *Visual Arts Review, 9,* 82–87.

Raven, J. (1981). The most important problem in education is to come to terms with values. *Oxford Review of Education, 7,* 253–272.

Roe, A. (1953). A psychological study of eminent psychologists and anthropologists and a comparison with biological and physical scientists. *Psychological Monographs 67*(2), (Whole No. 352).

Samson, G., Graue, M. E., Weinstein, T., & Walberg, H. J. (1984). Academic and occupational performance: A quantitative synthesis. *American Educational Research Journal, 21,* 311–322.

Schaefer, C. E., & Anastasi, A. (1968). A biographical inventory for identifying creativity in adolescent boys. *Journal of Applied Psychology, 52,* 42–48.

Schiller, D. P., & Walberg, H. J. (1982). Japan: The learning society. *Educational Leadership, 39,* 411–413.

Simon, H. A. (1954). Some strategic considerations in the construction of social science models. In P. Lazarsfeld (Ed.), *Mathematical thinking in the social sciences* (pp. 192–213). Glencoe, IL: Free Press.

Simon, H. A. (1981). *Sciences of the artificial.* Cambridge, MA: MIT Press.

Sternberg, R. J., & Davidson, J. E. (1985). Cognitive development in gifted and talented. In F. D. Horowitz & M. O'Brien (Eds.), *The gifted and talented* (pp. 103–135). Washington, DC: American Psychological Association.

Strykowski, B. F., & Walberg, H. J. (1983). Psychological traits and conditions of eminent writers. *Roeper Review: A Journal of Gifted Education, 6,* 102–104.

Taylor, C. W., & Ellison, R. L. (1967). Biographical predictors of scientific performance. *Science, 155,* 1075–1080.

Visher, S. S. (1955). Sources of great men. *Eugenics Quarterly, 21,* 103–109.

Walberg, H. J. (1969a). A portrait of the artist and scientist as young men. *Exceptional Children, 36,* 5–11.

Walberg, H. J. (1969b). Physics, femininity, and creativity. *Developmental Psychology, 1,* 45–54.

Walberg, H. J. (1971). Varieties of creativity and the high school environment. *Exceptional Children, 38,* 111–116.

Walberg, H. J. (1982). Childhood traits and environmental conditions of highly eminent adults. *Gifted Child Quarterly, 25,* 103–107.

Walberg, H. J. (1983). Scientific literacy and economic productivity in international perspective. *Daedalus, 112*(2), 1–28.

Walberg, H. J. (1984a). Families as partners in educational productivity. *Phi Delta Kappan, 65*(6), 397–400.

Walberg, H. J. (1984b). Improving the productivity of America's schools. *Educational Leadership, 41,* 19–27.

Walberg, H. J. (1984c). *National abilities and economic growth.* Paper read at the American Association for the Advancement of Science, New York.

Walberg, H. J. (1987). Learning and life-course accomplishments. In C. Schooler & K. W. Schaie (Eds.), *Cognitive functioning and social structure over the life course.* Norwood, NJ: Ablex.

Walberg, H. J., Rasher, S. P., & Hase, K. (1978). IQ correlates with high eminence. *Gifted Child Quarterly, 22,* 196–200.

Walberg, H. J., Rasher, S. P., & Parkerson, J. A. (1979). Childhood and eminence. *Journal of Creative Behavior, 13*(94), 225–231.

Walberg, H. J., Strykowski, B. F., Rovai, E., & Hung, S. S. (1984). Exceptional performance. *Review of Educational Research, 54,* 84–112.

Walberg, H. J., & Tsai, S.-L. (1984). Matthew effects in education. *American Educational Research Journal, 20,* 359–374.

Walberg, H. J., & Weinstein, T. (1984). Adult outcomes of connections, certification, and verbal competence. *Journal of Educational Research, 77,* 207–212.

Wallach, M. A. (1985). Creativity testing and giftedness. In F. D. Horowitz & M. O'Brien (Eds.), *The gifted and talented.* Washington, DC: American Psychological Association.

15   The possibility of invention

D. N. Perkins

The *ex nihilo* problem

It is axiomatic that what is "actual" is possible. Bumblebees actually fly, and therefore it is possible for them to fly, although classic aerodynamics supposedly would predict that they cannot. We need to figure out how. The same principle that applies to bumblebees applies to the entire universe: The universe is actual and therefore is possible, although, again, *how* is not so clear. Physicists building accounts of the first microseconds of the universe have made some progress in telling the story, but inevitable mysteries remain. What was the universe like at time zero? What about before time zero, or was there no time, making the question meaningless? Why should the universe have happened at all?

In between bumblebees and the universe, we human beings sit, pondering on occasion how bumblebees fly, how the universe came to be, and our own peculiar nature. One part of that nature is creativity. We are a species conspicuous for invention. To be sure, some other animals show, from time to time, a bit of inventiveness, but invention is the stock-in-trade of humankind. This creativity is actual and therefore, like the bumblebee's capacity for flight and the universe's existence, is possible. But, again, like both of those, *how* it is possible is harder to say.

Let us consider just what the mystery is. Our inventiveness often puzzles us as a particular example of what might be called an *ex nihilo* problem: Something comes out of nothing. The universe poses a similar dilemma on a far grander scale. Once there was no universe, and then there was. Where did it come from, and how? Every day, as human beings write poems, paint paintings, formulate new commercial products, discover theorems, and devise theories, novel objects and ideas come into being, *ex nihilo,* as it were. The question is: How is this novelty possible? How can any mechanism of mind produce something genuinely new, something that reaches beyond the boundaries of human achievement up to that point in time?

The main mission of this chapter is to offer some broad answers to that puzzling question. It will help if we dissociate the problem partly from the peculiarities of the human condition. Although human beings are the most conspicuously inventive systems around, they are not the only inventive systems. Nature, in the course of millennia, invents through the process of evolution. Certain computer programs developed by artificial-intelligence researchers show a modest degree of inventiveness. Finally, languages, customs, and other social constructs are invented by complex social processes that, although they involve human beings, do not necessarily yield invention through ground-breaking contributions of key individuals, but rather in more gradual and even mindless ways. By looking across these varied inventive systems, we can perhaps gain some insight into the fundamental principles that underwrite the possibility of invention.

Easy nonanswers

Some clearing of underbrush needs to be done before considering serious resolutions of the *ex nihilo* problem of inventive thinking. We human beings love easy answers, sometimes so much that we give them more credit than they deserve. The *ex nihilo* problem has attracted some easy nonanswers that cling with remarkable tenacity.

Not really ex nihilo

Perhaps the simplest response to the *ex nihilo* puzzle is to say that invention is not really *ex nihilo*. Human invention never produces something entirely out of nothing. Always the inventor brings to the occasion a host of concepts, facts, structures, and so on that fuel the process of invention. So there is no puzzle to explain. Invention is better seen as an act of combination rather than an act of *ex nihilo* creation.

A classic exemplar of this combinatorial account of invention appeared in John Livingston Lowes's *The Road to Xanadu,* in which Lowes offered a close analysis of the writing of Samuel Taylor Coleridge's *Kubla Khan* (Lowes, 1927). Coleridge reported composing the poem very quickly in a kind of opium daze and publishing it virtually untouched, a remarkable feat of the poetic imagination. In fact, later research disclosed that Coleridge was misrepresenting or, at best, seriously misremembering the circumstances, because he apparently undertook significant revisions of the "raw" *Kubla Khan* (Schneider, 1953). However that may be, Lowes focused on what happened before rather than after Coleridge's inventive epiphany, examining the origins of the poem's elements in Coleridge's life. Lowes showed how Coleridge's prior readings and writings filled his mind with the images that would coalesce into the poetic tide of *Kubla Khan.*

The point that the elements brought together in an invention are not *ex nihilo* is surely important. However, this point does not resolve the *ex nihilo* problem. The remaining gap is easily stated: Although the elements may have precedent, the combination achieved in an episode of invention does not. That novel combination at least is *ex nihilo*. To be sure, our recognition that the elements lie at hand makes it easier to understand how a creative outcome might emerge, for it is not as though the inventor had to invent everything from scratch. Nonetheless, for the results to count as genuinely inventive, the combination must go significantly beyond arbitrary combinatorial play, to achieve notable power, parsimony, and novelty. To phrase the matter, for emphasis, in extreme form: How much understanding of the making of a poem do we gain through recognizing that all the words were already in the dictionary? How much insight into the discovery of a mathematical theorem do we garner through recognizing that the mathematical operators and rules were already at hand?

Reductio ad absurdum

We turn now to another easy nonanswer to the *ex nihilo* question. This nonanswer urges that the question itself is logically flawed, and so it is senseless to try to resolve the question. The argument goes something like this. Imagine we had a scientific account of how invention was possible. This model, in turn, would allow forecasting what inventions would be made. But *genuine* inventive thinking, by definition, breaks boundaries in unexpected ways, implying that a forecast cannot be made. Accordingly, we can have no such scientific account. Hausman (1976, 1985) has argued somewhat in this manner.

Just to keep our Latin lively, it is worth pointing out that this argument has the form of *reductio ad absurdum,* in which one assumes the proposition one doubts and derives a contradiction, thereby negating the proposition. In the present case, we assume that we have a scientific account of invention, infer that this implies forecasting what inventions would be made, and note a contradiction with our concept of the boundary-breaking character of invention. Given this contradiction, we reject the initial assumption that we could have a scientific account of invention. Of course, the catch with this, as with any *reductio ad absurdum* argument, is that its soundness depends on the validity of the line of argument connecting the assumption to the contradiction. Although the line of argument laid out earlier may have some surface plausibility, in fact it suffers from at least two major faults.

First, the argument assumes that a sound scientific account of something yields predictions of just what will happen in the future. Comparison with various contemporary and respected scientific theories quickly shows that this is far too strong a criterion for a good scientific theory. An especially appropriate case in point is quantum mechanics, which not only does not allow precise prediction of events at the atomic level but also asserts the impossibility of such prediction by way of the irritating Heisenberg uncertainty principle. For an example from classic physics, thermodynamics yields only statistical forecasts of how a gas will behave under various circumstances. If these theories drawn from the hardest of the hard sciences fall short of perfect forecasting, then what can one expect in the field of psychology, where there is hardly any precedent for a theory of more than statistical predictiveness? It seems that we can freely seek a scientific account of invention so long as the resulting account does not make precise predictions about what will be invented. This limit is easily tolerated, because such predictiveness is not routinely achieved in science anyway.

However, we need not accept even that very acceptable limitation; a second flaw in the argument makes it unnecessary. The *reductio ad absurdum* argument says that the very concept of genuine invention implies that genuine inventions cannot be predicted. But does this unpredictability really follow from our concept of invention? Let us do a thought experiment. We usually count the development of the theory of relativity as an unquestionable case of invention. Now suppose that someone developed a scientific theory of the evolution of science that, applied retroactively, forecast the emergence of the theory of relativity from the historical milieu around 1900 and the youthful character traits of Einstein. Faced with this successful retroactive prediction, it seems that we have to reclassify the formulation of the theory of relativity as not creative after all. We were wrong in thinking that it was genuinely inventive.

What is the general point here? If we presume that our notion of genuine invention implies unpredictability, we may in the end have to reclassify certain discoveries we now consider inventive as not inventive after all. But this is very odd. Why should we have to defrock canonized instances of creativity for the sake of a questionable criterion of unpredictability? What we mean by "genuine invention" is defined at least as much by what world events we customarily call inventive as it is by any putative semantic analysis of "genuine invention." Although a fully predictive theory of invention seems exceedingly unlikely now or in the future, it is much too strong to say that our concept of genuine invention *forbids* a fully predictive theory.

In summary, the *reductio ad absurdum* argument itself verges on the absurd, depending on unreasonably strong assumptions about what a scientific account must do and what "genuine invention" implies. Although a good account of inventive thinking no doubt is hard to come by, nothing in the *logic* of the question appears to forbid such an account.

Deus ex machina

A final evasion of the *ex nihilo* problem merits a few words motivated not so much by the seriousness of the challenge as by historical tenacity. A nice metaphor for this nonanswer comes from the theatrical term *deus ex machina,* machinery of the gods. When a play presents a dilemma not readily sorted out by mortals, the gods may come down to mediate a resolution. Of course, to come down, they have to get delivered to the stage by some mechanical contraption of pulleys and platforms – the machinery in question. Metaphorically speaking, a *deus ex machina* solution resolves a problem by introducing an ad hoc element from outside the authentic context of the problem.

As venerable a person as Plato was not at all shy about offering a *deus ex machina* account of inventive thinking. He had Socrates articulate the following well-known poetic account of the poetic process (Cooper, 1961):

A poet is a light and winged thing, and holy, and never able to compose until he has become inspired, and is beside himself and reason is no longer in him . . . for not by art do they utter these, but by power divine.

Moreover, things have not changed that much in 2,500 years. Many thoughtful individuals still speak in somewhat similar terms about the process of invention. For example, an impressive poem by Ted Hughes entitled "The Thought Fox" describes the conceiving of an idea through the metaphor of a fox appearing at a distance in a dark wood, cautiously approaching until his green eyes begin to loom, and suddenly leaping into the reader's head (Hughes, 1969). In a recent essay, Doris Grumbach (1986) compares her process of creation to the bubbling up of gases from a compost heap. The compost heap metaphor resonates with Lowes's account of the writing of *Kubla Khan,* with his emphasis on finding the precedents in Coleridge's earlier life for the images that bubbled up during Coleridge's opium daze. Although neither the fox nor the compost heap involves the gods themselves, they both imbibe the *deus ex machina* spirit, treating the source of invention as something outside the center of conscious striving, something that enters in and delivers up the creative outcome. Invention is thus styled as a kind of sensitive and expectant waiting. The maker is a vessel rather than a cook.

There may be some truth some of the time in such images of the experience of creating, although it seems to me that creating much more often feels like vigorous exploration. However, what the experience of creating feels like is simply not the same question as what mechanisms account for creating. However true or untrue to the typical subjective experience of invention they may be, thought foxes and compost heaps describe the process of invention in ways that do not give us an explanatory hold on the *ex nihilo* problem.

Generation, selection, and preservation as a mechanism of invention

It seems that the *ex nihilo* problem is more than a mere nothing to be dismissed by a few logical or poetic maneuvers, but the challenge of offering a serious answer remains. It is natural to turn to examples of invention to garner insight into the underlying mechanism – the experience of Coleridge reconceived under some paradigm more subtle than that of Lowes, classic episodes of discovery such as those of Gutenberg with the printing press, Pasteur with vaccination, Fleming with penicillin, or Kekulé with the benzene ring, and whatever other resources history affords (Koestler, 1964). However, there is a double problem with this ploy. First, human behavior is notoriously complicated, and its intricacies may obscure important principles. Second, by examining only human beings as inventive systems, we might miss a more fundamental and cross-cutting insight into the sorts of mechanisms that can yield invention.

With these hazards in mind, a look at quite a different inventive system seems useful. Nature invents. Nature invented *Penicillium notatum,* the mold Fleming identified, along with ferns, oak trees, scorpions, elephants, and ourselves. Biological science sustains a long and agreeable tradition of marveling over the cleverness of nature – such instances as orchids in the shape of female bees that ensure their pollination by luring male bees, or spiders that cast their webs like nets, or ants that milk aphids. The writings of Lewis Thomas, for instance, routinely celebrate the creativity of nature. To be sure, nature does not know what it is doing in being so clever. Some might even prefer not to use a term like "invention" in association with nature, reserving it for application only to conscious human enterprise. However, in this discussion we use "invention" broadly and hope for illumination through comparing various systems that, at least in a loose sense, invent.

So how does nature do it? The classic answer was offered by Charles Darwin in his *Origin of Species*. Nature's mechanism of invention lies in the process of natural selection. Unpacked into its details, natural selection depends on three subprocesses: (1) genetic variation; (2) selection of adaptive results via the test of survival and reproduction; (3) inheritance of the adaptive results. According to the Darwinian perspective, this trio of subprocesses, over millennia, leads to the emergence of new species.

To see the general character of the Darwinian model, we can strip away the terms that make it specific to the biosphere, isolating these three subprocesses: (1) generation of alternatives; (2) selection of alternatives; (3) preservation of results. The generation, selection, and preservation need not occur through genetic or, more generally, biological mechanisms. There results an elementary problem-solving cycle that, repeated over many "generations," can yield snowballing results.

Viewed from a Darwinian perspective, the challenge of the *ex nihilo* problem yields up a simple solution. Mere generation, selection, and preservation are enough in the course of millennia to yield remarkable inventions, such as the opposable thumb and the human brain. The accomplishment of nature seems all the more impressive in light of what one might call the blindness of the process. Natural selection selects for mere survival, not anything more exalted, such as elegance, parsimony, or originality. Indeed, elegance, parsimony, and originality are properties we read into organisms from our human perspective because we are interested in such things, not properties evolution directly tries for. They emerge because the reductive criterion of mere survival yields them as secondary effects. Apparently, elegance, parsimony, and originality often serve survival well; so these characteristics appear in the course of evolution without being selected for as such.

It is worth noting here that some contemporary scientists see the need to apply various qualifications to the classic model of evolution. For instance, the process of genetic variation may not be entirely random, but may involve various "best-bet" paths that have themselves been selected for during the evolution of the genetic machinery. Usually conceived as a gradual process, evolution may occur in spurts, according to the theory of "punctuated equilibrium" (Gould, 1980, chap. 17–18). However that may be, for present purposes a straight Darwinian account will do, because generation, selection, and preservation presumably still figure in the modified models, and because our discussion will quickly get beyond the level of complexity of a simple generation, selection, and preservation mechanism in any case.

The pattern of generation, selection, and preservation appears in social evolution as well. Of course, some social evolution of technologies, customs, and ideas calls for attention to the inventiveness of particular human beings, because it occurs through the enterprise of a few individuals. One can trace, person by person, the history of the printing press or the ball-point pen. However, considerable social evolution occurs nearly as blindly as biological evolution; generation by generation, practices and customs of language and conduct change under subtle pressures, without any single individual playing a particularly pivotal role. As in the biosphere, sometimes remarkable invention results from this relatively blind process; for example, consider the languages spoken in the world today, each one a marvelously complex mechanism attributable not to one or a few inventors, but to a gradual process of social evolution.

Of course, the mechanisms of generation, selection, and preservation are different in the social and biological contexts. In the social context, accidents and individual efforts generate variations, social functionality and acceptability select, and a variety of social processes from storytelling to formal education preserve. In his insightful and amusing book *The Selfish Gene,* Richard Dawkins (1976) calls the conceptual entities that spring up and live or die in the petri dish of society "memes," in analogy to genes.

Thus, blind or fairly blind generation, selection, and preservation suffice for remarkable invention, given enough time. But it would be a mistake to see the fundamental pattern of exploration embodied in generation, selection, and preservation as intrinsically blind. Individual human invention routinely depends on the trio, but certainly not in a blind form. Poets, physicists, and other problem solvers routinely generate options and select among them mindfully, preserving the results to build up a complex product. The criteria of selection have nothing like the reductive character of "mere survival" – instead often involving directly such matters as elegance, parsimony, power, and originality. Of course, this does not imply that a working poet or physicist goes through a checklist with the items elegance, parsimony, and originality on it in sizing up candidate phrases or formulas. The judgments may be quite intuitive, merely tacitly and indirectly embodying such principles. However, the principles have a much stronger presence than in the case of biological evolution. Indeed, process-tracing studies of poets creating poems have disclosed that usually critical appraisals come with reasons for the judgments, rather than reflecting opaque intuitions (Perkins, 1981).

While it is apparent that humans select and preserve not blindly but mindfully, humans also generate in a much more strategic way than nature's rolling of genetic dice. For example, you can easily bias your memory retrieval processes to retrieve low-probability rather than high-probability responses. Here is a simple thought experiment: First list a few common color terms, and then list a few rare color terms, such as puce. You will find that the second list comes readily enough, although perhaps with an occasional intrusion of a more common color term. Or if you try to remember people you have not seen in some time, several will readily come to mind. As in elementary acts of memory retrieval, so in more complex circumstances, it is often rather easy to adopt a mental set that favors generation of options of a certain sort – for instance, imaginative options. *How* the mind does this we do not address here, but *that* the mind does it seems plain, supplementing mindfully directed selection and preservation with mindfully directed generation.

Let us take stock of our progress in addressing the *ex nihilo* problem. It seems that a quite elementary mechanism can account for some quite remarkable cases of invention: generation, selection, and preservation – *blind* at that. The same mechanism operating at a faster pace not locked into the cycle of birth operates in society, yielding a relatively blind process of social evolution. Generation, selection, and preservation also have a transparent relevance to individual human invention, in which they gain more pace and leverage through mindfully directed selection, preservation, and even generation. Although individual inventors cannot know exactly what they will end up with before they arrive at it, they can bias their generativity and selectivity in the direction of the *sort* of thing they want and preserve pieces of it as the pieces turn up. Recalling Dawkins's notion of memes, one might say that society is a kind of jungle in which memes spring up and propagate or die according to the vagaries of the society. But an individual creative mind is more like a tended garden, in which seeds of memes are sown with some calculation, and sprouting memes are subjected to selective weeding and cultivation.

A tale of three boundaries

Central to our informal notion of creativity is the notion that significant boundaries get crossed. Quantum mechanics made a sharp break with classical mechanics; the impressionists ushered in a philosophy of painting the light rather than the objects in a scene; modern poetry challenged the secure dominion of rhyme and regular meter. Yet, thus far in this discussion of generation and selection, nothing has addressed directly how boundaries get crossed *ex nihilo*. The question is worth asking, especially because it points to the need for elaborating the notion of generation, selection, and preservation in a crucial direction.

The flight of creatures originally terrestrial surely signals a boundary-breaking episode in the evolution of the animal kingdom. Recent paleontological inquiry and speculation have yielded accounts of how this might have come about (Gould, 1980, chap. 26). One possible version of the story goes something as follows: Current evidence suggests that the dinosaurs of long ago were warm-blooded, although today's reptiles are all cold-blooded. Any warm-blooded creature faces the problem of preserving body heat, a problem particularly acute in small creatures with a higher surface-to-volume ratio and hence a more rapid relative rate of heat loss. So small dinosaurs developed feathers as an insulating agent, under the pressure of natural selection.

It turned out that these insulating feathers provided a certain adaptive stability as the two-legged dinosaurs scurried along with their forelimbs upraised. The stability function commenced to improve through natural selection, the feathers growing larger along the forelimbs. This, in turn, led to the forelimb feathers providing some lift. The lift, like the stabilizing effect and the insulating effect before that, proved adaptive. Natural selection again went to work, extending the feathers and tuning them toward what they soon were to become: full-fledged (as it were) instruments of flight. Dinosaurs had become birds, a line of descent taken seriously enough by some that they have proposed that dinosaurs be rescued from extinction by tax-onomic legerdemain: Dinosaurs should not be classified as *Reptilia* nor birds as *Aves*. Instead, dinosaurs and birds should be grouped together under a new class: *Dinosauria*.

This tale of how birds came to flight involves the crossing of at least two notable boundaries – from insulation to stabilization, and from stabilization to flight. Yet a crucial point needs making about the manner of the crossing. In keeping with the blind character of natural selection, there was no explicit involvement of the boundary as such in the process. The process of generation, selection, and preservation just kept on doing its usual incremental work. To cast the matter in metaphor, imagine a person hiking inattentively across country. The crest of a particular hill may take the person from one enormous watershed to another quite different one. But to this traveler, concerned only with putting one foot in front of another, nothing special has happened.

A tale in some ways different and in some ways the same can be told about recent research in artificial intelligence. In the course of the last decade, certain investiga-tors have made serious efforts to program computers to accomplish tasks with some claim to creativity (Bradshaw, Langley, & Simon, 1983; Langley, Bradshaw, & Simon, 1983; Lenat, 1983). Perhaps the strongest claim of success comes from the work of Lenat (1983), whose AM program has generated significant mathematical discoveries, or, more precisely, rediscoveries. The program works on elementary set theory and number theory, starting with elementary properties of sets and build-ing toward more complex concepts and theorems about sets and numbers concepts.

Certain features of AM make the program atypical of most work in artificial intelligence, but perhaps more typical of much of human creative thinking. First, the program has what might be called an aesthetic. Incorporated into its functioning are criteria not just for what makes a proposition right or wrong but also for what makes a concept *interesting*. For instance, a relationship that sometimes, but only rarely, holds true gets points for interestingness. Second, the program has no specific problem to solve, but rather simply *ruminates,* seeking out new concepts and propositions that score high on interestingness, checking the truth of the propo-sitions, and continuing to build in this manner.

The analogy to Darwinian natural selection should be plain. Various heuristics for generating candidate concepts and propositions operate. The selection principles are truth and interestingness. Finally, the program preserves its interesting and true forays as the foundation for yet further rumination and construction. And the tactic works to a significant degree. For example, starting from a very primitive base of concepts, AM succeeded in rediscovering the concept of prime numbers, which counts as interesting, because a prime number satisfies the "holds-true-rarely" principle: A prime number is divisible only by itself and by 1.

As in the evolution of birds, boundaries get crossed here. A path from primitive notions of set theory to the construction of the concept of primes surely deserves some credit for boundary crossing. But what are the contrasts and commonalities with evolution? One contrast lies in the greater vision of AM. Not blind like evolution, AM "knows" what it is about in its efforts to ensure truth and interestingness, and it guides its search with attendant calculation. But one important commonality deserves mention as well: AM pays no more attention to boundaries than to evolution. Crossing a conceptual boundary is not an act of special significance for the program, but simply one more step that happens to carry the program into a new watershed.

Another observation brings out this point more strongly yet. AM does not challenge its own operating rules. *Human* mathematicians, physicists, poets, and painters do from time to time challenge their operating rules as such and revise them. This characteristic of AM should not be seen as vitiating its achievement, because its achievement is quite impressive in any case, nor should the characteristic be taken as a signal that machines never can think creatively in a genuine way. Although AM does not challenge its own rules, certainly computers can be programmed to challenge some of their own rules. So one should not take the point as implying more than it does. Nonetheless, the point certainly contrasts with an important aspect of human creative practice.

Let us tell a human tale, one of many that might be related. During the first years of the twentieth century, Einstein nourished the seeds of ideas that would grow into the general theory of relativity. His earliest paper with a plain connection to relativity began with an odd motivation. Einstein observed that a certain asymmetry occurred in classic electrodynamics (Holton, 1973). The details do not matter here. But it seems that in one situation a particular formula applied, and in another situation that seemed to differ merely in frame of reference another formula applied. Both yielded correct predictions in their contexts, and so there was no *real* problem; the theory worked. Nonetheless, Einstein found this asymmetry offensive. A neat universe and a neat theory would not tolerate two different accounts of essentially the same thing because of superficially different circumstances. Einstein's pique set him off on a program of challenging fundamental assumptions, and that program led to the body of work on relativity we know today.

The analogy with the ruminating of Lenat's AM program should be apparent. Einstein, like the program, was guided by an aesthetic that gave him an index of what was worthwhile and what was not. However, in another way, Einstein worked from a view of the matter differing sharply from that embodied in the AM program. Einstein knew that a whole theoretical paradigm was at stake. He referred to classic electrodynamics in sweeping terms. He worked with the double-edged advantage/disadvantage of realizing that a certain step might take him from one watershed into another entirely.

What was true of Einstein is widely true of human invention in contexts from the lofty to the mundane: We are mindful boundary crossers and indeed operate *on* the boundaries rather than blindly within them. We often map them out and challenge them, asking what other boundaries might be drawn. A profound change in perspective is involved in this maneuver. The inventions of biological and social evolution and even those of AM come about by a search process that most of the time proceeds within boundaries, occasionally crossing one by accident. But human invention quite commonly proceeds by direct attention to the boundaries themselves. Generation and selection still have relevance, but the objects operated on are the boundary rules. One generates and selects in terms of whole systems or paradigms, in Thomas Kuhn's term (1962) – or whole watersheds, to keep that metaphor alive – rather than by increments.

We see this mindful operating on boundaries at work in many of the notable syntheses of our time, for instance, psychology and biology cross-bred into psychobiology, or biology and physics into biophysics. We see it again in numerous historical episodes in which one or a few individuals have made a sharp conscious break with established paradigms: the poetry of Walt Whitman, the excursions of the surrealists, the toppling of the mathematical ideal of completeness by Gödel, the calculated construction of 12-tone music by Schönberg, and so on. To be sure, accidental passages also happen in human history with great frequency, for better or worse. For example, who ever forecast the transforming effects of the automobile on the life-styles of affluent countries? When the first Ford rolled off Henry Ford's assembly line, he set foot on a watershed with ramifications beyond his imagining. Indeed, perhaps he would have been dismayed instead of delighted. However, although much happens blindly in human society and human minds, much also happens with both insight about the boundaries we move within and foresight about the opportunities to cross them.

Why do people operate on boundaries?

It seems clear that we human beings often represent to ourselves and operate on the boundaries within which we have been thinking. But why? What lures us or drives us to do so? To understand the human knack for invention, we need to understand the roots of this inclination.

Intransigent problems

One commonplace reason is intransigent problems within the boundary. Classic physics is an apt example. Einstein worried about one sort of intransigence when he felt disillusionment with the elegance of the classic formulation. Experimental data that posed difficulties for the classic view also spurred developments. For instance, the phenomena ultimately accommodated by quantum mechanics were not easy to reconcile with a Newtonian world view. Likewise, on the modest scale of everyday affairs, when one's business management tactics or methods of studying for quizzes or socializing persistently lead to problems, one sometimes pulls back, reconsiders, and tries a new tack altogether. To be sure, people often perseverate instead, digging the same hole deeper, but they do not *always* perseverate.

Exhaustion of opportunities

Another important reason for boundary crossing is exhaustion of the opportunities within the boundaries. Certainly something like this came to be felt by those who gave direction to impressionist art and modern poetry and music. To these restless figures, the styles of the times felt worn and overworn, in fact, worn out. A striking case in point is Schönberg's invention of 12-tone music in the calculated belief that music needed a fresh idiom that offered opportunities entirely outside an arena already crowded with the likes of Beethoven and Mozart. Of course, one can argue that the opportunities in a rich paradigm of painting, poetry, or music are never really exhausted. Always there is something more powerful and at least a little fresh to be rendered. But, however that may be, certainly creators in these areas commonly feel the need for new vistas. Whether all the niches are really occupied is perhaps less relevant than the perception that they mostly are, a perception that sends inventive people hunting for the boundaries and vaulting over them.

Boundary fiddling

Besides these straightforward reasons of intransigent problems and exhaustion of opportunity, one should not neglect the enthusiasm of some members of the human species for just plain fiddling around. One sort of fiddling around is boundary fiddling – fiddling with the boundaries of things just to see what might turn up and where things might lead. Such fiddling shows up in many contexts. An apt example is humor, which generally depends on breaking rules in a manner that nonetheless sort of fits.

For example, when Woody Allen confesses to youthful disillusionment because he learns that the universe is expanding, or when he stages a television advertisement for New Testament cigarettes, with the priest saying "I smoke 'em; *He* smokes 'em," we recognize at once that unrealistic pictures are painted. But at the same time, we recognize that these pictures bear a discernible relation to reality. Sometimes some people do get upset about matters cosmological, and sometimes some religions do become overly commercial. Considering such cases, Koestler (1964) urges that humor invariably involves bringing together remote frames of reference such as religion and cigarettes in an unexpected fit. Minsky (1983) argues that humor reflects our efforts to police the cognitive boundaries of our meaning-making activities by playing with them.

Of course, boundary fiddling is hardly likely to be limited to humor. It can occur in the most serious of paradigms, even when no very severe problems mar the integrity of the paradigm and when ample room remains to undertake novel enterprises within the paradigm. Moreover, sometimes it is not so easy to tell what the real motivation might be. Was Einstein compulsively fussy about his theories, or an inveterate fiddler wanting a good excuse? Perhaps it does not matter that much, so long as time gets spent operating on the boundaries as well as within the boundaries.

Combinatorial corks

Our quest for solutions to the *ex nihilo* problem has led to thinking of inventive processes as matters of search. A short-range search process, like generation and selection coupled with some mechanism of preservation, can lead in the long term to startlingly inventive results. This proves all the more true when generation, selection, and preservation are not blind, but fine-tuned to concerns like parsimony, power, and originality. The mechanism of search becomes yet more potent when the search process operates on the boundaries that previously have governed searching, rather than crossing boundaries only by accident.

Although helping to make sense of how invention can occur *ex nihilo,* these mechanisms of search resurrect a phantom familiar to all serious efforts to model problem-finding and problem-solving processes – the hazard of a combinatorial explosion. A game of chess provides the classic example of this problem. In a theoretical sense, it is quite clear how you should think about what move to make. You consider all the possible moves you might make, all the possible replies your opponent might offer in response, all your possible moves in return, and so on, tracking each path of play out to its ultimate conclusion many moves away in a checkmate for one side or another, or in one of the official draw conditions specified for chess. Having enumerated each path, you need only select an immediate move that gives you the best opportunity to win as the game unfolds.

The catch, of course, lies in the number of paths that need exploring to make this strategy of exhaustive search work. There are far more possibilities than could be explored with a universe full of computers working at top speed. Although the case of exhaustive chess playing is extreme, the specter it raises applies quite generally to efforts to understand practical search processes. As soon as a process appears on the scene that explores options and "looks ahead," a combinatorial explosion becomes a risk. To do its job, a search process must, on the one hand, look far enough ahead to avoid dead ends and disasters, but, on the other hand, it must look selectively, avoiding anything like a genuinely exhaustive search by choosing, on the basis of one or another criterion, those branches for exploration that are most likely to be important in the long run.

The account of invention given here certainly faces such a problem. Particularly when a search process starts challenging the very rules that normally govern and constrain search, a combinatorial explosion threatens. With boundaries challenged, it would seem that all combinations of old and new rules would have to be explored to arrive at a new and better paradigm. In this sense, the point about generation, selection, and preservation operating on boundaries makes the occurrence of invention harder to understand, not easier. How can any process cope with such radical uncertainty in a manageable and productive way?

Here is a good occasion to remember the principle announced at the beginning: What is actual is possible. Because people actually do operate on the boundaries and get productive results, it must be possible. There must be principles that contain the combinatorial explosion, preventing it from getting out of hand. With the encouragement that these combinatorial corks must exist, it does not prove so difficult to see what they might be.

Hill climbing

This classic search strategy corks the combinatorial explosion by taking it a step at a time. A hill-climbing strategy assumes that there is some rough measure of local progress: The process in question can gauge which of two neighboring states, X or Y, lies closer to an acceptable solution, even if both fall well short of acceptability. In such circumstances, search can proceed by increments. Starting at state A, for example, the search process generates neighbors of A and selects the "highest"; call it B. The search process repeats this cycle of generation and selection on B, and by continuing in like manner it gradually converges on an acceptable solution. There is no combinatorial explosion because the search process considers only neighbors of the current position at any given point along the way, and there are not very many of those neighbors.

Of course, the hill-climbing strategy has its weaknesses. One is the well-known problem of local maxima. There may be "low hills" in the search space where the measure of height takes on a maximum not high enough to count as an adequate resolution. The search process will hang there unless there is some provision for taking a leap and starting over from a new origin. Another problem is that the domain in question may not afford any reasonable measure of height. To be sure, such a measure need not be terribly pure; the poet's or mathematician's intuitive "nose" for what is a good bet may provide an adequate criterion for hill climbing. Nonetheless, nothing guarantees in any particular case that a sound or even roughly sound measure of height exists.

Despite these cautions, the power of hill climbing is plain. Virtually all human invention depends blatantly on hill climbing, as makers in diverse domains "home in" on final products from rough-and-ready beginnings. The role of hill climbing in nature is no less apparent. Darwinian natural selection is basically a hill-climbing process, as variations around the genetic norm of a species occur and get selected by the criterion of viability.

Parallel processing

The combinatorial explosion gets corked somewhat if multiple options are explored in parallel rather than solely serially. This is the rule in nature, of course. The many representatives of a particular life form across a considerable geographic range create ample opportunity for the process of natural selection to explore various options at the same time. Human society functions much the same way. At any given time, dozens of people may be engaged in the same enterprise. For instance, we remember Edison as the inventor of the light bulb, but although he devised the solution, he did not devise the problem. The possibility of getting efficient lighting out of electricity was widely recognized and widely pursued by dozens of inventors of his era (Conot, 1979). To be sure, this parallel processing does the individual inventor little good; in fact, it simply creates competition that may be unwelcome. Think of all the ambitious inventors who failed to invent the light bulb. But from the standpoint of the technological advancement of society, the parallel independent endeavors of many individuals plainly pay off in a brisker pace of technological progress.

Invention by inference

As emphasized earlier, inventive people often operate self-consciously on the boundaries of a discipline. The risk of a combinatorial explosion depends on a simple assumption: These inventive people are being inventive most of the time, upsetting a boundary rule here and a boundary rule there and yet another somewhere else at every turn. But perhaps sometimes invention occurs through a series of fairly methodical inferences. The individual breaks the boundary not through a haphazard exploration of what rules to change but through willingness to follow through on the logic and let what follows follow, never mind the rules.

A suggestive case in point is the well-known incident of the discovery of the principle of natural selection. Whereas Darwin gave a fairly terse account of the actual moment, Alfred Russell Wallace, who discovered the same principle some 20 years later, but before Darwin had published, offered more details. Like Darwin, Wallace achieved the key insight while reading Malthus's well-known essay on human population and the threat of exponential growth. Boiled down a bit, Wallace's thoughts ran something as follows (Perkins, 1981, pp. 54–55):

1. There are many checks to human increase, according to Malthus.
2. The same causes act in the case of animals. (Wallace's interest as a naturalist appears.)
3. Because animals breed faster, this implies constant and enormous destruction. (Wallace realizes a straightforward implication, which will turn out to be the selection mechanism.)
4. "Why do some die and some live?" Wallace asks. (The lucky question, prompted perhaps by the habit of a scientific thinker to seek causes.)
5. The best fitted live. (The obvious answer.)
6. The race is improved. (Wallace recognizes the best fitted as the most adapted and realizes he has an explanation for how species become adapted.)

Two points about this episode invite emphasis. First, Wallace had been puzzling over the mechanism of evolution, and so his mind was prepared to take steps such as those laid out. As Gruber (1974) has compellingly argued, such leaps of discovery can hardly be expected in an unprepared mind. Second, no step in the sequence is particularly startling. One could not say that each step was logically entailed by the prior, but each one follows comfortably and naturally enough from the prior. To be sure, Wallace makes a boundary-crossing move by comparing mechanisms that limit human population growth and mechanisms that limit animal population growth. But the crossing is a highly plausible one. The episode indeed reminds us that boundary crossing does not necessarily involve boundary discarding or rearranging.

To generalize, sometimes a sequence of reasonable steps can lead to a surprising conclusion, especially if the reasoner is ready to accept it. We should remind ourselves repeatedly that a surprising conclusion simply does not have to imply a startling step along the way. To think otherwise is to embrace a kind of magical thinking in which effects must resemble their causes.

Radical/conservative thinking

In cases of inference such as that outlined earlier, no combinatorial explosion results because each step in a relatively short chain is relatively conservative. Perhaps each is not actually forced logically by the prior steps, but at least it comes naturally, and not that many other steps would come naturally. As the example illustrates, even boundary-crossing steps can come fairly naturally, so long as one does not fastidiously recoil from the boundary. But what about cases of invention that absolutely require a direct challenge to the boundary? How does the search process there evade a combinatorial explosion?

One likely answer is that most of the steps in even a boundary-challenging sequence of thought may be relatively conservative. A case in point is Einstein's development of the theory of relativity. Einstein, by means of thought experiments, reached the conclusion that the speed of light should be the same when measured in any frame of reference. Experimental results accumulating at the time pointed in the same direction (A. I. Miller, 1984). The question remained what to make of this, how to come to terms with it. Einstein chose a radical solution: He challenged the notion that time works the same way in any frame of reference and that events simultaneous in one frame of reference are necessarily simultaneous in another frame of reference. Now this was a peculiar challenge to make, because the invariance of time certainly is one of our deep intuitions about the world. Nonetheless, the questioning of temporal invariance offered a way out of the otherwise paradoxical idea that the speed of light would measure the same in any frame of reference. Once this radical step was taken, then (so I understand) further ramifications of relativity followed conservatively, a matter of working out the implications of the revised assumption.

In summary, several combinatorial corks help to control the combinatorial explosion that otherwise would result in the search processes that mediate invention. We have the help at least of hill climbing, parallel processing, conservative inference that nonetheless crosses boundaries, and radical/conservative sequences of steps in which one radical step is followed up conservatively. Indeed, an important moral can be drawn from this examination of the problem of combinatorial explosions. Invention is not as radical as one might think. Inventive processes, including human thought, cannot be wildly radical most of the time, challenging prior assumptions willy-nilly. That sort of functioning would lead to a combinatorial explosion in which most of the possibilities explored would have little likelihood of paying off. Instead, processes of invention are by and large selective in their radicalism, salting conservative inferential and hill-climbing maneuvers with an occasional radical revision of one or two assumptions.

Human creativity

The discussion to this point has ranged across biological evolution, social evolution, and invention by machine as well as invention by individual human beings. But after this steadfast exercise in evenhandedness, perhaps a little ethnocentrism is permissible. Then what can be said about human creativity from the standpoint of the general solution to the *ex nihilo* problem outlined here?

First of all, when we speak of creativity and not a particular episode of invention, we refer to an abiding trait in a person. A creative person, by definition, does not simply achieve one breakthrough episode at the age of 27, but more or less regularly produces outcomes in one or more fields that appear both original and appropriate. We need not be narrow about what an "outcome" is. The outcomes in question may be scientific theories, jokes, paintings, flower arrangements, advertising campaigns, parties, or most anything else. To say all this is to characterize loosely what one might call the "outer meaning" of creativity, the symptoms by which we know it when we see it in people. We know that a person is creative when we see that person regularly producing original appropriate outcomes.

Of course, what we really want to understand is what might be called "inner creativity," the psychological traits and mechanisms that lead to regular production of creative outcomes. Psychologists, philosophers, and other scholars have offered various accounts of inner creativity. I have recently reviewed some of their thinking in other contexts (Perkins, in press-a,b) and will not repeat the details here, but the literature does support some broad conclusions. First of all, efforts to relate real-world creativity (using track-record measures of various sorts) to basic abilities of various sorts have, by and large, been unsuccessful. For instance, measures of ideational fluency and flexibility apparently do not relate reliably to real-world creative achievement within a discipline (Mansfield & Busse, 1981; Wallach, 1976a, 1976b). IQ likewise does not forecast creativity, nor indeed achievement in general, within a discipline (Baird, 1982; Barron, 1969; Wallach, 1976a, 1976b).

There is more reason to think that the *way* people deploy their abilities has something to do with creativity. For instance, Getzels and Csikszentmihalyi (1976) present evidence that creative artists tend to engage in problem finding, a pattern of behavior in which they explore many options flexibly at the outset before settling on a particular artistic problem to pursue, and also remain open to the possibility of changing directions even after they are well under way with a particular project. It seems likely that problem finding is an important pattern of creative thinking in any field. Finally, real-world creativity relates quite strongly to values and personality characteristics. Creative individuals tend to be autonomous, independent, and self-reliant, as one would expect. They value originality, tolerate ambiguity and uncertainty, have an aesthetic appreciation for things rather than just a pragmatic mind-set, and reveal strong intrinsic motivation in pursuing their projects (Amabile, 1983; Barron, 1969; Getzels & Csikszentmihalyi, 1976; Mansfield & Busse, 1981). To generalize, one might say that creativity is more a matter of values and personality than particular ways of deploying abilities, and more a matter of ways of deploying abilities than of having particular mental abilities. Of course, some repertoire of abilities is a necessary condition for creativity, but far from a sufficient condition.

What sense does this make in terms of the view of inventive systems outlined here? Invention depends on the ability to do such things as generate with a relevant bias, select according to criteria (including originality), assess local progress to achieve hill climbing, and represent to oneself the boundaries in a situation so that one can operate directly on those boundaries rather than cross or revise boundaries only by accident. The negligible relationship between ability measures, such as flexibility and fluency, and human creativity suggests that these abilities per se are not major limiting factors in human creativity within a discipline. For instance, less creative physicists, as well as more creative ones, are quite capable of discriminating what is more or less original and are capable of identifying boundaries in a situation in the sense of having the raw ability to do so.

Invention requires not simply the raw ability to do the sorts of things listed, but a molar organization of behavior in that direction. For instance, the physicist, poet, or painter who makes a revolution by revising boundaries not only needs to have enough raw ability to represent and ponder the boundaries but also needs to have patterns of deploying that ability that can lead to such representing and pondering. Although this may seem paradoxical, having an ability and having a pattern of deployment are two quite different things. I may be able to identify boundary assumptions if someone prompts me, for example, but such a quest as a personal maneuver of thought may simply not be in my repertoire. The results on problem finding mentioned earlier at least suggest that having certain patterns of deployment prominent in their repertoires may make practitioners within a discipline more creative.

Inventive processing calls not only for ability and patterns of deployment but also for the inclination to so deploy one's ability. The creative business person, dancer, or engineer needs curiosity about boundaries, restlessness concerning their limits, and toughness in tolerating the ambiguity that inevitably appears when boundaries are challenged. Here, more than anywhere else, psychological traits emerge that differentiate the more creative from the less creative individuals within a field.

In summary, the needs of an inventive system relate to human psychology as follows: Invention requires such processes as boundary representing. The raw ability, patterns of deployment, or motivation to do such things might be in question. In fact, within a discipline, motivation seems to be more at issue than patterns of deployment, and patterns of deployment more at issue than raw ability. Presumably, what this means is that to gain entry to a discipline – to become a physicist or poet at all – one needs enough raw ability to function adequately in the discipline and that raw ability is enough also to support whatever inventive thinking one might like to do. However, one may lack the patterns of deployment that lead to inventive results and the values that drive the process. It is reasonable to suspect that values may be more important than the patterns of deployment, at least in a developmental sense, because a person with the right profile of values will tend to evolve the patterns of deployment. For instance, a person who delights in originality and tolerates ambiguity most likely will eventually bootstrap himself or herself into operating on boundaries.

At least two qualifications to this broad picture need airing. First, what characterizes creativity within a discipline may not hold so strongly when we pull back to view the broader panorama of human achievement. Whereas among physicists, ability may not function to limit creativity in physics, among the population in general ability plainly does. Not all individuals are able to master the basic skills of physics, and so many of them cannot be creative in physics. So the conclusion is not that abilities have nothing to do with creativity, but rather that, beyond the basics, they may not figure that strongly.

The second qualification concerns the general coarseness of the net we cast here. In discussing abilities, we refer to the basics in a discipline along with such broad traits as fluency, flexibility, and general intelligence. It is possible that someone might identify finer-grained abilities that do differentiate more from less creative persons within a discipline. For instance, perhaps the most creative poets are those who can judge poetry best, as to both its originality and its excellence otherwise. Perhaps the most creative physicists are those with the strongest visual imagery, a possibility encouraged by Miller's writings on the role of imagery in the development of modern physics (A. I. Miller, 1984). Such possibilities must be allowed.

Keeping these cautions in mind, this general picture has implications for both the testing and the teaching of creativity. As to testing, the overview argues that we certainly can test for creativity with some validity, but the ways we most often try may be off-center. Whereas testing for creativity typically emphasizes flexibility, fluency, and similar indices, values and patterns of deployment seem to offer the best predictors of creativity. Investigators would do well to keep this in mind, because reliance on flexibility and fluency measures of creativity and an emphasis on creativity as an ability persist in the contemporary literature despite considerable evidence to the contrary. I have discussed the problems of testing at more length elsewhere (Perkins, in press-a,b).

As to instruction, this profile suggests that values and patterns of deployment deserve emphasis. Flexibility and fluency training, as such, appears misguided. My own suspicion is that sometimes it has good effects, not so much through boosting people's ability to generate ideas flexibly and fluently but by inducing related values of exploration and originality and by putting organized molar patterns of deployment like formal brainstorming into people's behavioral repertoires. Such spinoffs are welcome, of course, but if it is the spinoffs that really do the job, the instruction should focus on them directly. Finally, although considerable creativity instruction does focus not just on flexibility and fluency but on various patterns of deployment – strategies of creativity, if you like – attention to building creative values typically plays much less of a role. Creativity is treated as a matter of technique rather than a matter of attitude. It is both, of course, but perhaps even more a matter of attitude than of technique. Therefore, efforts to foster creativity should pay at least as much attention to building creative attitudes as imparting technical resources. Again, these comments are shorthand for more thorough explorations of these themes offered elsewhere (Perkins, 1981, 1984, in press-a,b).

The inevitability of invention

We began with the premise that what is actual is possible. Invention is actual; so, *ex nihilo* though it looks, it must somehow be possible. But knowing that it is possible is not to grasp *how* it is possible. The discussion of generation, selection, and preservation, biasing toward originality, operating on boundaries, and so on, offered an account of the possibility of invention.

Now that we know how invention is possible, we can return full circle to ask, How come invention is actual? Why does invention actually occur, given that it is possible in the ways outlined? That it is actual is plain, but is there anything inevitable about this actuality, or have we inventive human beings somehow lucked out?

The broad answer seems to be this: Given certain prevailing conditions, invention becomes not only possible but also more or less inevitable. Consider again the case of evolution. For evolution to occur at all, certain conditions are required; according to the classic Darwinian profile, one needs variation, selection, and inheritance. Given these, evolution should proceed at least at a slow pace, inventing in its blind and uncaring way. Invention under those conditions is a mechanical consequence of the situation.

Some might argue that the trio of conditions does not suffice to account for the inventiveness of evolution. The contemporary notion of "punctuated equilibrium" suggests that evolution may come in bursts (Gould, 1980, chaps. 17–18). Such bursts might be triggered by periods of intense radiation leading to greater variation or by massive extinction due to natural disasters that open up an array of ecological niches for the survivors to fill. Whatever the case, these accounts still lie within the broad spirit of generation, selection, and preservation, and they still see nature's invention following more or less inevitably when certain conditions are met, albeit somewhat more refined conditions.

What about social evolution? The evolution of ideas within a society again appears more or less inevitable. Societies provide the key conditions for the elementary mechanism of variation, selection, and preservation to operate, and so operate it will. Again, a qualification somewhat in the spirit of punctuated equilibrium may be in order. Certainly some societies have proved much more inventive in much briefer periods than others. This can perhaps be traced back to analogues of radiation-inducing genetic variation. For instance, the contact between different cultures can yield a rich crop of mutant ideas. The opening up of new domains, physical or intellectual, can trigger a burst of social evolution, just as with biological evolution. Consider, for example, the flood of inventions following the development of the assembly line or, more recently, the transistor.

Whereas it is not so difficult to think of biological or social evolution as the mechanical consequence of certain conditions, we only reluctantly see individual human invention in that light. Yet such a view certainly can be taken. I am far from being a behaviorist, but I have always admired an engaging essay by B. F. Skinner (1972): "A Lecture on 'Having' a Poem." Skinner paints a picture of poetry writing from a behaviorist perspective, urging that a poet "has" a poem as inevitably and naturally as a hen lays an egg. We should think of the poet not as a mindful, active, striving organism with all that mentalistic paraphernalia that good behaviorists do without, but rather as a locus of causation, where the contingencies of reinforcement conspire to bring a poem about.

A confirmed mentalist, I *do* think of the poet as a mindful, active, striving organism with as much awareness and will as anyone could want. Nonetheless, this is not at all incompatible with viewing the existence of poets and poetry as an inevitable consequence of circumstances. Of course, what particular poem gets written, or even what human poetry is like, is not in any narrow way determined. But the fact that human beings involve themselves in inventing something as "impractical" as poems seems to follow from our status as sapient beings who communicate and can represent boundaries to ourselves. Let us look at the argument.

Given the power to symbolize, and in particular to represent and operate on boundaries, *practical* invention certainly follows. With the power of operating on boundaries come the advantages of doing so. Plainly, sometimes people solve vexing and important problems having fairly direct survival value by discovering what the boundaries are that previously have constrained and undermined efforts to resolve the problems. This does not mean that all boundary breaking yields positive outcomes, of course. Anything from social ostracism to a laboratory explosion can result from unwise or unlucky operations on boundaries. But this does not change the fact that the payoffs are real enough and frequent enough to fuel the process of exploration.

Although such an account may explain pragmatic invention, it falls short of explicating "impractical" inventive activities like poetry writing. Why bother with such stuff? For a first cut at an answer, we have to recognize that human beings in fact respond aesthetically to language. Given that responsiveness, it is hardly surprising that some human beings will exercise their talents, including their talents for operating on boundaries, to explore the aesthetic possibilities of language. Indeed, "impractical" language acts such as poetry writing are not all that impractical in a human social context, because people will pay for them for the pleasure they afford and for their use by religious and other organizations in which they can reinforce the institution in question. So the question is not why people invent poetry, given that poetry has its rewards; the question becomes why poetry is rewarding in the first place.

Let me argue that in a sapient communicating species, aesthetic responsiveness to language is nearly as inevitable as fear, hunger, and passion. Let us grant that human beings have evolved to be language users. Let us also grant what one always presumes of evolution: The process of natural selection "cares" about the payoff of an adaptation only as gauged by survival and reproduction. Under these circumstances, a motivational system will have evolved associated with language, a system that encourages its use because of its survival value. Likewise, there are motivational systems associated with such primary activities as eating and reproduction.

Now there are two possibilities to entertain. Option 1: The development of this motivational system for language use is perfectly attuned to the practical survival-oriented applications of language and nothing else. Option 2: The motivational system misses somewhat the precise pragmatics of language use. That is, there are some motivated language behaviors that do not serve survival directly and some unmotivated language behaviors that do. It seems virtually certain that option 2 obtains. Consider the following reasons.

First, there is no ready way an evolutionary process could tune an adaptation precisely to the survival payoffs in the long term; after all, how could biological evolution, blind process that it is, "know" that millions of years later, in societies far removed from the original context of evolution, people might waste their time writing poetry? To put it another way, at the time the motivational system evolved, there was no information available in the biosphere concerning survival-irrelevant preoccupations with language such as poetry writing; so evolution could hardly guard against such preoccupations.

Second, it is plain that other motivational systems have associated with them behaviors largely irrelevant to or even counter to survival, behaviors that were not anticipated by evolution. The use of birth control is a good example. It reminds us that human beings are most strongly motivated to make love rather than to reproduce per se. Our love-making motivation only roughly matches evolution's "real purpose," and so we manage to find technical ways of separating the one from the other.

Finally, we can easily see something of how the motivational system sustaining language use works and how that makes it somewhat independent of direct survival concerns. Language and other symbol systems allow us to symbolize matters involving primary drives – how to avoid danger, secure food, seek mates, and so on. Uses of language directly in the service of survival therefore can occur. However, the same power of language that allows us to represent to ourselves real survival circumstances also allows us to represent surrogate circumstances that tap into the survival reward system. Note that poetry, and literature in general, typically deals with matters concerning primary drives – love, death, acquisition and defense of territory, and the like.

This last argument notwithstanding, it is important to note that our responsiveness to literature does not lie solely in its power to deliver surrogate experiences involving primary drives. We also find pleasure in the rhythm of language, in its music, in the surprise of startling metaphors. These sorts of responsiveness might also connect in roundabout ways to primary drives. Or they might prove rewarding for other reasons buried in the history of human evolution. We need not see exactly what the causes are to conclude that our responsiveness to varied dimensions of language represents aspects of the imperfect match one can expect between the motivational system for language and sheer survival factors.

To underscore the form of the argument, let us recast it for Martians. Let us imagine that Martians are sapient and have one or more principal channels of communication – speech, hand signals, blinkers on foreheads, whatever you like. Then Martians will have poetry, or Martian analogues of it. That is, they will have artistic forms associated with their principal channels of communication that go well beyond direct survival applications. Why? Because for Martians, as for us, evolution will have made an imperfect match between the motivational system promoting the use of these modes of communication and survival. In particular, Martians will symbolize surrogate experiences that have no immediate or even long-term survival payoffs, but excite primary drives. Moreover, Martian poetry, like human poetry, will overshoot even this indirect connection to pragmatics, displaying a concern with rhythm and rhyme or other formal features that tickle Martians. What those features would be is difficult to predict, but that there would be such "extra" features of importance follows from the general mismatch phenomenon. So Martians will have Martian poetry.

It is a long path from the original *ex nihilo* question to Martian poetry. Perhaps a quick reminder of some landmarks along the way is in order. Invention is actual. Invention is therefore possible. We can appreciate in broad terms how it is possible and even fairly efficient – through generation, selection, and preservation, mindfully directed, involving representing and operating on boundaries, with various factors corking the problem of a combinatorial explosion. Seeing how it is possible and efficient, we can further see that it pretty much has to be actual, given the conditions that exist. Even "impractical" invention, as in poetry, has to be actual – for us and for any sapient communicating Martians there may be. The froth of particular invention, unpredictable in its details, rides on a tide of inexorable causation. Far from being exceptional, invention under certain broad and prevailing conditions becomes inevitable. At this very moment, poets and physicists are sitting down at their desks to upset the way we think things are, and although we cannot say just what they will devise, that they will create some upsets follows from the way things are.

References

Amabile, T. M. (1983). *The social psychology of creativity*. New York: Springer-Verlag.

Baird, L. L. (1982). *The role of academic ability in high-level accomplishment and general success* (College Board Report No. 82-6). New York: College Entrance Examination Board.

Barron, F. (1969). *Creative person and creative process*. New York: Holt, Rinehart & Winston.

Bradshaw, G. F., Langley, P. W., & Simon, H. A. (1983). Studying scientific discovery by computer simulation. *Science, 222*(4627), 971–975.

Conot, R. (1979). *A streak of luck*. New York: Seaview.

Cooper, L. (Trans.); Hamilton, E., & Cairns, H. (Eds.). *The collected dialogues of Plato*. Princeton, NJ: Princeton University Press.

Dawkins, R. (1976). *The selfish gene*. New York: Oxford University Press.

Getzels, J., & Csikszentmihalyi, M. (1976). *The creative vision: A longitudinal study of problem finding in art*. New York: Wiley.

Gould, S. J. (1980). *The panda's thumb: More reflections in natural history*. New York: Norton.

Gruber, H. (1974). *Darwin on man: A psychological study of scientific creativity*. New York: E. P. Dutton.

Grumbach, D. (1986). The literary imagination. In R. M. Caplan (Ed.), *Exploring the concept of mind* (pp. 121–131). Iowa City: University of Iowa Press.

Hausman, C. R. (1976). Creativity and rationality. In A. Rothenberg & C. R. Hausman (Eds.), *The creativity question* (pp. 343–351). Durham, NC: Duke University Press.

Hausman, C. R. (1985). Can computers create? *Interchange, 16*(1), 27–37.

Holton, G. (1973). On trying to understand scientific genius. In G. Holton (Ed.), *Thematic origins of scientific thought: Kepler to Einstein* (pp. 353–380). Cambridge, MA: Harvard University Press.

Hughes, T. (1969). The thought fox. In *The New Yorker Book of Poems* (p. 718). New York: Viking Press.

Koestler, A. (1964). *The act of creation*. New York: Dell.

Kuhn, T. (1962). *The structure of scientific revolutions*. University of Chicago Press.

Langley, P., Bradshaw, G. L., & Simon, H. A. (1983). Rediscovering chemistry with the BACON system. In R. S. Michalski, J. G. Carbonell, & T. M. Mitchell (Eds.), *Machine learning: An artificial intelligence approach* (pp. 307–330). Palo Alto, CA: Tioga Publishing.

Lenat, P. B. (1983). Toward a theory of heuristics. In R. Groner, M. Groner, & W. Bischof (Eds.), *Methods of heuristics* (pp. 351–404). Hillsdale, NJ: Lawrence Erlbaum.

Lowes, J. L. (1927). *The road to Xanadu*. Boston: Houghton Mifflin.

Mansfield, R. S., & Busse, T. V. (1981). *The psychology of creativity and discovery*. Chicago: Nelson-Hall.

Miller, A. I. (1984). *Imagery in scientific thought: Creating 20th-century physics*. Boston: Birkhauser.

Miller, J. G. (1984). Culture and the development of everyday social explanation. *Journal of Personality and Social Psychology, 46*, 961–978.

Minsky, M. (1983). Jokes and the logic of the cognitive unconscious. In R. Groner, M. Groner, & W. F. Bischof (Eds.), *Methods of heuristics* (pp. 171–194). Hillsdale, NJ: Lawrence Erlbaum.

Perkins, D. N. (1981). *The mind's best work*. Cambridge, MA: Harvard University Press.

Perkins, D. N. (1984). Creativity by design. *Educational Leadership, 42*(1), 18–25.

Perkins, D. N. (in press-a). Creativity and the quest for mechanism. In R. S. Sternberg & E. Smith (Eds.), *The psychology of human thought*. Cambridge University Press.

Perkins, D. N. (in press-b). The nature and nurture of creativity. In Jones, B. F. (Ed.), *Dimensions of thinking: A review of research*. Hillsdale, NJ: Lawrence Erlbaum, in press.

Schneider, E. (1953). *Coleridge, opium and Kubla Khan*. University of Chicago Press.

Skinner, B. F. (2972). A lecture on "having" a poem. In *Cumulative record: A selection of papers* (3rd ed.) (pp. 345–355). New York: Meredith Corporation.

Wallach, M. A. (1976a). Psychology of talent and graduate education. In S. Messick & Associates (Eds.), *Individuality in learning*. San Francisco: Jossey-Bass.

Wallach, M. A. (1976b). Tests tell us little about talent. *American Scientist, 64*, 57–63.

16   Creativity, leadership, and chance

Dean Keith Simonton

Let me begin this chapter with two fundamental propositions about the nature of creativity.

Proposition 1: Creativity is a form of leadership in that it entails personal influence over others.

For the most part, the diverse approaches to defining creativity can be grouped into four distinct categories – what I call the "four p's" of creativity research (cf. Stein, 1969). First, we can focus on creativity as a *process*. Under this definition, researchers want to discern the patterns of thought or information-processing habits that underlie creativity. Such is the central orientation of Koestler's *The Act of Creation* (1964), as well as Ghiselin's *The Creative Process* (1952), which gathers together introspective reports by "thirty-eight brilliant men and women." It is equally the chief interest of cognitive psychologists fascinated with "problem solving" and gestalt psychologists intrigued with "insight."

Second, the emphasis, alternatively, can be placed on the creative *product*. The creative process presumably should result in some concrete entity – whether a poem, painting, invention, or theory – that can be deemed creative in some clear sense. In abstract terms, it is often said that a product demonstrates creativity if it is simultaneously "original" and "adaptive." In practice, however, it has proved difficult to gauge such dimensions, except in the realm of artistic products. Several researchers in empirical aesthetics have attempted to pinpoint what accounts for the differential success of literary, visual, and musical art objects (Martindale, 1975; Simonton, 1980d, 1980e), and new methods have been devised to assess how products vary in aesthetic impact (Amabile, 1982; Simonton, 1983a, 1986a).

Third, we may conceive creativity in terms of the *person*. This is the favored attack of personality psychologists who study what individual-difference variables, whether cognitive or motivational, distinguish creative people from those less so (Barron & Harrington, 1981). Much of the research conducted since the 1950s has adopted this conception, with the result that we now have a cornucopia of personality measures that purport to identify creative individuals.

Fourth and last, we can view creativity as an act of *persuasion;* that is, individuals become "creative" only insofar as they impress others with their creativity (Albert, 1975). From this viewpoint, creativity becomes an interpersonal or social

386

phenomenon. Indeed, it emerges as a particular type of leadership. Social psychologists are accustomed to label that group member a "leader" whose influence over group performance or decision making far exceeds that projected by the average member of the group (Simonton, 1985a). By the same token, one who is part of a sociocultural world, or at least an intellectual or aesthetic discipline, becomes a "creator" to the degree that one displays an impact on others that amply surpasses the norm. Just as a leader must have followers to be counted a leader, so must a creator claim appreciators or admirers to be legitimatized as a true creator (Simonton, 1984a). Needless to say, this notion of creativity has been most favored by sociologists and anthropologists, though recently some social psychologists have in various ways come around to this point of view (Amabile, 1983; Simonton, 1984c; Sternberg, 1985).

Now, in an ideal state of affairs, it should not matter which one of the four p's our investigations target, for they all will converge on the same underlying phenomenon. The creative process should yield creative products, those products should emerge from the hands of creative persons with characteristic personalities, and those same persons should, through the merits of their offered products, convince potential appreciators of their creative worth. But reality is not so simple, needless to say. The creative process need not arrive at a creative product, nor must all creative products ensue from the same process or personality type; and others may ignore the process, discredit the product, or reject the personality when making attributions about creativity. If we cannot assume that all four aspects cohesively hang together, then it may be best to select one single definition and subordinate the others to that orientation. As a social psychologist who has devoted over a dozen years to the understanding of exceptional personal influence, I naturally opt for creativity as persuasion (Simonton, 1984c, 1985a, 1987c, in press).

This choice has two distinct assets. In the first place, viewing creativity in social terms permits us to link the phenomenon with the subject of leadership, on which there has been an abundance of quality research (Bass, 1981). Even if creators and leaders differ in many respects, they also share a large number of personological, developmental, and social correlates (Simonton, 1984c, 1987c).

Second, requiring that creators be sociocultural leaders allows us to merge experimental and correlational investigations of the usual everyday subject pools (mostly college students) with historiometric inquiries into the notable geniuses of the past (Cox, 1926; Goertzel, Goertzel, & Goertzel, 1978; Simonton, 1984c). It is self-evident that creators of the stature of Newton, Descartes, Shakespeare, Michelangelo, or Beethoven have exerted tremendous influence over the course taken by human culture, just as Napoleon, Lenin, Lincoln, Gandhi, and Luther have held comparable sway over the direction taken by human society. Because any theory of creativity that is to claim any explanatory power must account for these universally recognized creative figures, it is an advantage, not a limitation, that the persuasion definition obliges us to begin our studies with precisely those persons who have forced the most people for the longest period of time to acknowledge the magnitude of their creative accomplishments. Furthermore, I argue that the difference between history-making creativity and more mundane forms is a contrast of degree only, and thus the separate research traditions should converge on a single picture of creative phenomena (Simonton, 1986b). In particular, I insist that the bulk of the literature, historiometric or psychometric, directs us to the next affirmation.

Proposition 2: Creativity involves the participation of chance processes both in the origination of new ideas and in the social acceptance of those ideas by others.

This statement is far more complicated than first meets the eye. I am certainly not claiming that creative people are merely "lucky," but rather that probabilistic or stochastic mechanisms operate at fundamental levels to generate original conceptions and to isolate that subset of these ideas that are judged adaptive by others – and hence deserving of the designation "creative." Chance intervenes in the process, product, person, and persuasion sides of creativity. To make this case requires that I allot a sizable portion of this chapter to describing what I call the "chance-configuration" theory, a sociopsychological interpretation of creativity (Simonton, in press, chap. 1). After I present the essential concept, I shall elaborate it by bringing together a considerable body of empirical research. I shall then close with a brief discussion of the theory's main implications for fostering and identifying creativity.

The theory

There is nothing original about the chance-configuration theory, for I have merely built on the ideas of my predecessors. In particular, my theoretical outlook can be said to have taken its start from Donald Campbell's blind-variation and selective-retention model of creative thought (Campbell, 1960), albeit with considerable elaboration and shift in nomenclature. Accordingly, I should enumerate the three core propositions of Campbell's model before I offer my version:

1. The solution of novel problems requires some means of generating ideational *variation.* Campbell argued that this variation, to be truly effective, must be fully "blind," but many alternative qualifiers might be placed on the variations, such as chance, random, aleatory, fortuitous, and haphazard (Campbell, 1974, p. 147).

2. These heterogeneous variations are subjected to a consistent *selection* process that deletes all but those that feature adaptive fit. In other words, there must exist somewhat stable criteria by which variations that offer viable solutions to the problem at hand are separated from those that embody no advance and hence are useless.

3. The variations that have been selected must be preserved and reproduced by some mechanism; without such *retention,* a successful variation cannot represent a permanent contribution to adaptive fitness.

Campbell (1960) noted the fundamental contradiction between the first and third proposition: Blind variation implies a departure from retained knowledge. Any society can boast a rich repertoire of skills and concepts that enable its members to survive and prosper, and, accordingly, cross-generational preservation and transmission of these adaptive features are high priorities; but without any provision for variation, for creativity, the sociocultural system will eventually stagnate, lose adaptive advantages, and in the end emerge defeated in the competition with rival systems. In the specific realm of scientific creativity, Kuhn (1963, p. 343) has referred to this contradiction as an "essential tension," for "very often the successful scientist must simultaneously display the characteristics of the traditionalist and of the iconoclast."

Campbell's model (1960) continues a long philosophical tradition. One notable case in point is the essay "Great Men, Great Thoughts, and the Environment," by William James, which affirmed "that the relation of the visible environment to the great man is in the main exactly what it is to the 'variation' in the Darwinian philosophy" (James, 1880, p. 445). In particular, "the new conceptions, emotions, and active tendencies which evolve are originally *produced* in the shape of random images, fancies, accidental outbirths of spontaneous variation in the functional activity of the excessively unstable human brain, which the outer environment simply confirms or refutes, adopts or rejects, preserves or destroys – *selects,* in short, just as it selects morphological and social variations due to molecular accidents of an analogous sort" (James, 1880, p. 456). The chance-configuration theory builds further on this tradition by introducing three sets of key concepts: (a) the chance permutation of mental elements, (b) the formation of configurations, and (c) the communication and social acceptance of those configurations.

Chance permutations

The creative process entails operations on what I choose to call *mental elements.* These psychological entities are the fundamental units that can be manipulated in some manner, such as the sensations that we attend to, the emotions that we experience, and the diverse cognitive schemata, ideas, concepts, or recollections that we can retrieve from long-term memory. These elements must be free to enter into various combinations. Indeed, the fundamental generating mechanism in creativity involves *chance permutation* of these elements. To clarify my meaning, let us start with the term "permutation." I favor this term over the alternative that is more often employed, namely, "combination," for the term "permutation" connotes that we must discriminate among combinations that, though containing identical elements, differ in how those elements are arranged. Thus, for musical creativity, two or more melodies may feature the same notes arranged in distinguishable sequences (Simonton, 1984f), and "a mathematical demonstration is not a simple juxtaposition of syllogisms, it is syllogisms *placed in a certain order,* and the order in which these elements are placed is much more important than the elements themselves" (Poincaré, 1921, p. 385).

In general, to claim that the permutations are generated by chance is equivalent to saying that each mental element is evoked by myriad determinants. Chance is a measure of ignorance, a gauge of the circumstance when the number of causes is so immense as to defy identification. Though chance implies unpredictability, it does not necessitate total randomness. We are under no compulsion to argue that all permutations of a specific set of elements are equiprobable. We must merely insist that a large number of potential permutations exist, all with comparably low, but nonzero, probabilities. Later I shall describe how chance permutations can come about.

Configuration formation

Some principle of selection must be introduced, for not all chance permutations should be retained. The primary selection procedure is here predicated on the fact that chance permutations vary appreciably in *stability*. On one extreme are transitory juxtapositions of mental elements that lack sufficient coherence to form a stable permutation, so that the permutation process continues without pause. These unstable permutations we may call mental *aggregates*. On the other extreme are permutations whose elements, though brought together by a chance confluence of multiple determinants, seem to hang together in a stable arrangement or patterned whole of interrelated parts. These stable permutations I label *configurations*. Of course, aggregates and configurations are permutations of mental elements that fall along a continuum from the highly unstable to the highly stable, with many graduations between. Nonetheless, of the innumerable chance permutations, only the most stable are retained for further information processing; the greater the stability, the higher the odds of selection. Further, on a subjective plane, the more stable a permutation, the more attention it commands in consciousness; the unstable permutations are too fleeting to rise above unconscious levels of processing.

I picked the word "configuration" advisedly, over the many alternatives that offered themselves (schemata, associative fields, constructs, concepts, ideas, matrices, etc.), according to etymology and common applications. The origin is a Latin word meaning to shape after some pattern. A configuration is a conformation or structural arrangement of entities, implying that the relative disposition of these entities is central to the configuration's identity. In the sciences, the spatial placement of atoms in a molecule is often called a configuration, a term also used for the characteristic grouping of heavenly bodies. More specifically, in gestalt psychology, a configuration is taken to be a collection of sensations, emotions, motor patterns, and concepts organized in such fashion that the collection operates as a unit in thought and behavior. Indeed, if a configuration becomes sufficiently refined, it converts into a new mental element that can enter into further permutations. That is, if the diverse elements that make up the configuration become strongly connected, they all become "chunked," so that they function as a single element, taking up less space in limited attention.

It may seem contradictory to assert that mental elements thrown together by happenstance can nevertheless feature a cohesion that prevents disintegration, but what jumbled the elements together is different from what glues them together. Even if two elements are tossed together by haphazard juxtaposition, those elements may stick together because of mutually compatible properties. Indeed, because certain elements possess intrinsic affinities for each other, a chance linkage of two elements can produce a stable pairing, and large clusters of elements can form themselves spontaneously into highly ordered arrangements out of utter chaos. Campbell (1974) offered the striking example of crystal formation, in which, under the proper conditions, a dissolved chemical will not merely precipitate into amorphous aggregates, but rather fine crystals. A specific crystalline structure is implicit in the ions or molecules leaving solution, such that a more organized spatial pattern is actually more stable than one less organized, yielding a specific configuration from the mere random collisions of the ions or molecules.

Configuration acquisition. To appreciate how chance permutations may generate stable collections of elements, we first must note that extremely few configurations arise in this way. On the contrary, the overwhelming majority of configurations consist of elements that have been linked on either a posteriori or a priori grounds.

A posteriori configurations establish a correspondence between perceived events and their cognitive representations. If, for example, we have a set of events A_1, A_2, . . . , A_n represented by a set of mental elements A_1', A_2', . . . , A_n', and if the conditional probability of any one event given any one of the others is much greater than zero, such as $p(A_i/A_j) \gg 0$ for all $i \neq j$, we would expect the mental elements to be configured such that the association strengths approximate the conditional probabilities (i.e., the rank order of conditional probabilities positively correlates with the rank order of association strengths). In some manner, a posteriori configurations are internal images of the world, mental expectations approximating the observed co-occurrences of events.

Whereas a posteriori configurations derive from experience, a priori configurations emerge from given conventions. These conventions define a set of mental elements and the rules by which these elements can be combined into a proper order. In mathematical disciplines, for instance, the members of a given tradition are provided with rules for the correct manipulation of numbers and certain abstract symbols defining constants, variables, and operations. Logic, too, regulates how verbal propositions of a specified kind can be combined so that we can determine when a set of statements is consistent or inconsistent. Likewise, grammars define the proper arrangements of words, morphemes, and phonemes that yield linguistic communication, and stylistic traditions determine what kinds of word combinations define a literary composition. Syntactic rules also prevail in music and the visual arts, such as painting and ballet. It is highly characteristic of a priori configurations that decisions of rightness or wrongness, truth or falsity, beauty or ugliness, are absolute within a given body of rules. The adequacy of a posteriori configurations, in contrast, is decided on probabilistic grounds, based on the degree of congruence between observation and cognitive representation.

Earlier we observed that configurations can undergo "consolidation," in which the elements can be so compacted that the configuration as a whole can function as a single unit in mental manipulations. This can occur for a posteriori and a priori configurations as well as for chance configurations. In the case of a posteriori configurations, certain events co-occur with such high frequency that they become definitive elements of a particular concept (e.g., birds as feathered egg-layers). For a priori configurations, particular operations may undergo refinements such that what once was a complicated procedure becomes conveniently simple. For instance, using algebraic rules and the concept of limits, one can demonstrate how various functions are differentiated, yielding a new set of rules that allow a mathematician to circumvent the original derivations. Once a priori and a posteriori configurations become sufficiently consolidated that they can be manipulated as mental elements, they can enter the process by which chance permutations emerge.

Self-organization. We are now in a position to indicate why some chance permutations often are more stable than others. Sometimes two configurations, of whatever origin, will harbor compatible structures such that the elements can line up more or less one-on-one. In other words, an approximate one-to-one correspondence can be fixed between the two configurations such that the elements of one set are mapped onto the elements of the other set. One example of this matching of elements across configurations is when one chance permutation produces a close analogy between two hitherto unrelated phenomena (cf. Sternberg, 1977). In science, for example, when light is conceived as a wave phenomenon, equivalences are set up between two a posteriori configurations, one encoding the diverse behaviors of light in experimental studies, the other the known behavior of waves; thus, different colors correspond to distinct wavelengths, color intensity to wave amplitude, and complex hues to mixtures of various wavelengths and amplitudes; and reflection, refraction, diffraction, and interference are effects with counterparts in both light and wave attributes. In the arts, a stable permutation usually involves a striking simile or, better yet, a metaphor that unifies hitherto unrelated domains of experience; in Shakespeare's sonnet 73, as an example, three successive images of winter's onset, dusk, and a dying fire are made to highlight, in accelerating urgency, the message of the final couplet that one's love, too, will pass away.

Frequently in scientific creativity an a posteriori configuration is paired with one derived a priori. For instance, a particular mathematical formula may describe relations between two or more abstract variables that fit the observed associations between a similar number of concrete variables. Hence, Balmer found by "induction" a relatively simple equation that could predict the location of the spectral lines of hydrogen, where the wavelengths are expressed as functions of integers.

What is gained by merging two or more configurations? One answer is that frequently one configuration is better consolidated than the other, which is less well defined. A good model of light, for instance, allows us to connect a vast range of phenomena that before would have been deemed isolated facts. We link together the diversity of light phenomena and place the visual spectrum within a single, uni-dimensional scale (wavelength) that stretches from X-rays and ultraviolet down to infrared and radiowaves, all with the same set of definitive behaviors (viz., reflection, refraction, diffraction, interference, etc.). A tight analogy or model permits us to know more about the world with less work. The same gain in informational efficiency is seen in the application of an arbitrary formula to empirical data. It takes less mental space to remember Balmer's equation than it does to memorize all the wavelengths appearing in the hydrogen spectrum. In aesthetic types of creativity, a vivid sensory image often stands in for the far more diffuse emotions that punctuate the significant events of human life – love, death, dreams, striving, and despair. Many of Shakespeare's sonnets employ concrete images that convey quite graphically the inexorable flow of time and the losses to love and beauty that such passage entails. In music, a melody, or a harmonic progression, may sound the way that certain fundamental emotions feel, an isomorphism of structure permitting the listener to translate subjective experience to a more objective or overt form (Simonton, 1980d, 1986a). Speaking in more general terms, integration of configu-rations renders our thoughts and feelings more coherent, more organized, for the number of unrelated elements we must cope with is dramatically reduced.

This gain becomes especially conspicuous when configurations are united in a hierarchical fashion, that is, when mental elements are ordered in an optimal man-ner for the retrieval of information or the anticipation of events. This asset is perhaps most conspicuous in biological taxonomy, where each living form is as-signed to a kingdom, phylum, class, order, family, genus, and species. Knowledge of how a particular species falls in each category immediately ushers forth a collec-tion of relevant data about morphology, physiology, and behavior. Likewise, in aesthetic compositions, a definite structure may coordinate the material into a hierarchical arrangement. Thus, classical music contains forms, such as sonata-allegro, fugue, and theme variation, that guide the expectancies of the appreciator and encapsulate the corresponding emotions in an ordered scheme. Whatever the specific example, we postulate that the human intellect is programmed to self-organize its cognitions and emotions into hierarchical structures such that experi-ence is most efficaciously organized. On the plane of subjective experience, we may posit that the mind receives pleasure from noticeable enhancements in mental order, where pleasure is merely the marking of an adaptive event. In other words, cognitive events that reduce mental "entropy," by joining configurations together into more comprehensive hierarchical formations, receive intrinsic reinforcement. Yet, however adaptive and pleasurable intellectual organization may be, configura-tions cannot become ordered into higher-order configurations unless they are suffi-ciently consolidated. Otherwise each component of a hierarchical structure will connect with so many other components that organization is, in fact, missing. That is why there was some wisdom in the decision of Descartes to ground his philoso-phy solely on ideas "clear and distinct."

Communication and acceptance

Although we now possess the rudiments of a chance-permutation and selective-retention theory, creativity cannot be fully explicated without adding two additional selective-retention processes, one intrapsychic and the other social.

Communication configurations. Once a configuration has been isolated and proves useful for structuring experience, that discovery remains only personal until it is successfully expressed to others. In the arts, for example, the chance configuration may be nothing more than a sketch for a painting, the outlines of thematic material and formal structure for a music composition, or the germinal idea for a plot or character in fiction – which then must undergo considerable development before something is presentable to the public. This conversion of a chance configuration from the ineffable to the articulate yields another entity altogether, the *communication* configuration. This new creation consists of symbols, whether verbal, mathematical, visual, or auditory, that permit the initial idea to be conveyed to fellow human beings. A communication configuration may be a scientific journal article, a philosophical treatise, an essay, novel, or poem, a painting, sculpture, or architectural design, or a song, string quartet, symphony, or opera, just to name a few of the myriad possibilities.

Given that a workable communication configuration has been devised and has been made available to the community of potential appreciators, the selection mechanisms cease to be merely intrapsyhic and become fully social – which brings us to the last selection procedure.

Social acceptance. The offered creative product must succeed in the domain of interpersonal influence; that is, it must be accepted by others with an active involvement in the same area of creative endeavor. Here we are brought back to the first fundamental proposition of this chapter, namely, that creativity ultimately must be viewed as a form of leadership entailing overt exercise of personal influence. Although the specific criteria by which communication configurations are judged vary from field to field, in general, potential appreciators must be able to exploit the articulated idea to restructure their own thinking habits in approximately the same manner as experienced by the originator. Hence, social acceptance signifies that a group of people have found the suggested configuration to be of value in their own personal endeavors toward self-organization, toward augmented cognitive effectiveness – whether the idea be a scientific or philosophical viewpoint that makes the objective world appear more coherent or an artistic, literary, or musical composition that helps render subjective experience more sensible or meaningful. Several requirements have to be met before social acceptance can be achieved, four perhaps standing out:

1. Each member of the community must have available a similar repertoire of mental elements, such as a shared body of facts, experiences, methods, techniques, concerns, values, emotions, and enigmas.

2. Those mental elements must be in comparative disarray within the minds of potential acceptors, so that a need exists for a more efficient approach to structuring experience. In the case of science, for instance, Darwin (1952/1860, p. 240) noted in the last chapter of his *Origin of Species:* ''Although I am fully convinced of the truth of the views given in this volume . . . I by no means expect to convince experienced naturalists whose minds are stocked with a multitude of facts all viewed, during a long course of years, from a point of view directly opposite to mine.''
3. A consensus must exist on the meanings of symbols composing the communication configuration; this consensus enables each member of the community to reconstruct the original configuration from its social representation.
4. The originator must have successfully translated the initial conception into a form that permits others to perform the requisite reverse translation.

All four of these requirements presuppose that the creator's psychological constitution is somewhat representaive of others within the same endeavor. To the extent that a creator is unrepresentative of others on these matters, personal impact will lessen. At the same time, for reasons that will become clear later, the efficacy of the chance-permutation process depends heavily on the creative individual's fundamental uniqueness. Hence, the essential tension mentioned earlier reappears: Chance permutations require an iconoclastic disposition, whereas the formation of viable communication configurations demands more of a traditionalist orientation. As a result, the ultimate success of a creation in the sphere of personal influence often ends up being a curvilinear, inverted-U function of its originality, revealing a trade-off between these two contradictory components of the creativity equation. In classical music, for example, how often a composition is likely to be heard in the concert hall or recording studio is a concave-downward, nonmonotonic function of its melodic originality (Simonton, 1980e, 1986a).

Empirical elaboration

To place more flesh on the foregoing skeleton, I shall later discuss several key aspects of creativity, namely, the creative process, personality correlates, productivity, developmental antecedents, and the multiples phenomenon. Along the way, it should become clear that the theory deals with all the four p's of creativity (for more detailed documentation, see Simonton, in press).

The creative process

In the essay mentioned earlier, William James (1880, p. 456) described the thinking patterns of ''the highest order of minds'' in this way:

Instead of thoughts of concrete things patiently following one another in a beaten track of habitual suggestion, we have the most rarefied abstractions and discriminations, the most unheard of combination of elements, the subtlest associations of analogy; in a word, we seem suddenly introduced into a seething caldron of ideas, where everything is fizzling and bobbling about in a state of bewildering activity, where partnerships can be joined or loosened in an instant, treadmill routine is unknown, and the unexpected seems only law.

This quotation describes, in a far more concrete fashion, the chance-permutation process that we hypothesized in a more abstract form earlier. To further document this description, let us look at anecdotes and introspective reports regarding the act of creation.

Anecdotes. Often, creative persons have left us stories about the circumstances that led to some significant innovative idea (Ghiselin, 1952), and many of these anecdotes reveal quite strikingly the prominent role that chance plays in origination. The best illustrations probably can be taken from the great many instances of scientific and technological "serendipity," a term established by Walter B. Cannon in his classic 1940 paper "The Role of Chance in Discovery." The numbers of scientists and inventors who have so benefited from "lady luck" are quite large and impressive, including Arago, Becquerel, Bernard, Columbus, Dam, Edison, Fleming, Foucault, Galvani, Grimaldi, Hauy, Kirchhoff, Mayer, Nobel, Oersted, Perkin, Pasteur, Richet, Roentgen, and Schönbein (Beveridge, 1957; Cannon, 1940; Koestler, 1964; Mach, 1896). Serendipitous creativity fits with the chance-configuration theory in two ways:

1. This phenomenon is really nothing more than a special case of the more universal chance-permutation procedure. The sole distinction of note is that at least one of the mental elements composing the new stable permutation is provided by outside experience. Rather than confine the permutations to cognitive elements, such as concepts and images retrieved chaotically from memory, one or more elements entail a sensation or perception of a present event, an external stimulus that often provides the scientist with the keystone for constructing a novel configuration.

2. A chance encounter with an environmental event acquires significance only when incorporated into a stable permutation: "In fields of observation, chance favors only the prepared mind," said Pasteur. Daily life is replete with unexpected events that might insert the lacking element into a striking configuration; yet these stimuli stimulate nothing, passing through consciousness without linking up with other elements. As the physicist Ernst Mach observed in his notable 1896 article "On the Part Played by Accident in Invention and Discovery," the fortuitous facts that inspired many critical discoveries "were *seen* numbers of times before they were *noticed*" (p. 169). A creative scientist is primed to spot the larger implications of otherwise trivial events.

The foregoing two points are illustrated in the thinking patterns of Charles Darwin, as recounted by Francis Darwin (1958/1892, p. 101), who served as his father's laboratory assistant for many years. Francis described his father's

instinct for arresting exceptions: it was as though he were charged with theorizing power ready to flow into any channel on the slightest disturbance, so that no fact, however small, could avoid releasing a stream of theory, and thus the fact became magnified into importance. In this way it naturally happened that many untenable theories occurred to him; but fortunately his richness of imagination was equalled by his power of judging and condemning the thoughts that occurred to him. He was just to his theories, and did not condemn them unheard; and so it happened that he was willing to test what would seem to most people not at all worth testing. These rather wild trials he called "fool's experiments," and enjoyed extremely.

Hence, Darwin projected the chance-permutation procedure onto his experimental activities, actively seeking serendipitous results rather than passively waiting for them to happen. An analogous disposition can be found in aesthetic types of creativity as well. For instance, the surrealist painter Max Ernst described the method of "frottage" by which haphazard forms in everyday objects are developed into artistic ideas, and the modern sculptor Henry Moore noted how he expanded his visual sensitivity by walking along the seashore, picking up curious pebbles and shells that fed his current form interests (Ghiselin, 1952).

Introspective reports. Einstein clearly described a two-stage process in some introspections published by the French mathematician Jacques Hadamard (1945). The first stage involves the free permutation of mental elements: "The psychical entities which seem to serve as elements in thought are certain signs and more or less clear images which can be 'voluntarily' reproduced and combined. . . . [T]his combinatory play seems to be the essential feature in productive thought" (p. 142). These "elements are . . . of visual and some of muscular type" (p. 143). In fact, even though "the desire to arrive finally at logically connected concepts is the emotional basis of this rather vague play with the above mentioned elements," the combinatory play takes place "before there is any connection with logical construction in words or other kinds of signs which can be communicated to others" (p. 142). Because "the words or the language, as they are written or spoken, do not seem to play any role in my mechanism of thought" (p. 142), "conventional words or other signs have to be sought for laboriously only in a secondary stage, when the mentioned associative play is sufficiently established and can be reproduced at will" (p. 143). This second stage is only weakly aided by the presence of "a certain connection between those elements and relevant logical concepts" (p. 142).

A fuller discussion of the "vague . . . combinatory play" is offered by Henri Poincaré (1921), the mathematician and philosopher of science. Poincaré began by defining mathematical creation: "It does not consist in making new combinations with mathematical entities already known [for] the combinations so made would be infinite in number and most of them absolutely without interest. To create consists precisely in not making useless combinations and in making those which are useful and which are only a small minority. Invention is discernment, choice" (p. 386). The most useful combinations "are those which reveal to us unsuspected kinship between other facts, long known, but wrongly believed to be strangers to one another" (p. 386). Accordingly, "among chosen combinations the most fertile will often be those formed of elements drawn from domains which are far apart. Not that I mean as sufficing for invention the bringing together of objects as disparate as possible; most combinations so formed would be entirely sterile. But certain among them, very rare, are the most fruitful of all" (p. 386). He maintained that "the sterile combinations do not even present themselves to the mind of the inventor. Never in the field of his consciousness do combinations appear that are not really useful, except some that he rejects but which have to some extent the characteristics of useful combinations" (p. 386). Later he qualifies the criterion of usefulness by saying that combinations, to enter full consciousness, must appeal to the mathematician's "emotional sensibility," the sense of "beauty and elegance" (p. 391). Thus, "among the great numbers of combinations blindly formed by the subliminal self, almost all are without interest and without utility; but just for that reason they are also without effect upon the esthetic sensibility. Consciousness will never know them; only certain ones are harmonious, and, consequently, at once useful and beautiful" (p. 392). Every so often, "a sudden illumination seizes upon the mind of the mathematician [that] does not stand the test of verification; well, we almost always notice that this false idea, had it been true, would have gratified our natural feeling for mathematical elegance" (p. 392). Another of Poincaré's introspections features more vivid imagery regarding the creation of configurations from chance permutations, or "random collisions." One evening he found himself unable to sleep: "Ideas rose in crowds; I felt them collide until pairs interlocked, so to speak, making a stable combination. By the next morning I had established the existence of a class of Fuchsian functions" (p. 387). Later he explicitly compares these colliding ideas to "the hooked atoms of Epicurus" that move about "like the molecules of gas in the kinematic theory of gases" so that "their mutual impacts may produce new combinations" (p. 393).

Even though the foregoing introspections came from scientists, compatible reports have emerged from those in more artistic endeavors (Ghiselin, 1952). Mach (1896, p. 174) provided a thumbnail sketch of how chance permutations yield stable configurations, a sketch that applies just as well to aesthetic metaphors and forms as to scientific theories and discoveries: "From the teeming, swelling host of fancies which a free and high-flown imagination calls forth, suddenly that particular form arises which harmonizes perfectly with the ruling idea, mood, or design."

Individual differences

Individuals probably vary substantially in their capacity for generating chance permutations, and individual differences in this ability likely will correlate with other personal attributes due to some causal nexus, whether as antecedent or consequent. Let us draw a picture, then, of the creative person and indicate how this portrait merges with our larger theoretical scheme. This picture has two main features, one cognitive and the other motivational.

Cognition. F. C. Bartlett (1958, p. 136) made the critical distinction between original and routine information processing, holding that "the most important feature of original experimental thinking is the discovery of overlap and agreement where formerly only isolation and difference were recognized." Speaking more broadly, Carl Rogers (1954, p. 255) observed that the creation of this "novel relational product" requires the "ability to toy with elements and concepts." The cognitive style characteristic of creative persons apparently entails the ability to play with ideas until unexpected concordances are discerned – a conclusion that has support in empirical research. For example, high scores on the Barron-Welsh Art Scale, a measure of the preference for complexity and a good predictor of creativity (Stein, 1969), are associated with originality, flexibility, verbal fluency, independence of judgment, impulsiveness, and breadth of interests (Barron, 1963). Fluency of thought, whether verbal, associational, expressive, or ideational, has been linked with creativity as well (Guilford, 1963), along with the capacity to produce remote associations to various stimuli (Mednick, 1962). Highly creative individuals tend to display greater willingness to take intellectual risks, and they tend to be wide categorizers (Cropley, 1967). Versatility may also be an important trait of eminent achievers (White, 1931). Finally, just as intelligence is the single best person-ological predictor of leadership in general (Simonton, 1983c, 1984e, 1985a, 1986e, 1987c), creative individuals are noticeably more intelligent than average (Cattell, 1963; Roe, 1952b).

It is evident that a person is more likely to see congruence between hitherto isolated elements if that person boasts broad interests, versatility, intellectual fluency and flexibility, the capacity for remote associations that can connect disparate ideas, and an orientation to wide categories that oblige substantial overlap between ideas. The tendency to play with ideas would be aided, too, by independence, and a risk-taking orientation. An impressive intellect, lastly, would make it possible for an individual to acquire the copious supply of richly interconnected mental elements for such combinatory gymnastics. In brief, these diverse traits, which help define the cognitive style of the creative individual, probably form a constellation of interrelated attributes. To comprehend the causal foundation for this set of attributes, let me adapt a model published some years ago (Simonton, 1980a). The model starts by differentiating persons along two dimensions. First, people can be distinguished on the basis of sheer volume of mental elements, which determines the potential number of associations among those elements. Some individuals have few elements, others a great many. Second, persons differ in the distribution of association strengths among these elements. At the one extreme are those persons so cognitively constituted that the overwhelming majority of their associations are quite strong, and at the other extreme are those in whom the majority of associations are far weaker, albeit still prominent enough to have behavioral and emotional consequences. On the basis of these two dimensions we can advance a fourfold typology of ideal types, each with a characteristic distribution of associations. Figure 16.1 depicts this typology. The vertical axis on each of the four graphs represents the number of mental elements, whereas the horizontal axis, labeled

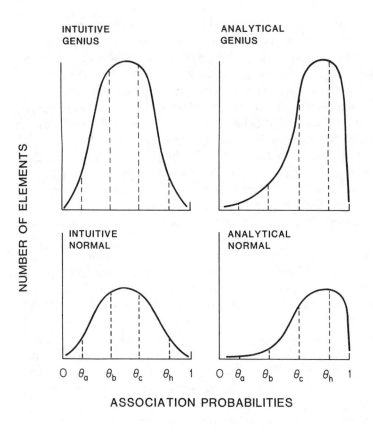

Figure 16.1. Four hypothetical personality types based on the probability distributions of conditional probabilistic associations (Simonton, 1980a).

"association probability" (because the model was conceived in terms of the distribution of conditional probabilities), registers the distribution of strength for the associations connecting these elements. This latter axis is subdivided into regions by four thresholds that demarcate the psychological repercussions of an association having a given strength. These are the thresholds of attention, behavior, cognition, and habituation that determine, respectively, when an association can direct the perception of environmental stimuli (θ_a), support an "infraconscious" motor or visceral behavior (θ_b), be consciously manipulated via symbolic representations (linguistic, logical, or mathematical) (θ_c), and become habituated and hence "ultra-conscious" in execution (θ_h). The "normals" have a considerably smaller supply of elements than do the "geniuses," and consequently fewer mental elements are

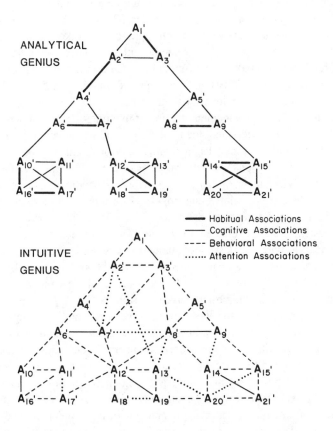

Figure 16.2. Typical associative connections among mental elements for analytical and intuitive geniuses.

available for chance permutations in normals than in geniuses. Nonetheless, being a "genius" does not suffice to guarantee that the mental elements have the potential to undergo chance permutation, for this capacity depends on the distribution of association strengths (or probabilities). Whereas the "intuitive genius" has a great many elements linked by numerous infraconscious but behaviorally and emotionally active associations, the "analytical genius" has a comparable number of elements linked by a smaller set of conscious and ultraconscious cognitions and habits. The implications of these opposed probability distributions can be better grasped if we examine Figure 16.2, which shows a typical cross section of the mental organization for each of the two cognitive styles.

On the one hand, the analytical genius has mental elements clustered into compact configurations arranged in a hierarchical order. The configurations are highly consolidated in that the elements within a configuration are linked by strong (cognitive or habitual) associations, and the elements within a configuration have minimal links with elements in other configurations. Configurations must be both "clear" (i.e., consist of strong associations among defining elements) and "distinct" (i.e., have minimal associations with elements outside the configuration) in order to form a hierarchical arrangement that might maximize the efficient distribution of knowledge. On the other hand, the intuitive genius, while having roughly the same quantity of mental elements, has a dramatically different way of retrieving information. Fewer connections are habitual or even properly symbolized, with a rich infusion of behaviorally active but infraconscious associations. Configurations are less clear and distinct, and thus knowledge is distributed in a more egalitarian fashion. Because mental elements are more richly interconnected, appreciably more ways exist of passing from one element to another. This is immediately apparent in Figure 16.2 when we trace all possible paths between any two randomly selected elements. For instance, an analytical genius is very limited in the means by which element A_{21}' can be evoked by element A_1', and that route is well ingrained by strong associations, whereas the possible avenues from A_1' to A_{21}' in the intuitive genius are far more numerous, and these are both weak and largely equiprobable. *This associative richness provides the mechanism for chance permutations.* Mach (1896, p. 167), after admitting the virtues of "a powerfully developed *mechanical* memory, which recalls vividly and faithfully old situations," claimed that "more is required for the development of *inventions*. More extensive chains of images are necessary here, the excitation by mutual contact of widely different trains of ideas, a more powerful, more manifold, and richer connection of the contents of memory."

The model just abstracted, besides offering an account of the chance-permutation process, facilitates explanation of the cognitive style of creative persons (Simonton, 1980a). The distribution of associative strengths seen in the upper-left-hand quadrant of Figure 16.1 would necessarily be related to the ability to generate remote associations. Given that configurations are less distinct, the corresponding concepts or schemata will be more inclusive, and thus the intuitive genius should feature wide categories. With such profusely interrelated thoughts, we would also expect more prominent fluency, flexibility, and independence, and perhaps even a risk-taking orientation. In addition, the intuitive genius has a much larger pool of associations that have just barely passed the threshold of attention, signifying a more impressive alertness to novel or unusual stimuli on the fringe of focused attention. This proclivity toward curiosity or inquisitiveness may explicate the breadth of interests and preference for complexity displayed by creative individuals. Impulsive openness to experience could also supply that "*sharpened attention, which detects the uncommon features of an occurrence*" (Mach, 1896, p. 168) and thereby renders a person more susceptible to serendipity. Obviously, the intuitive genius, having a larger reservoir of infraconscious associations to draw on, will arrive at chance configurations by routes not totally open to core awareness, a capacity as important to science as it is to the arts. The physicist Max Planck (1949, p. 109) claimed that the pioneer scientist "must have a vivid intuitive imagination, for new ideas are not generated by deduction, but by an artistically creative imagination."

This model presumes a high correlation between clarity and distinctness. Configurations range from small, tidy collections of elements that act as a unit (because all elements are strongly connected and minimally linked with outside configurations) down to more diffuse configurations, or near aggregates, with weak associative bonds between elements and with minimal separation from kindred configurations so that one concept easily flows into another. The act of consolidation serves as a sharpening process, accentuating the "in-group" elements at the expense of the "out-group" elements, producing configurations that are progressively more clear and distinct. Consolidation counts as an intellectual asset, for configurations, when sufficiently refined, can enter hierarchical structures for the most efficacious organization of information; consolidation initially facilitates the permutation process insofar as configurations must behave more or less as a unit in order to be freely recombined. Yet, ironically, the end result of this self-organization is a population of configurations that do not lend themselves to chance permutations, because of the dearth of interconnections among ideas.

Motivation. According to Mach (1896, p. 170): "Supposing, then, that such a rich organic connexion of the elements of memory exists, and is the prime distinguishing mark of the inquirer, next in importance certainly is that *intense interest* in a definite object, in a definite idea, which fashions advantageous combinations of thought from elements before disconnected, and obtrudes that idea into every observation made, and into every thought formed, making it enter into relationship with all things." Hence, in Cox's classic historiometric inquiry (1926, p. 187) into 301 geniuses, an exceptional IQ did not, by itself, suffice to assure distinction, for intellect had to be accompanied by a tenacity of purpose: "High but not the highest intelligence, combined with the greatest degrees of persistence, will achieve greater eminence than the highest degree of intelligence with somewhat less persistence." Distinguished contributors to science, for example, are exceptionally hard-working, and a commitment to work is positively correlated with both the number of their publications and the frequency that those publications are cited by others (McClelland, 1963; Manis, 1951; Simonton, in press, chap. 4). Anne Roe (1952a, p. 25) concluded from extensive interviews with 64 eminent scientists that "driving absorption in their work" characterized them all. The distinguished researcher "works hard and devotedly at his laboratory, often seven days a week. He says his work is his life, and has few recreations, those being restricted to fishing, sailing, walking or some other individualistic activity" (p. 22). As a group, "they have worked long hours for many years, frequently with no vacations to speak of, because they would rather be doing their work than anything else" (p. 25).

Roe's remarks hint that the drive to create obliges competing drives to assume subsidiary roles, thereby inducing a distinctive motivational profile. Creative personalities prefer time for reflection, and thus they avoid interpersonal contact, social affairs, administrative responsibilities, and political activities (Helmreich, Spence, Beane, Lucker, & Matthews, 1980; McClelland, 1963; Manis, 1951; Roe, 1952b; Terman, 1955). Cattell (1963) found that both historical and contemporary scientists tended to be "schizothymic" (i.e., withdrawn and internally preoccupied) and "desurgent" (i.e., introspective, restrained, brooding, and solemn). The following three reasons may be offered for the introverted personality of creative individuals:

1. The creator does not arrive at truth or beauty directly in some momentous flash of insight, but rather must sift through a long and laborious parade of chance permutations before the solution to a scientific or aesthetic problem is found. John Dryden, in his dedication to *The Rival Ladies,* spoke of his play beginning as "only a confused mass of thoughts tumbling over one another in the dark; when the fancy was yet in its first work, moving the sleeping images of things towards the light, there to be distinguished, and then either chosen or rejected by the judgment" (Ghiselin, 1952, p. 80). And the economist William S. Jevons (1900, p. 577) claimed the following:

It would be an error to suppose that the great discoverer seizes at once upon the truth, or has any unerring method of divining it. In all probability the errors of the great mind exceed in number those of the less vigorous one. Fertility of imagination and abundance of guesses at truth are among the first requisites of discovery; but the erroneous guesses must be many times as numerous as those that prove well founded. The weakest analogies, the most whimsical notions, the most apparently absurd theories, may pass through the teeming brain, and no record remain of more than the hundredth part.

Highly extroverted creators simply will not have adequate time for this process to take place, and, to paraphrase Euclid's response to the Ptolemy I Soter of Egypt, there is no royal road to creativity.

2. Social interaction may elicit a social-interference effect, as would be predicted by Zajonc's theory (1965) of social facilitation: The mere presence of others tends to raise arousal, which in turn increases the likelihood that highly probable responses will be emitted at the expense of responses less probable. Because the chance-permutation process demands access to low-probability associations, such socially induced arousal would necessarily inhibit creativity (Simonton, 1980a). To the extent that the presence of others implies the possibility of evaluation, this interference effect would be heightened all the more (Dentler & Mackler, 1964).

3. Amabile (1983) has amply documented how extrinsic motives – whether evoked by evaluation, social approval, or expectation of material rewards – tend to vitiate creativity; the creator must focus on the intrinsic properties of the task, not on

potential rewards or criticisms that await the outcome. Indeed, extrinsic motivation probably deflects any chance permutations toward the wrong goal: An individual might waste too much time generating chance permutations about the wrong things, such as fantasies about all the benefits of becoming "rich and famous" or worries about the adverse repercussions of failing to get tenure or a pay raise. Consequently, a creative person must retain an "internal locus of evaluation" (Rogers, 1954, p. 254). Recognition of the need to spurn extrinsic pressures toward conforming to social expectations may be partly responsible for the insistence on independence often displayed by creative persons (Cattell, 1963). "The pervasive and un-stereotyped unconventionality of thought which one finds consistently in creative individuals is related generically to a tendency to resist acculturation, where acculturation is seen as demanding surrender of one's personal, unique, fundamental nature" (Barron, 1963, p. 151).

The intrinsic motive to engage in acts of creative synthesis ultimately ensues from the more fundamental drive toward self-organization. Because a creator has a mental structure lying closer to the "intuitive genius" end of the spectrum, but instinctively seeks ultimately to attain the information-processing efficiency of the "analytical genius," tremendous personal satisfaction, or subjective pleasure, attends the successive discovery of chance configurations that move the creator ahead toward order. So the quest for self-organization provides a powerful incentive that shoves other motives aside.

Productivity

The distinguishing characteristic of genius is immense productivity (Simonton, 1984c, chap. 5). Frank Barron (1963, p. 139) said that "there is good reason for believing . . . that originality is almost habitual with persons who produce a really singular insight. The biography of the inventive genius commonly records a lifetime of original thinking, though only a few ideas survive and are remembered to fame. Voluminous productivity is the rule and not the exception among the individuals who have made some noteworthy contribution." The chance-configuration theory explicates three aspects of this feature of abundant creativity: (a) the distinctive cross-sectional distribution of productivity, (b) the relation between age and productive output, and (c) the association between quantity and quality.

Cross-sectional distribution. The distribution of output in any creative endeavor is highly elitist, with a small proportion of the total contributors accounting for the majority of the published contributions. Dennis (1955), in a study of several disciplines, found that the top 10% more prolific contributors were responsible for about half of the total work, whereas the bottom 50% least productive can be credited with only about 15% of the contributions. According to Price's law, if n is taken to represent the total number of contributors to a given field, then $n^{1/2}$ is the predicted number of contributors who will generate half of all contributions (Price, 1963, chap. 2). To illustrate, about 250 composers are responsible for the works that make up the classical repertoire (Moles, 1968), so $(250)^{1/2}$, or around 16, should account for half of these pieces, and such is indeed the case. Not only does this law imply a highly skewed distribution, but additionally a distribution that becomes ever more elitist as the discipline expands (Simonton, 1984c, chap. 5). Lotka's law describes the shape of the distribution, which decreases monotonically at a decelerating rate, yielding a long upper tail (Lotka, 1926). If n is now the number of published papers and $f(n)$ is the number of scientists who publish n papers, then $f(n)$ is inversely proportional to n^2, where the proportionality constant varies from discipline to discipline.

Many theories have been proposed to explain this distinctive distribution, each suffering from some theoretical or empirical difficulty (Simonton, 1984c, chap. 5, 1987a, in press, chap. 4). However, a plausible explanation can be derived directly from our theory. Suppose that the number of mental elements available for chance permutations is proportional to an individual's native intelligence, and hence this attribute is normally distributed. It follows that the total supply of potential chance permutations of those elements will be characterized by a highly skewed curve with an extremely stretched-out upper tail – for the number of permutations of n items increases as an accelerating function of n. Unfortunately, we cannot specify precisely what this function is, but let us assume that if n is the number of mental elements, e^n is the number of potential chance permutations. Even if n is normally distributed in the population of scientists, e^n definitely will not be.

To illustrate, I ran an exploratory Monte Carlo simulation. Ten thousand random normal deviates were generated by a computer to represent the distribution of the quantity of mental elements across individuals. A second set of random scores was created by taking the exponential of the first set. To render comparisons more concrete, both sets of numbers were standardized to a mean of 100 and a standard deviation of 16, as if they were IQ-like scores, and then these standardized scores were truncated to integer values. The first set of scores, which are taken to reflect the supply of mental elements, ended up with a distribution not all that different from what is normally found for IQ: The minimum was 37, the maximum 155, for a range of 118 points, and the distribution was highly symmetric and normally peaked (skewness -0.02 and kurtosis -0.09). The second set of scores, in contrast, had a low of 87 and a high of 341, for a spread of 254 points, and the distribution was highly skewed right, featuring a long flat upper tail (skewness 4.20 and kurtosis 31.37). The lowest score was much closer to the mean (100) than was the highest score, and the distribution monotonically decreased at a decelerating rate throughout almost the entire range of scores, rendering the outcome extremely elitist. The upper tail of the second curve, in fact, is indistinguishable from the distribution usually observed for productivity (Simonton, in press, chap. 4).

Age and output. A considerable amount of empirical work on the relation between age and productivity is summarized in Harvey C. Lehman's *Age and Achievement* (1953). Despite frequent methodological criticisms of Lehman's chief inferences, his conclusions have been substantiated and extended in more recent research that has exploited more sophisticated analytical techniques (Simonton, 1975a, 1977a, 1977b, 1980b, 1980e, 1983a, 1984b). The principal generalizations are that (a) creative productivity within any field is a curvilinear, concave-downward function of age, with a shape approximately that of an inverted backward J, (b) the specific form of the age curve, especially the points defining the onset, peak, and degree of post-peak decline in productivity, varies in a predictable fashion from discipline to discipline, and (c) exceptional lifetime output is correlated with precocity, longevity, and high productivity rates. These key conclusions can be deduced from the change-configuration theory.

The theory maintains that creativity, on the intrapsychic level, involves a two-step cognitive process, a conception compatible with a recent mathematical model of creative productivity (Simonton, 1984b). It, too, is predicated on a two-step process: One, each creator begins with a supply of "creative potential" (i.e., the degree of rich associative interconnections among numerous elements) that during the course of the creator's career becomes actualized in the form of "creative ideations" (i.e., chance configurations). Two, the ideas produced in the first step are progressively translated into actual "creative contributions" (i.e., communication configurations). We can then proceed to derive a set of linear differential equations based on two rates. The first corresponds to step 1 and is called the *ideation rate,* which assumes that a "law of mass action" operates such that the rate at which creative potential is converted into creative ideations is proportional to the size of that potential at a given time (i.e., the more free mental elements, the more possible "collisions," to use Poincaré's molecular analogy). The second rate corresponds to step 2 and is called the *elaboration rate,* which is proportional to the quantity of ideations that await articulation. The solution to these differential equations yields the following equation:

$$p(t) = c(e^{-at} - e^{-bt}).$$

Here, $p(t)$ is creative productivity at time t, a is the ideation rate, b the elaboration rate, and e the exponential constant (2.718 . . .). The integration constant c is a function of a, b, and m, where m is the initial creative potential, that is to say, the maximum number of contributions that a creator is theoretically capable of producing given an infinite life-span (i.e., m should be roughly proportional to e^n, where n is the number of mental elements not yet tied down in a hierarchical structure of strongly consolidated configurations). Significantly, t is taken to represent not chronological age, but rather professional age or career age, for this is an information-processing model in which $t = 0$ at the moment that the ideation (i.e., chance-permutation) process begins. Figure 16.3 presents a typical age curve according to

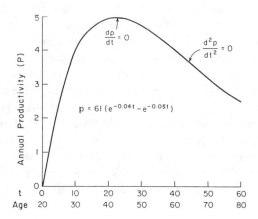

$$\frac{dp}{dt} = 0$$

$$\frac{d^2p}{dt^2} = 0$$

$$p = 61\,(e^{-0.04t} - e^{-0.05t})$$

Figure 16.3. Predicted productivity as a function of age under typical parameters (Simonton, 1984b).

the model, assuming that $t = 0$ at age 20 and that $a = 0.04$, $b = 0.05$, and $c = 61$ (i.e., $m = 305$). Creative productivity increases rapidly up to a single peak (in a decelerating curve) and soon thereafter begins a gradual decline, reaching the zero point asymptotically – yielding an inverted backward-J curve, as found in the empirical literature. The average correlation between predicted and observed values is .95.

Significantly, the parameters must be adjusted to comply with the particular information-processing needs of each discipline. In some fields, such as lyric poetry and pure mathematics, both the ideation and the elaboration rates are faster (i.e., circa 0.09 and 0.1, respectively), resulting in a curve that peaks much sooner (in the early 30s) and drops off much more quickly. Other disciplines, such as scholarship, feature slower ideation and elaboration rates (i.e., circa 0.03 and 0.04, respectively), creating an age curve that peaks out later and declines rather slowly afterward. The ideation constant a is perhaps the most interesting, for this determines the rate at which creative potential is used up. We may define the typical "creative half-life" in any discipline as the natural logarithm of 2 divided by a. In lyric poetry and pure mathematics, then, the half-life is as small as 8 years, meaning that half of the initial creative potential will normally be consumed in the production of chance configurations. In more scholarly endeavors, the half-life may be as long as 35 years. This concept of a creative half-life projects an optimistic picture for the later years of a creator's life. Because creative potential is lost at a decelerating rate, a creator who works for 60 years, under the typical parameters, can still accomplish more in that last decade than was achieved in the first decade. Furthermore, at the end of that final career decade, about one-quarter of the initial creative potential will remain unrealized.

Besides accounting for the overall age curve and interdisciplinary contrasts, the foregoing model explains the final key generalization to emerge from Lehman's work (1953), this regarding cross-sectional variation in creative productivity. There are three principal ways that creators can attain an impressive lifetime corpus of contributions: they can exhibit creative *precocity* by beginning to produce at an exceptionally young age; they can display extraordinary creative *longevity* by continuing to produce until quite late in life; they can produce at high *rates of output* per unit of time. From a purely mathematical standpoint, these three components are quite distinct and can comprise orthogonal determinants of the final contribution count. Yet empirically these three variables are positively correlated with each other (Simonton, 1977b, 1984c, chap. 5). The two-step cognitive model actually *predicts* a high positive relation among all three components. The source of this prediction is the constant c that we specified was a function of a, b, and m. Now the first two constants, the ideation and elaboration rates, are presumed to be characteristic of a given creative endeavor, but m directly gauges creative potential. With a and b fixed, c is directly proportional to m, and accordingly stands for a creator's potential output. Because all age curves are similar for a given enterprise, c describes the height of the curve. It immediately follows that the higher the creative potential, the earlier a career will begin, the higher the rate of productive flow, and the later the career will terminate (Simonton, 1984b). At the same time, contributors in the same domain should exhibit the same productive peaks no matter how they differ in initial creative potential, which turns out to be the case (Simonton, 1975a, 1984b).

To say that the foregoing implications arise from human information processing should not be taken as a dogmatic assertion that extrinsic events do not impinge on the intrinsic working out of creative potential. Certainly anything that reduces time investment in permutation generation will depress productivity, and thus it comes as no surprise that administrative duties (Roe, 1972) and increased parental responsibilities (Hargens, McCann, & Reskin, 1978) cause creative output to drop somewhat more than predicted by the model. Inferior physical health can have an adverse impact as well (Simonton, 1977a). Furthermore, because the chance-permutation process depends on having access to the network of infraconscious associations, any environmental stressor of sufficient strength to appreciably raise the emotional level will inherently undermine creativity (Simonton, 1980a). Therefore, it is consistent with the theory to find that major wars lower the probability of notable creative contributions (Simonton, 1976b, 1980c).

Quality and quantity. Thus far we have been speaking of "productivity" rather than "creativity" per se. Actually, on both empirical and theoretical grounds, these two concepts can be used almost interchangeably; total quantity of output is intertwined with selective quality of output. Those creators who can claim the longest bibliographies or inventories of products equally tend to boast the biggest lists of notable contributions, and hence the most impressive ultimate fame (Simonton, 1977b, 1984c, chap. 5). Furthermore, this consistent link between quantity and quality holds not just across careers, but within careers (Simonton, 1977a, 1984c, chap. 6, 1985b). Those periods in which a creator is the most productive also tend to be those in which the most exceptional contributions are made. Both major and minor works tend to covary within any given career even after partialling out the overall age trend, and the "quality ratio" of major to minor offerings exhibits no systematic change over time, whether linear or curvilinear.

Dennis (1954, p. 182) ventured "that the correlation between fame and fecundity may be understood in part in terms of the proposition that the greater the number of pieces [of] work done by a given man, the more of them will prove to be important." Hence, "quantity and quality are correlated, although they are not identical" (p. 183). This basic idea has been developed into the "constant-probability-of-success model," which simply holds that the odds of making a contribution are probabilistic consequences of total output, this whether we are scrutinizing cross-sectional or longitudinal data (Simonton, 1977a, 1985b). Moreover, because this model follows as an essential corollary of Campbell's model (1960), the covariation between quality and quantity can be derived from the chance-configuration theory as well.

To be sure, exceptions do apparently exist regarding the close link between quantity and quality, for the correlation is by no means perfect. As regards individual differences, even if the majority of members of any discipline fall along the continuum connecting the "silent," who produce little and that of minimal value, and the "prolific," who generate an impressive collection of contributions, two sorts of outliers appear in the graph as well: "perfectionists," who devote all their efforts to a handful of supreme contributions, and "mass producers," who churn out hundreds of valueless items (Cole & Cole, 1973, chap. 4). Even so, the exceptions are nothing more than departures from a pervasive rule and would be expected anyway according to theory. The more communication configurations made available for social selection, the higher the odds that one will earn acceptance, but those odds function only on the average. If we compared samples of contributors with equal productivity levels, their contribution levels would not be equal, but rather would be randomly scattered around some central value. Furthermore, a portion of the residuals around the regression line can be ascribed to individual differences in the efficacy of variation generation. Many mass producers are not exploiting chance permutations at all, but rather are engaged in totally routine applications of fixed techniques or heuristics. On the other hand, many perfectionists generate a few highly distinct configurations that cannot be considered merely as minor variations on the same theme.

The constant-probability-of-success model and the chance-configuration theory from which it can be derived have a couple of additional implications. In the first place, the model facilitates explanation of the notable durability of creative reputation over time, even in the hindsight of centuries (Farnsworth, 1969; Over, 1982; Rosengren, 1985; Simonton, 1976a, 1984g). Notwithstanding occasional exceptions, those who attain fame in their own day tend also to be highly regarded by posterity, and the initially obscure remain so. Creative persons with enduring reputations are those who have staked their claims to eminence on a respectable body of varied contributions, and accordingly their status does not rise or fall with the fate of single contributions. Beethoven's fame rests on far more than the Fifth Symphony, Michelangelo's on much more than the Sistine Chapel, and Shakespeare's on more than his *Hamlet;* according to Max Born, Einstein "would be one of the greatest theoretical physicists of all times even if he had not written a single line on relativity" (Hoffman, 1972, p. 7). It often happens that the contributions for which creators are best known today are not the contributions that earned them renown in their own time: Einstein was honored with the Nobel Prize – 16 years after he began publishing on special relativity and 6 years after his work on general relativity appeared – not for relativity theory at all, but rather for his paper on the photoelectric effect. Furthermore, the creators themselves are not the best judges of what will be most favorably received by posterity: Beethoven's favorite compositions are not the ones most often heard today. The transhistorical stability of creative reputations far surpasses that of single creative products on which those reputations are based.

Second, if we can expect prolific creators to enjoy high odds of success, they should experience fairly high opportunities for failures as well. Not all chance configurations, not even all those selected for conversion into communication configurations, will earn social acceptance, whether in the short or long run. It is a myth to assert that genius has privileged access to truth or beauty. Beethoven's *Wellington's Victory,* Michelangelo's Pauline Chapel, and Shakespeare's *Pericles* are universally considered inferior to the better creations of their less illustrious colleagues; and Einstein persevered in advocating a totally deterministic unified theory that ignored the advances made by the Copenhagen school of quantum mechanics. What W. H. Auden said of poets applies equally to creators of any stripe: "The chances are that, in the course of his lifetime, the major poet will write more bad poems than the minor," simply because major poets "write a lot" (Bennett, 1980, p. 15).

Developmental antecedents

How does one acquire the creative potential requisite for a long and productive career? Mach (1896, p. 171) hinted at an explanation when he said that "if the psychical life is subjected to the incessant influences of a powerful and rich experience, then every representative element in the mind is connected with so many others that the actual and natural course of the thoughts is easily influenced and determined by insignificant circumstances, which accidentally are decisive." Research has in fact demonstrated the central importance of diversified, enriching environments in the emergence of individuals who attain eminence (Simonton, 1987a). Let me cite illustrations from five domains, namely, family background, role models, formal education, marginality, and the zeitgeist.

Family background. The early childhood of the future creator is characterized by events that should raise the effectiveness of any chance-permutation mechanism. May the following three examples suffice:

1. Achieving individuals usually display a higher incidence of parental loss, especially orphanhood, relative to any reasonable baseline (Simonton, 1987a). For example, Roe (1952b) found, in her examination of notable contemporary scientists, that 15% had lost a parent by death before age 10. It is evident that such loss would seriously disrupt the usual socialization practices, producing a youth who may perceive the world in a less than fully conventional manner.

2. Eminent persons are more likely to have been firstborn children in the family (Helmreich et al., 1980; Roe, 1952b; Simonton, 1987a). According to Zajonc's "confluence model" (1976) of intellectual development, ordinal position in the family determines the amount of environmental stimulation available during childhood. If valid, the confluence model would explain the preeminence of firstborns, for an exceptional intelligence is no doubt requisite for a richly interconnected and vast collection of mental elements (Simonton, 1987a).

3. The household environment of a prospective creative genius is replete with intellectually and culturally stimulating materials (Simonton, 1987a). Parents are more likely to have intellectual and cultural interests, as revealed by respectable home libraries, magazine subscriptions, and artistic or mechanical hobbies. Accordingly, very early in life, future achievers acquire numerous stimulating hobbies, including omnivorous reading (Simonton, 1984c, chap. 4). This picture of a stimulating home environment holds for those who attain distinction in virtually all domains of creativity or leadership (Roe, 1952b; Schaefer & Anastasi, 1968).

Role models. In broad terms, adulthood achievement is dependent on the availability of role models during the early, formative years of a person's life (Simonton, 1987a). For instance, the odds of an eminent figure emerging in generation g have been shown to increase with the number of eminent figures in the same endeavor in generations $g - 1$ and $g - 2$, an autoregressive function that apparently holds for both creativity and leadership (Simonton, 1975b, 1983c). Moreover, these role models can be either impersonal "paragons" who are admired at a distance or personal "mentors" who affect the emerging genius in a far more direct fashion (Simonton, 1984a). Nonetheless, role models can have a negative rather than purely positive consequence for creative development (Segal, Busse, & Mansfield, 1980; Simonton, 1976b, 1976c). Even if the availability of role models improves the prospects for exhibiting creative precocity (Simonton, 1977b), the long-term impact on lifetime productivity can be negative, likely because of excessive imitation of models (Simonton, 1987a). There are at least three ways to augment the utility of models while concomitantly diminishing any tendency toward debilitating imitation (Simonton, 1984a). First, the larger the number of models, the harder it is to imitate any one. Second, in the instance of paragons, if one must admire just one or two predecessors, more benefit accrues from modeling oneself after those who are temporally most distant and thus less able to provide an exact template for guiding contemporary creativity. Third, in the case of mentors, it is probably more advantageous to study under someone still in the prime of a career rather than in the later stages of self-organization (Sheldon, 1980; Simonton, 1984c, chap. 2).

The equivocal influence of role model illustrates the "essential tension" mentioned by Kuhn (1963). On the one hand, the creator must to some extent be a "traditionalist," mastering the repertoire of problems, techniques, and standards, thereby becoming representative of other colleagues in the field. Insofar as identification with accomplished predecessors provides this sort of cognitive congruence, some degree of exposure to suitable role models must be developmentally healthy. On the other hand, to become a revolutionary who utterly transforms the foundations of a discipline demands that the creator be an "iconoclast." Otherwise, severe constraints will be placed on the chance-permutation process: The repertoire of mental elements that enter into the combinatory play will be more specialized, and the interconnections between these elements will be rather more limited and more firm. This tension between traditionalists and iconoclasts implies a curvilinear, inverted-U curve between the magnitude of influence of role models on a prospective innovator and that person's ultimate contribution to human culture. Just such a curve has been demonstrated (Simonton, 1984a).

Formal education. Einstein once condemned current educational methods with these words: "It is, in fact, nothing short of a miracle that the modern methods of instruction have not yet entirely strangled the holy curiosity of inquiry; for this delicate little plant, aside from stimulation, stands mostly in need of freedom; without this it goes to wreck and ruin without fail" (Schlipp, 1951, p. 17). Several studies have indeed found evidence that creativity is a curvilinear, inverted-U function of the level of formal education (Simonton, 1976a, 1983b, 1984c, chap. 4). As educational level increases, the probability of achieving eminence in a creative endeavor also increases up to a certain optimum, and thereafter declines so that further formal training diminishes the odds of achieving the highest eminence. The turnaround point usually appears somewhere between the junior and senior year of undergraduate education. This nonmonotonic function suggests that the essential tension that mediates the impact of role models also moderates the repercussion of formal education. On the one side, the traditionalist aspect of creativity is clearly reinforced by extensive formal training. Education, after all, is society's method of preserving and passing down to future generations the cultural variations that have shown adaptive value in the past history of sociocultural evolution. On the other side, the iconoclastic facet of creativity – the capacity to produce genuinely original chance configurations – quite obviously requires that the young creator not be excessively socialized into a single, narrow-minded way of associating ideas. Hence, the peak of the curve expressing achievement as a function of formal education may reveal the point at which the iconoclastic component begins to be sacrificed for the sake of the traditionalist component.

Of course, the optimal mix of iconoclasm and traditionalism may vary across distinct creative endeavors. Thus, artistic creativity may stress the iconoclastic side more, scientific creativity the traditionalist side, suggesting that the optimal level of formal training appears later in the sciences than in the arts, and such is indeed the case (Simonton, 1984c, chap. 4). In addition, it is conceivable that the proper combination depends on whether one plans to be an "advancer" who merely extends the endeavors of one's predecessors or a true "revolutionary" who utterly transforms the scientific or artistic paradigm. Hence, a revolutionary scientist, such as Einstein, might actually require less formal training for full success than an academic artist who pursues totally traditional themes and techniques.

Marginality. Campbell (1960, p. 391) noted that "persons who have been uprooted from traditional cultures, or who have been thoroughly exposed to two or more cultures, seem to have the advantage in the range of hypotheses they are apt to consider, and through this means, in the frequency of creative innovation." The Goertzels offered more contemporary endorsement when they pointed to the respectable percentage of first- and second-generation immigrants among distinguished twentieth-century personalities (Goertzel et al., 1978). Such individuals are provided with a heterogeneous array of mental elements, permitting combinatory variations unavailable to those who reside solely in one cultural world.

Professional marginality can have much the same effect as sociocultural marginality. Koestler (1964, p. 230) proclaimed that "all decisive advances in the history of scientific thought can be described in terms of mental cross-fertilization between different disciplines." Likewise, Bartlett (1958, p. 98) observed that "it has often happened that critical stages for advance are reached when what has been called one body of knowledge can be brought into close and effective relationship with what has been treated as a different, and a largely or wholly independent, scientific discipline." Kuhn (1970, p. 90) elaborated this point a bit further when he asserted that "almost always the men who achieve these fundamental inventions of a new paradigm have been either very young or very new to the field whose paradigm they change." A scientist exposed to more than one discipline can combine elements in a truly unique fashion. And, speaking more generally, important innovations in any given field frequently are introduced by those who either changed fields or were largely self-taught (Hughes, 1958).

Unfortunately, little empirical work has been done on professional marginality, albeit some evidence exists on behalf of this hypothesis (Simonton, 1984c). However, research has been carried out on yet a third kind of marginality, namely, geographic marginality, but this has been shown to have an adverse impact on creative development. Those creators born and raised far away from the cultural center of their day may face an uphill struggle for recognition (Simonton, 1977b, 1984a, 1986a). So-called provincials are likely deprived of the extremely diversified and stimulating environments to be found in the metropoli of civilization, with corresponding losses in the creative potential that they can develop.

Zeitgeist. Generational analyses have revealed that the zeitgeist, or the "spirit of the times," exerts an independent influence on creative development (Simonton,

1984d). Most intriguing are the instances in which the political milieu in generation *g* shapes the path taken by creativity in generation *g* + 1. For one thing, creativity increases whenever a civilization area is fragmented into a large number of sovereign nations, the growth of empire states signaling the forthcoming decline of cultural innovation (Simonton, 1975b, 1976c, 1984c, chap. 8). Such political fragmentation apparently augments cultural and ideological diversity, which condition best promotes the emergence of individuals with exceptional creative potential (Simonton, 1987a). Moreover, the collapse of controls during periods of political upheaval prepares the ground for fruitful creativity later on. For example, nationalistic revolts and rebellions directed against the hegemony of empires tend to increase creativity after a one-generation lag, an effect likely due to the resurgence of cultural heterogeneity against the homogenizing impositions of imperial systems (Simonton, 1975b). And civil disturbances generally tend to mix up the cultural broth, thereby resuscitating the zeitgeist most friendly to the creative growth (Simonton, 1976d, 1984c, chap. 9).

Nonetheless, not all violent events in the political sphere have this pleasant outcome. Wars between states, for instance, tend to produce an ideological zeitgeist that may not welcome innovation, and creativity is definitely unlikely to come forth after a political system crumbles into total anarchy, as registered by military revolts, dynastic conflicts, political assassinations, coups d'état, and other exemplars of chaos among the power elite (Simonton, 1975b, 1976c). The essential tension between traditionalism and iconoclasm offers a basis for interpreting these findings. On the one hand, wartime propaganda and patriotism may excessively reinforce traditionalism at the expense of iconoclasm; war indeed discourages the emergence of individualism and empiricism, for instance (Simonton, 1976d). On the other hand, an era of utter political instability may instill in the forthcoming generation a debilitating iconoclasm, a distrust of tradition that may verge on nihilism. The more rational and systematic endeavors, like science and philosophy, are more inhibited by political anarchy than are artistic activities, like painting and sculpture, where iconoclasm is probably more desirable.

Multiples

I close this empirical elaboration of the chance-configuration theory by treating a specific phenomenon, that of multiple discovery and invention. This phenomenon occurs whenever two or more scientists, working independently and often even simultaneously, offer the exact same contribution. Classic illustrations are the devising of calculus by Newton and Leibniz, the prediction of the planet Neptune by J. C. Adams and LeVerrier, the production of oxygen by Scheele and Priestley, the proposal of a theory of evolution by natural selection by Darwin and Wallace, and the invention of the telephone by Bell and Gray. Investigators have compiled extensive lists of such multiples, some running into the hundreds of separate cases (Merton, 1961b; Ogburn & Thomas, 1922).

The traditional interpretation of multiples was promulgated largely by sociologists and anthropologists, especially Kroeber (1917), Ogburn and Thomas
(1922), and Merton (1961a, 1961b): Briefly expressed, multiples have been thought
to prove that the source of scientific advance lies outside the individual, for the
zeitgeist determines when the time has come for a given contribution. At a specific
moment in history, particular discoveries or inventions become absolutely inevitable, in a supreme illustration of sociocultural determinism. Scientific progress,
therefore, does not depend on acts of genius, for individual scientists are epi-
phenomenal to the course of history. In the words of Merton (1961a, p. 306),
"discoveries and inventions become virtually inevitable (1) as prerequisite kinds of
knowledge accumulate in man's cultural store; (2) as the attention of a sufficient
number of investigators is focused on a problem – by emerging social needs, or by
developments internal to the particular science, or by both."

Clearly, if the traditional explanation were valid, the theoretical scheme offered
here would be very much mistaken. In the first place, this position holds that at
some level, the chance permutations must be predetermined to come out a specified
way – an apparent contradiction. In addition, this view suggests that scientific
creativity differs substantially from artistic creativity, and thus one theory cannot
cover all varieties of creativity. No one would claim, for example, that at a specific
moment in history Beethoven's Fifth Symphony became absolutely inevitable, and
thus would still have been heard in the concert halls had Ludwig died in the crib!
Nevertheless, by scrutinizing the logical and empirical issues, I shall show that
multiples actually offer some of the best data available for bolstering the present
theory (Simonton, 1987b, in press, chap. 6).

Logical issues. Merton (1961b, p. 477) maintained that "it is the singletons –
discoveries made only once in the history of science – that are the residual cases,
requiring special explanation" and that "all scientific discoveries are in principle
multiples, including those that on the surface appear to be singletons." Even so,
counterarguments are easily proposed that render multiples the truly exceptional
events and singletons the normal state of affairs. Schmookler (1966, p. 191) scrutinized the list of nearly 150 multiples published by Ogburn and Thomas (1922) and
concluded that this collection "is based on a failure to distinguish between the
genus and the individual." For example, in the enumeration of technological multiples, generic terms such as "telegraph," "steamboat," and "airplane" are permitted to obscure the fact that the putative "duplicates" were often completely different conceptions. It is possible to define artistic contributions in such a generic way
that multiples become possible: Try "a four-movement symphony in C minor."

Furthermore, even if independent discoveries or inventions may have some components in common, very often one contribution is more fully developed than
another. Ogburn and Thomas (1922, p. 93) themselves confessed, in a footnote,
that "the most serious difficulty in making the list is the fact that the contribution of
one person is in some cases more complete than that of another." They gave the

example of the nebular hypothesis of the origin of the solar system, Laplace's treatment being far more advanced and sophisticated than Kant's earlier speculation. In a similar vein, Patinkin (1983) has argued that two scientists should not be credited with the same contribution unless the idea in question is the "central message" of both claimants. Any scientist capable of generating a massive corpus of publications will in all likelihood incorporate a great many parenthetical remarks or tangential speculations. To assign these ideational fragments the same status as a completely elaborated and documented contribution is to trivialize the scientific enterprise. Darwin was not the first scientist to discuss evolution, but he was the first to fully develop the idea of natural selection into a comprehensive and convincing treatise. In a similar vein, Goethe was by no means the first to handle the story of Faust, but his treatment firmly established that theme in one of the enduring monuments of world literature.

Enumerations of multiples often overlook another significant fact, namely, that supposed duplicates often are far from simultaneous. In the Merton (1961b) compilation of 264 multiples, only 20% occurred within a 1-year period, whereas in fully 34% of these cases, a decade or more elapsed before the last duplicate appeared. This magnitude of temporal separation casts a dark shadow over the traditional account as an explanation of scientific creativity. If at a given moment in history the laws of genetics had to be discovered, why were they discovered first by Mendel in 1865 and then rediscovered by DeVries, Correns, and Tchermak in 1900? Mendel could not have been "ahead of his time" if the times define the generative mechanism. Obviously, the traditional interpretation failed to distinguish between scientific creativity taking place within the individual mind (process) and the social acceptance of an idea by the larger scientific community (persuasion). In the words of James (1880, p. 448), "social evolution is a resultant of the interaction of two wholly distinct factors: the individual, deriving his peculiar gifts from the play of physiological and infra-social forces, but bearing all the power of initiative and origination in his hands; and, second, the social environment, with its power of adopting or rejecting both him and his gifts." In some instances, a proffered finding will be "premature" in the sense that "its implications cannot be connected by a series of simple logical steps to canonical, or generally accepted, knowledge" (Stent, 1972, p. 84). In an analogous fashion, in aesthetic endeavors we have instances of the "precursor genius" whose experiments with new forms and techniques are in advance of the times, but whose ideas anticipate those that later become successfully embedded in the artistic mainstream.

A final definitional problem concerns the doctrine of "inevitability." Properly speaking, inevitability implies that at some designated time the probability of a specified event occurring becomes unity, or nearly so. Hence, Kroeber (1917, p. 199) emphatically maintained that genetics "was discovered in 1900 because it could have been discovered only then, and because it infallibly must have been discovered then." Yet closer inspection of how the word is employed in practice reveals that the advocates of zeitgeist confused necessary causes with necessary and sufficient causes: Rather than use the adverb "inevitably," they should have employed the weaker word "eventually." The accumulation of prerequisite knowledge in the cultural repertoire does not *make* a discovery happen, but only *allows* it to happen. Given all the mental elements needed for a given scientific synthesis, and granted sufficient time, chance permutations will eventually generate all possible configurations of those elements, including the desired synthesis – but that is not equivalent to saying that such an outcome is inevitable, except in the loosest sense. Scientific history is replete with discoveries that could just as well have been created much earlier than they were as far as prerequisites are concerned (Simonton, 1987b), as the common occurrence of rediscoveries conclusively proves.

Hence, we must question the traditional view that scientific history unfolds in a foreordained sequence of events. If discoveries and inventions, even when the prerequisite elements are present and the social need is manifest, take place only eventually rather than inevitably, the course of subsequent events for which those contributions are required is vulnerable to capricious chance. Further, the unique character of so-called duplicates signifies that it is not immaterial which particular scientist succeeds first in making a given contribution (Stent, 1972). We must not ignore how much of a scientist's own personality individualizes a contribution. Boltzmann said that "a mathematician will recognize Cauchy, Gauss, Jacobi, or Hemlholtz, after reading a few pages, just as musicians recognize, from the first few bars, Mozart, Beethoven, or Schubert" (Koestler, 1964, p. 265). The set of elements that supply the creative potential for each scientist is idiosyncratic, especially for revolutionary scientists whose backgrounds place them outside the mainstream. The creative process grows "out of the uniqueness of the individual on the one hand, and the materials, events, people, or circumstances of his life on the other" (Rogers, 1954, p. 251). By the same token, it was bound to happen, eventually, given the existence of the requisite forms and instrumental resources, that some composer would create a symphony having the general properties of the Fifth – C-minor, sonata-allegro outer movements, thematic integration, triumphant C-major finale, and so forth – but it was Beethoven's work that provided the specific model admired and imitated by subsequent generations of composers.

Empirical issues. Logical issues aside, the raw facts support the inference that multiples ensue from stochastic processes. Let us simply accept the compilations of multiples on face value, or at the minimum assume that a subset of the candidates for multiple status are indeed legitimate. Then we must observe two essential features about the appearance of multiples.

First of all, tremendous variation exists across scientists in the odds that they will participate in a multiple. Merton (1961b, p. 484), in providing some latitude in his theory for the operation of individual creators, said that "men of great scientific genius will have been repeatedly involved in multiples . . . because the genius will have made many scientific discoveries altogether." If scientists are all subjecting

Table 16.1. *Observed multiple grade and predicted Poisson values for three data sets*

Grade	Ogburn-Thomas		Merton		Simonton	
	Observed	Predicted	Observed	Predicted	Observed	Predicted
0	—	132	—	159	—	1,361
1	—	158	—	223	—	1,088
2	90	95	179	156	449	435
3	36	38	51	73	103	116
4	9	11	17	26	18	23
5	7	3	6	7	7	4
6	2	1	8	2	0	0
7	2	0	1	0	0	0
8	1	0	0	0	1	0
9	1	0	2	0	0	0
μ	1.2		1.4		0.82	

Source: Adapted from Simonton (1987b).

more or less the same collection of mental elements to chance permutations, then those who produce the most total configurations will be more prone to generate the most configurations that are similar to those conceived by colleagues. By comparison, less prolific scientists will be responsible for fewer total configurations, and thus will participate in multiples less often. More eminent scientists are indeed more likely to become involved in multiples, a positive association almost entirely attributable to the higher productivity of the more distinguished contributors (Simonton, 1979). This phenomenon may be seen as nothing more than an extension of the constant-probability-of-success model – the "constant-odds-of-duplication" model.

Second, we must recognize that multiples can be distinguished according to their "grade" (Simonton, 1978). A multiple's grade is simply the number of independent investigators who are reputed to have made a given contribution. Hence, we can talk of multiples of grades 2 (doublets), 3 (triplets), 4 (quadruplets), 5 (quintuplets), 6 (sextuplets), and so on. We can equally speak, albeit loosely, of "multiples" having grades of 1 (singletons) and even 0 (nulltons). Now the frequency distribution of grades for true multiples displays a distinctive pattern: the lower the grade, the higher the frequency. This monotonically decreasing, concave-upward function can be readily discerned in Table 16.1, which exhibits the grade frequencies for the three most extensive tabulations of multiples (Merton, 1961b; Ogburn & Thomas, 1922; Simonton, 1979).

Derek Price (1963, chap. 3) first suggested that the empirical distribution of multiple grades could be interpreted as the consequence of a Poisson process. What renders this suggestion especially provocative is that the Poisson distribution applies best to events that are extremely rare, events so unlikely that an unusual number of trials must be expended before those events have any reasonable opportunity of occurrence. The single parameter of the Poisson distribution, μ, can be conceived in terms of the two parameters of the binomial distribution, namely, the probability that a single trial will successfully generate the event (p) and the number of attempts assigned to achieving that same event (n) (Simonton, 1978). The Poisson distribution then becomes the exponential limit of the binomial distribution as p approaches zero and n approaches infinity, wherein $\mu = np$. This conception of multiples origination dovetails more tightly with a chance-configuration theory than it does with the traditional viewpoint. In the chance permutation of elements, a huge succession of unstable mental aggregates must be sifted through before a stable permutation emerges, and there is no guarantee that the desired chance configuration will appear at all, given how improbable are stable permutations to begin with. Besides the close fit between the present theory and the hypothesized stochastic mechanism, the Poisson distribution yields expected frequencies for multiple grades that match the observed values almost perfectly, as is also apparent in Table 16.1.

Chi-square goodness-of-fit tests reveal that any discrepancies between the observed and expected frequencies can be ascribed to sampling error (Simonton, 1987b). Moreover, the congruence between data and theory persists even when the tests are confined to only the most secure cases of multiples (Simonton, 1979) or when the samples of multiples are broken down by discipline (Simonton, 1978, 1979). The estimated values of μ have an apparent central tendency of around unity, which suggests binomial parameters falling somewhere between $p = .1, n = 10$ and $p = .01, n = 100$ (Simonton, 1978, 1979). Given this value, only about one-third of all potential contributions end up becoming multiples, whereas another third become only singletons, and yet another third nulltons. Thus, the existence of multiples cannot contradict the statement that a respectable proportion of potential discoveries and inventions fail to get made at all! In addition, this implication would still hold even if the inventory of multiples were considerably expanded. Indeed, the model actually predicts that the absolute number of multiples is tremendously underestimated in all the published lists (Simonton, 1978).

Needless to say, the Poisson model is a blatant first approximation to a complete treatment of the multiples phenomenon. In a series of mathematical elaborations, Monte Carlo simulations, and Gedanken experiments, I have shown how allowance can be made for communication among scientists (i.e., personal influence), necessary but not sufficient a priori causal ordering of a subset of discoveries and inventions, and other more realistic features of scientific creativity – all without compromising the fundamental stochastic basis for the multiples (Simonton, 1986c, 1986d, 1986f, 1987b, in press, chap. 6). The case is strong, therefore, that the empirical data seem inconsistent with the traditional interpretation of multiples, and instead endorse the theory developed here. Thus, scientific and artistic creativity likely emerge from the same fundamental chance-permutation process.

Implications

The foregoing empirical elaboration should firmly establish the case for the two propositions announced at the outset of this chapter. Creativity cannot be properly understood in isolation from the social context, for creativity is a special form of personal influence: The effective creator profoundly alters the thinking habits of other human beings by making a contribution to their quest for enhanced self-organization. Moreover, chance intervenes at several distinct points throughout the conversion of creative potential into demonstrated creative leadership, including the role of chance permutations in the introduction of innovative ideas, the probabilistic nexus between quantity and quality of output, and the stochastic basis for the generation of multiple discoveries and inventions. I maintain, in fact, that the chance-configuration theory explicates a great many critical features of all four key facets of creativity, whether we are looking at process, product, person, or persuasion. For example, we have witnessed how the theory is compatible with the introspective reports about the act of creation, the constellation of personality traits associated with creative persons, and the developmental antecedents of creative achievement. Furthermore, this explanatory power is frequently accompanied by unusual predictive precision. From the chief tenets of the theory, for instance, we can directly predict the highly skewed cross-sectional distribution of creative productivity, the longitudinal fluctuations in output over the course of a career (including interdisciplinary contrasts), and the observed probability distribution of multiple grades.

Beyond these explanatory and predictive assets, I believe the chance-configuration theory has practical applications as well. To begin with, the theory suggests the most suitable approach to measuring creativity. On the negative side, the theory does not hold much hope for highly generalized "creativity" tests. The capacity to generate chance permutations is domain-specific, although we would expect some overflow across kindred domains (cf. Amabile, 1983). The associative richness requisite for arriving at worthwhile configurations concerns the mental elements characteristic of a particular artistic or scientific endeavor. Hence, it is understandable that psychometric measures of creativity can claim only rather modest validity coefficients. Moreover, because creativity is conceived as a form of leadership, we cannot speak of this phenomenon in the absence of the social context. At best, we can devise domain-specific indicators of creative potential. On the positive side, the theory provides a number of clues to how to identify those individuals who have the greatest creative potential. Biographical inventories can be derived from the known developmental antecedents (Schaefer & Anastasi, 1968). And certain character traits should generalize across creative endeavors, permitting the use of personality indices. Especially important is an individual's cognitive and motivational capacity to generate a cornucopia of ideas in the domain of interest. The prospective creative genius is revealed by an extraordinary fascination in a chosen enterprise and by a fruitful imagination that seems unceasing (Albert, 1975). This orientation will ultimately manifest itself in an impressive list of offered creative products. Accordingly, the best gauge of creative potential is perhaps productive fertility, indicated by high rates of output, precocity, and, for decreased creators, longevity (Hocevar, 1981).

A more significant practical implication of the chance-configuration theory is that it outlines the general conditions that favor creativity. As Campbell (1960, p. 397) summarized them, "a creative solution is more likely the longer a problem is worked upon, the more variable the thought trials, the more people working on the problem independently, the more heterogeneous these people, the less the time pressure, etc." Any developmental, personological, or sociocultural variable that impinges on one or more of the favorable conditions will affect the prospects for creative contributions to a given discipline. In the section on developmental antecedents we inventoried some of these advantageous conditions, such as family background, role-model availability, formal education, and marginality. However, the theory may contribute to the fostering of creativity in a far more direct fashion as well – by demystifying the creative genius. Campbell (1974, p. 155) noted that "too many potential creators are inhibited by a belief that gifted others solve problems directly." What distinguishes the genius is merely the cognitive and motivational capacity to spew forth a profusion of chance permutations pertaining to a particular problem. "Genius," Edison professed, "is one percent inspiration and ninety-nine percent perspiration." Even "Newton, when questioned about his methods of work, could give no other answer but that we was wont to ponder again and again on a subject" (Mach, 1896, p. 174). Notable creators do not have any direct access to truth or beauty, but attain success and influence only by betraying a willingness to accept failure – by taking intellectual or aesthetic risks. This is the primary lesson of the constant-probability-of-success model. To be sure, from the Lotka and Price laws we know that there are immense numbers of mediocre creators in the world; so by chance alone a significant number will experience a stroke of luck. As Campbell (1960, p. 393) again observed, it is "likely that many important contributions will come from the relatively untalented, undiligent, and uneducated, even though on an average contribution per capita basis, they will contribute much less." Nevertheless, it remains best to exploit the odds by being prolific. Chance mediates the conversion of potential to actual creative influence; so those who buy the most lottery tickets have a higher likelihood of winning.

References

Albert, R. S. (1975). Toward a behavioral definition of genius. *American Psychologist, 30*, 140–151.
Amabile, T. M. (1982). Social psychology of creativity: A consensual assessment technique. *Journal of Personality and Social Psychology, 43*, 997–1013.
Amabile, T. M. (1983). *The social psychology of creativity*. New York: Springer-Verlag.
Barron, F. (1963). The needs for order and for disorder as motives in creative activity. In C. W. Taylor & F. Barron (Eds.), *Scientific creativity* (pp. 153–161). New York: Wiley.
Barron, F., & Harrington, D. M. (1981). Creativity, intelligence, and personality. *Annual Review of Psychology, 32*, 439–476.

Bartlett, F. C. (1958). *Thinking*. New York: Basic Books.

Bass, B. M. (1981). *Stogdill's handbook of leadership*. New York: Free Press.

Bennett, W. (1980). Providing for posterity. *Harvard Magazine, 82*(3), 13–16.

Beveridge, W. I. B. (1957). *The art of scientific investigation* (3rd ed.). New York: Vintage.

Campbell, D. T. (1960). Blind variation and selective retention in creative thought as in other knowledge processes. *Psychological Review, 67,* 380–400.

Campbell, D. T. (1974). Unjustified variation and selective retention in scientific discovery. In F. J. Ayala & T. Dobzhansky (Eds.), *Studies in the philosophy of biology* (pp. 139–161). London: Macmillan.

Cannon, W. B. (1940). The role of chance in discovery. *Scientific Monthly, 50,* 204–209.

Cattell, R. B. (1963). The personality and motivation of the researcher from measurements of contemporaries and from biography. In C. W. Taylor & F. Barron (Eds.), *Scientific creativity* (pp. 119–131). New York: Wiley.

Cole, J. R., & Cole, S. (1973). *Social stratification in science*. University of Chicago Press.

Cox, C. (1926). *The early mental traits of three hundred geniuses*. Stanford, CA: Stanford University Press.

Cropley, A. J. (1967). *Creativity*. London: Longmans, Green.

Darwin, C. (1952). *The origin of species* (2nd ed.). In M. J. Mortimer (Ed.), *Great books of the western world* (Vol. 49). Chicago: Encyclopaedia Britannica. (Original work published 1860.)

Darwin, F. (Ed.). (1958). *The autobiography of Charles Darwin and selected letters*. New York: Dover. (Original work published 1892.)

Dennis, W. (1954). Bibliographies of eminent scientists. *Scientific Monthly, 79,* 180–183.

Dennis, W. (1955). Variations in productivity among creative workers. *Scientific Monthly, 80,* 277–278.

Dentler, R. A., & Mackler, B. (1964). Originality: Some social and personal determinants. *Behavioral Science, 9,* 1–7.

Farnsworth, P. R. (1969). *The social psychology of music* (2nd ed.). Ames: Iowa State University Press.

Ghiselin, B. (Ed.). (1952). *The creative process*. Berkeley: University of California Press.

Goertzel, M. G., Goertzel, V., & Goertzel, T. G. (1978). *Three hundred eminent personalities*. San Francisco: Jossey-Bass.

Guilford, J. P. (1963). Intellectual resources and their values as seen by scientists. In C. W. Taylor & F. Barron (Eds.), *Scientific creativity* (pp. 101–118). New York: Wiley.

Hadamard, J. (1945). *An essay on the psychology of invention in the mathematical field*. Princeton, NJ: Princeton University Press.

Hargens, L. L., McCann, J. C., & Raskin, B. F. (1978). Productivity and reproductivity: Fertility and professional achievement among research scientists. *Social Forces, 57,* 154–163.

Helmreich, R. L., Spence, J. T., Beane, W. E., Lucker, G. W., & Matthews, K. A. (1980). Making it in academic psychology: Demographic and personality correlates of attainment. *Journal of Personality and Social Psychology, 39,* 896–908.

Hocevar, D. (1981). Measurement of creativity: Review and critique. *Journal of Personality Assessment, 45,* 450–464.

Hoffman, B. (1972). *Albert Einstein*. New York: Plume.

Hughes, E. C. (1958). *Men and their work*. Glencoe, IL: Free Press.

James, W. (1880). Great men, great thoughts, and the environment. *Atlantic Monthly, 46,* 441–459.

Jevons, W. S. (1900). *The principles of science* (2nd ed.). London: Macmillan.

Koestler, A. (1964). *The act of creation*. New York: Macmillan.

Kroeber, A. (1917). The superorganic. *American Anthropologist, 19,* 163–214.

Kuhn, T. S. (1963). The essential tension: Tradition and innovation in scientific research. In C. W. Taylor & F. Barron (Eds.), *Scientific creativity* (pp. 341–354). New York: Wiley.

Kuhn, T. S. (1970). *The structure of scientific revolutions* (2nd ed.). University of Chicago Press.

Lehman, H. C. (1953). *Age and achievement*. Princeton, NJ: Princeton University Press.

Lotka, A. J. (1926). The frequency distribution of scientific productivity. *Journal of the Washington Academy of Sciences, 16,* 317–323.

McClelland, D. C. (1963). The calculated risk: An aspect of scientific performance. In C. W. Taylor & F. Barron (Eds.), *Scientific creativity* (pp. 184–192). New York: Wiley.

Mach, E. (1896). On the part played by accident in invention and discovery. *Monist, 6,* 161–175.

Manis, J. G. (1951). Some academic influences upon publication productivity. *Social Forces, 29,* 267–272.

Martindale, C. (1975). *Romantic progression.* Washington, DC: Hemisphere Publishing.

Mednick, S. A. (1962). The associative basis of the creative process. *Psychological Review, 69,* 220–232.

Merton, R. K. (1961a). The role of genius in scientific advance. *New Scientist, 12,* 306–308.

Merton, R. K. (1961b). Singletons and multiples in scientific discovery: A chapter in the sociology of science. *Proceedings of the American Philosophical Society, 105,* 470–486.

Moles, A. (1968). *Information theory and esthetic perception* (Trans. J. E. Cohen). Urbana: University of Illinois Press.

Ogburn, W. K., & Thomas, D. (1922). Are inventions inevitable? A note on social evolution. *Political Science Quarterly, 37,* 83–93.

Over, R. (1982). The durability of scientific reputation. *Journal of the History of the Behavioral Sciences, 18,* 53–61.

Patinkin, D. (1983). Multiple discoveries and the central message. *American Journal of Sociology, 89,* 306–323.

Planck, M. (1949). *Scientific autobiography and other papers* (Trans. F. Gaynor). New York: Philosophical Library.

Poincaré, H. (1921). *The foundations of science.* New York: Science Press.

Price, D. (1963). *Little science, big science.* New York: Columbia University Press.

Roe, A. (1952a). A psychologist examines 64 eminent scientists. *Scientific American, 187*(5), 21–25.

Roe, A. (1952b). *The making of a scientist.* New York: Dodd, Mead.

Roe, A. (1972). Maintenance of creative output through the years. In C. W. Taylor (Ed.), *Climate for creativity* (pp. 167–191). New York: Pergamon.

Rogers, C. R. (1954). Toward a theory of creativity. *ETC: A Review of General Semantics, 11,* 249–260.

Rosengren, K. E. (1985). Time and literary fame. *Poetics, 14,* 157–172.

Schaefer, C. E., & Anastasi, A. (1968). A biographical inventory for identifying creativity in adolescent boys. *Journal of Applied Psychology, 58,* 42–48.

Schlipp, P. A. (Ed.). (1951). *Albert Einstein.* New York: Harper.

Schmookler, J. (1966). *Invention and economic growth.* Cambridge, MA: Harvard University Press.

Segal, S. M., Busse, T. V., & Mansfield, R. S. (1980). The relationship of scientific creativity in the biological sciences to predoctoral accomplishments and experiences. *American Educational Research Journal, 17,* 491–502.

Sheldon, J. C. (1980). A cybernetic theory of physical science professions: The causes of periodic normal and revolutionary science between 1000 and 1870 AD. *Scientometrics, 2,* 147–167.

Simonton, D. K. (1975a). Age and literary creativity: A cross-cultural and transhistorical survey. *Journal of Cross-Cultural Psychology, 6,* 259–277.

Simonton, D. K. (1975b). Sociocultural context of individual creativity: A transhistorical time-series analysis. *Journal of Personality and Social Psychology, 32,* 1119–1133.

Simonton, D. K. (1976a). Biographical determinants of achieved eminence: A multivariate approach to the Cox data. *Journal of Personality and Social Psychology, 33,* 218–226.

Simonton, D. K. (1976b). Interdisciplinary and military determinants of scientific productivity: A cross-lagged correlation analysis. *Journal of Vocational Behavior, 9,* 53–62.

Simonton, D. K. (1976c). Philosophical eminence, beliefs, and zeitgeist: An individual-generational analysis. *Journal of Personality and Social Psychology, 34,* 630–640.

Simonton, D. K. (1976d). The sociopolitical context of philosophical beliefs: A transhistorical and causal analysis. *Social Forces, 54,* 513–523.

Simonton, D. K. (1977a). Creative productivity, age, and stress: A biographical time-series analysis of 10 classical composers. *Journal of Personality and Social Psychology, 35,* 791–804.

Simonton, D. K. (1977b). Eminence, creativity, and geographic marginality: A recursive structural equation model. *Journal of Personality and Social Psychology, 35,* 805–816.

Simonton, D. K. (1978). Independent discovery in science and technology: A closer look at the Poisson distribution. *Social Studies of Science, 8,* 521–532.

Simonton, D. K. (1979). Multiple discovery and invention: Zeitgeist, genius, or chance? *Journal of Personality and Social Psychology, 37,* 1603–1616.

Simonton, D. K. (1980a). Intuition and analysis: A predictive and explanatory model. *Genetic Psychology Monographs, 102,* 3–60.

Simonton, D. K. (1980b). Land battles, generals, and armies: Individual and situational determinants of victory and casualties. *Journal of Personality and Social Psychology, 38,* 110–119.

Simonton, D. K. (1980c). Techno-scientific activity and war: A yearly time-series analysis, 1500–1903 A.D. *Scientometrics, 2,* 251–255.

Simonton, D. K. (1980d). Thematic fame and melodic originality: A multivariate computer-content analysis. *Journal of Personality, 48,* 206–219.

Simonton, D. K. (1980e). Thematic fame, melodic originality, and musical zeitgeist: A biographical and transhistorical content analysis. *Journal of Personality and Social Psychology, 39,* 972–983.

Simonton, D. K. (1983a). Dramatic greatness and content: A quantitative study of 81 Athenian and Shakespearean plays. *Empirical Studies of the Arts, 1,* 109–123.

Simonton, D. K. (1983b). Formal education, eminence, and dogmatism: The curvilinear relationship. *Journal of Creative Behavior, 17,* 149–162.

Simonton, D. K. (1983c). Intergenerational transfer of individual differences in hereditary monarchs: Genes, role-modeling, cohort, or sociocultural effects? *Journal of Personality and Social Psychology, 44,* 354–364.

Simonton, D. K. (1984a). Artistic creativity and interpersonal relationships across and within generations. *Journal of Personality and Social Psychology, 46,* 1273–1286.

Simonton, D. K. (1984b). Creative productivity and age: A mathematical model based on a two-step cognitive process. *Developmental Review, 4,* 77–111.

Simonton, D. K. (1984c). *Genius, creativity, and leadership.* Cambridge, MA: Harvard University Press.

Simonton, D. K. (1984d). Is the marginality effect all that marginal? *Social Studies of Science, 14,* 621–622.

Simonton, D. K. (1984e). Leaders as eponyms: Individual and situational determinants of monarchal eminence. *Journal of Personality, 52,* 1–21.

Simonton, D. K. (1984f). Melodic structure and note transition probabilities: A content analysis of 15,618 classical themes. *Psychology of Music, 12,* 3–16.

Simonton, D. K. (1984g). Scientific eminence historical and contemporary: A measurement assessment. *Scientometrics, 6,* 169–182.

Simonton, D. K. (1985a). Intelligence and personal influence in groups: Four nonlinear models. *Psychological Review, 92,* 532–547.

Simonton, D. K. (1985b). Quality, quantity, and age: The careers of 10 distinguished psychologists. *International Journal of Aging and Human Development, 21,* 241–254.

Simonton, D. K. (1986a). Aesthetic success in classical music: A computer content analysis of 1935 compositions. *Empirical Studies of the Arts, 4,* 1–17.

Simonton, D. K. (1986b). Biographical typicality, eminence, and achievement style. *Journal of Creative Behavior, 20,* 14–22.

Simonton, D. K. (1986c). Multiple discovery: Some Monte Carlo simulations and Gedanken experiments. *Scientometrics, 9,* 269–280.

Simonton, D. K. (1986d). Multiples, Poisson distributions, and chance: An analysis of the Brannigan-Wanner model. *Scientometrics, 9,* 127–137.

Simonton, D. K. (1986e). Presidential personality: Biographical use of the Gough Adjective Check List. *Journal of Personality and Social Psychology, 51,* 1–12.

Simonton, D. K. (1986f). Stochastic models of multiple discovery. *Czechoslovak Journal of Physics B, 36,* 138–141.

Simonton, D. K. (1987a). Developmental antecedents of achieved eminence. *Annals of Child Development, 5,* 131–169.

Simonton, D. K. (1987b). Multiples, chance, genius, and zeitgeist. In D. N. Jackson & J. P. Rushton (Eds.), *Scientific excellence* (pp. 98–128). Beverly Hills, CA: Sage Publications.

Simonton, D. K. (1987c). *Why presidents succeed.* New Haven, CT: Yale University Press.

Simonton, D. K. (in press). *Scientific genius.* Cambridge University Press.

Stein, M. I. (1969). Creativity. In E. F. Borgatta & W. W. Lambert (Eds.), *Handbook of personality theory and research* (pp. 900–942). Chicago: Rand McNally.

Stent, G. S. (1972, December). Prematurity and uniqueness in scientific discovery. *Scientific American, 227,* 84–93.

Sternberg, R. J. (1977). Component processes in analogical reasoning. *Psychological Review, 84,* 353–378.

Sternberg, R. J. (1985). Implicit theories of intelligence, creativity, and wisdom. *Journal of Personality and Social Psychology, 49,* 607–677.

Terman, L. M. (1955). Are scientists different? *Scientific American, 192*(1), 25–29.

White, R. K. (1931). The versatility of genius. *Journal of Social Psychology, 2,* 460–489.

Zajonc, R. B. (1965). Social facilitation. *Science, 149,* 269–274.

Zajonc, R. B. (1976). Family configuration and intelligence. *Science, 192,* 227–235.

Part IV

Integration and conclusions

17   What do we know about creativity?

Twila Z. Tardif and Robert J. Sternberg

Integration and conclusions: creating a field of creativity

The preceding chapters discussed creativity in many different ways. Different levels of analysis were used to address the concepts; within levels, different components were put forth; and even when similar components were discussed, differences were seen in how these components were defined and how crucial they were claimed to be for the larger concept of creativity. Given these differences, which are as varied as creative expression itself, one might ask if there is any consensus whatsoever, if we know anything at all about creativity, or if it is even a useful concept for scientific theory and research. Our response, parallel to those of the preceding authors, is that despite the differences, there exist major areas of agreement, and although many refinements are necessary, creativity is an essential concept for psychology and holds enormous potential for scientific investigation.

What we shall attempt to provide in this closing chapter, therefore, is a consensual summary of these many varied explanations of creativity, listing the major agreements and highlighting some of the more controversial issues. The organization of this summary will follow Stein's general approach (1969, as cited by Simonton) to dissecting the problem of creativity. That is, views of creative processes, persons, products, and places (problem domains and socially organized fields of enterprise) will be discussed separately, as these really are separate levels of analysis, and it is from comparisons within levels that coherent statements about our knowledge of creativity can be made.

Creative processes

In general, psychologists have viewed creativity as a process existing in a single person at a particular point in time. Some of the authors in this volume, however, present a new alternative to this view. Csikszentmihalyi, Gardner, Gruber and Davis, and Hennessey and Amabile represent the new view and discuss creativity as existing in the larger system of social networks, problem domains, and fields of enterprise, such that the individual who produces products that are judged to be creative is only one of many necessary parts. This systems view of creative pro-

429

cesses does not preclude the individual view, however. Rather, it provides additional insights regarding creative persons and products and their function in society as a whole. Our initial focus, therefore, will be to outline some understandings of the process within the individual before going on to the systems approach.

By far the greatest amount of agreement is with the statement that creativity takes time. In fact, some authors (Csikszentmihalyi; Gruber & Davis; Johnson-Laird) believe that the very nature of creativity depends on the time constraints involved and the opportunity to revise, or nurture, the outcomes once produced. Although not all theorists emphasize time to the same extent, the creative process is not generally considered to be something that occurs in an instant with a single flash of insight, even though insights may occur.

Instead of focusing on instantaneous insights, then, Barron and Torrance compare the process of creativity to procreation and emphasize the long gestation period that is required after the initial conception of an idea. Another process to which creativity has been compared (which also emphasizes time) is the more general and even lengthier process of evolution, in which the surviving products are determined through natural selection from a multitude of random variations; see Perkins and Simonton, in particular.

The view that creative processes take time, however, does not mean that insight is no longer thought to be an important aspect of creativity. Rather, insights are acknowledged by most of the authors in this volume. What is of issue in this hotly debated area is how "insight" is defined and the specific role that it plays in creative processes. The range of viewpoints presented in this volume, as might be expected, spans the entire spectrum from those who imply that creativity is little more than building on an initial insight (Feldman; Taylor) to those who deny that moments of insight have any importance whatsoever for creative processes (Gruber & Davis; Simonton; Weisberg). The majority view, however, falls in between, with flashes of insight discussed as small but necessary components of creativity (Gardner; Langley & Jones; Sternberg; Torrance).

Returning to the comparison between creativity and procreation or evolution, one might be inclined to ask, Where does it all begin? In other words, what is the big bang, the fusion, or impetus for the process of creation that psychologists refer to? There are disagreements on this point, particularly regarding the role of chance and random deviations from traditional norms versus mindful planning to produce something creative. Barron, Csikszentmihalyi, Gardner, Gruber and Davis, Perkins, Sternberg, and Walberg all suggest that creative processes involve an active search for gaps in existing knowledge, problem finding, or consciously attempting to break through the existing boundaries and limitations in one's field. On the other hand, Feldman, Johnson-Laird, Langley and Jones, Simonton, and Taylor suggest that creative products are outcomes of random variations at either the generative or selection stage in creative processes. A further alternative, intermediate between chance-dependent and completely intentional processes, is an approach that is also taken by several of the authors in this volume. Specifically, creative processes may be seen as initiating from a previous failure to find explanations for phenomena or to incorporate new ideas into existing knowledge (Barron; Feldman; Gardner; Schank; Simonton; Torrance; Weisberg), or from a general drive toward self-organization through the reduction of chaos (Barron; Feldman; Gruber & Davis; Simonton; Taylor; Torrance).

In addition to asking about origins, one might also ask about differences between the products of creative processes. Does the particular product or the domain in which creativity occurs affect the process itself, just as different children or different species may develop at different rates and perhaps go through unique series of stages? Although several authors (Csikszentmihalyi; Gardner; Johnson-Laird; Langley & Jones) claim that creativity is domain-specific, there are some claims for universals in creativity, as there are for development and evolution. Thus, several general characteristics of creative thinking, regardless of domain, have been proposed.

For example, creative thought processes, regardless of the problem on which they are focused, are claimed to involve the following: transformations of the external world and internal representations by forming analogies and bridging conceptual gaps (Barron; Feldman; Gardner; Gruber & Davis; Johnson-Laird; Langley & Jones; Schank; Simonton; Sternberg; Taylor; Torrance; Weisberg); constant re-definitions of problems (Sternberg; Torrance; Weisberg); applying recurring themes and recognizing patterns and images of wide scope to make the new familiar and the old new (Barron; Feldman; Gardner; Gruber & Davis; Langley & Jones; Sternberg; Taylor; Torrance); and nonverbal modes of thinking (Gruber & Davis; Sternberg).

Further, in six of the chapters, the authors (Barron; Feldman; Gardner; Gruber & Davis; Simonton; Torrance) also agree that irrespective of particular content, the processes involved in creation require tension. Even though the authors agree on the role of tension in creativity, however, there are at least three different ways in which tension can be observed in creative processes. First, one may be faced with conflict between staying with tradition and breaking new ground at each step in the process. Second, tension may lie in the ideas themselves, such that different paths to a solution or different products are suggested. Finally, it may exist in the constant battle between unorganized chaos and the drive to higher levels of organization and efficiency within the individual, or the society at large. It is likely that all three conceptions of tension are involved at some stage in the creative process, but whether or not different domains elicit more of one type than another is yet an empirical question.

In addition to time requirements, some element akin to insight, and the generality of processes across domains, a further issue on which several authors agree is that different levels of creative expression may occur. Although not all authors have addressed the levels issue explicitly, the general belief is that the processes responsible for varying levels of creativity may differ, if not in kind, at least in degree; see Feldman for a more detailed discussion. Thus, both within a domain and within the same individual at different points in time, there may be differences with respect to the amount of creative processing in which individuals engage. Einstein, in this view, may have attained a high level of creativity, or often have engaged creative thought processes, whereas a less influential scientist in his time may not have achieved such a high level, or simply did not apply creative processes to the same extent that Einstein did. Different levels of creativity may exist, therefore, in an analogous fashion to the idea that species differ in their complexity along the phylogenetic scale. However, this issue of levels brings up yet another area of controversy: the availability and accessibility of creative processes, both between and within individuals.

First, let us address the availability question, as it pertains to different individuals. Creativity, according to some authors, occurs only in special individuals (the Edisons, Einsteins, Freuds, Mozarts, and Picassos of the world) at rare moments in time. Other authors believe creativity to be a much more normative process, available to every thinking instrument – adult expert, growing child, or programmed computer. Thus, creative processes can be trained and improved, as far as Langley and Jones, Schank, Taylor, and Torrance are concerned, because their concept of creativity is in line with this latter, "available-to-everyone" view. Training is not possible, however, according to the theories of authors such as Barron, Csikszentmihalyi, Gruber and Davis, and Hennessey and Amabile, who maintain that creativity is achieved only when the "right" combination of particular problems, skills, individual, and social milieu comes together.

Related to the issue of the availability of creative processes between individuals is the matter of the absoluteness and uniqueness of creative processes that may be ascribed to each individual. Many of the authors in this volume (Csikszentmihalyi; Gruber & Davis; Johnson-Laird; Schank; Simonton; Torrance; Weisberg) agree that the processes that result in creative products are absolute. In other words, multiple creations of the same product, such as simultaneous invention of the calculus by Newton and Leibniz, as discussed by Simonton, for example, cannot occur. Rather, creativity is said to be relative to the particular person who produces the product, and each production is therefore considered to be absolute. Thus, some products may be the results of processes that are uncreative for some individuals, yet creative for others, and the process of creation itself is unique to an individual and is an emergent property of one's interaction with the problem domain, past history, and the societal state as a whole.

The alternative, discussed to some extent by Perkins, is that multiples do occur: The reason true multiples occur is because the creation was, in some form, predictable and inevitable; all that was required was the necessary combination of ideas within a particular individual. There is nothing special about the individual or the individual's unique context in this view. Thus, when more than one person produces essentially the same product, all are deemed equally responsible (or not responsible, to be more accurate) for the creation, even though credit for the discovery typically is reserved for the first or best-publicized individual.

Finally, there is controversy over the accessibility of creative processes within individuals. Disagreement on the accessibility issue ensues when the role of the unconscious and semiconscious elements in creative processing are brought up. As with insight, the expression of the unconscious is sometimes conceived of as the key to creativity (Feldman; Torrance). Thus, creativity, according to these authors, is accessible only by bringing unconscious elements into conscious awareness. In other views, however, the role of the unconscious and the question of accessibility are ignored completely. Once again, the consensus lies in between, with unconscious elements existing and being important for creativity, but not the essence of creative thought processes. Langley and Jones, for instance, provide a particularly interesting discussion of the unconscious in the memory-activation processes. In the Langley and Jones proposal, the memories relevant to a creative insight are not accessible until just the right cue activates them. Thus, they propose that such unconscious processes are involved in, but are not central or unique to, creativity.

The issues addressed when one considers creative processes, therefore, include the following: the time required for such processes; the role of insight and the sparks that set off creative thinking; how closely processes are tied to their products; general characteristics of creative thought across different domains; levels of creative processing; the need for the products of such processes to be unique in order for them to be labeled as "creative"; and how accessible and controllable the processes are in conscious awareness. Although there exists much agreement on the need to address these issues, the authors in this volume, and, indeed, creativity researchers in general, have yet to reach a consensus on the particular positions adopted for each issue. That such a consensus appears to be attainable with respect to the processes involved in creativity, however, is an exciting possibility, but one that will require much empirical research in the interim.

Creative persons

Descriptions of the creative person typically fall into three general categories: cognitive characteristics; personality and motivational qualities; special events or experiences during one's development. We shall discuss each category in turn.

It is generally acknowledged that people are creative within particular domains of endeavor, even though people who are creative in different domains may share common traits. Thus, one may be a creative biologist, but a very uncreative novelist, or vice versa. This is a curious statement, given that when the issue of domain specificity occurs in discussions of creative processes, much less agreement ensues. Nonetheless, domain specificity is a major consideration when describing creative persons (Csikszentmihalyi; Gardner; Johnson-Laird; Langley & Jones; Perkins; Simonton; Sternberg; Walberg; Weisberg), and it goes along with other characteristics such as using one's existing knowledge in the domain as a base to create new ideas (Csikszentmihalyi; Feldman; Gruber & Davis; Johnson-Laird; Langley & Jones; Perkins; Schank; Sternberg; Torrance; Walberg; Weisberg), being alert to novelty, and finding gaps in domain knowledge (Barron; Perkins; Schank; Simonton; Sternberg; Torrance; Walberg; Weisberg). Although it is generally agreed that creative individuals are creative within limited domains, various explanations have

Table 17.1. *Cognitive characteristics of creative persons, by author*

Characteristics	Barron	Csikszentmihalyi	Feldman	Gardner	Gruber & Davis	Hennessey & Amabile	Johnson-Laird	Langley & Jones	Perkins	Schank	Simonton	Sternberg	Taylor	Torrance	Walberg	Weisberg
Originality	•										•			•	•	
Articulate and verbally fluent	•										•			•	•	
High intelligence	•										•				•	
Good imagination	•											•		•		
Creative in a particular domain		•		•			•	•	•		•	•			•	•
Thinks metaphorically	•		•		•							•		•		
Uses wide categories and images					•						•			•		
Flexible and skilled decision maker		•						•			•	•	•	•		
Makes independent judgments	•										•			•	•	
Copes well with novelty											•	•				
Thinks logically	•							•								
Escapes perceptual set and entrenchment	•										•	•				
Builds new structures	•										•				•	
Finds order in chaos	•				•						•					
Asks "Why?"									•		•					
Questions norms and assumptions	•								•		•					
Alert to novelty and gaps in knowledge	•						•	•	•		•			•	•	•
Uses existing knowledge as base for new ideas		•	•		•		•	•	•	•		•		•	•	•
Prefers nonverbal communication												•		•		
Creates internal visualizations					•									•		

been offered for why individuals differ in their propensities toward and abilities in their domains of specialty. Csikszentmihalyi, Gardner, Perkins, and Walberg, for instance, attribute such specificities to inborn sensitivities to particular types of information or modes of operation. Gardner and Gruber and Davis, however, discuss unique combinations of "intelligences," whereas Walberg emphasizes highly practiced skills as a factor.

A list of cognitive characteristics that are shared by creative people, regardless of domain, can be grouped into three sets: traits, abilities, and processing styles that creative individuals use and possess. The most commonly mentioned of these characteristics, along with the authors who discussed them, are listed in Table 17.1. Let us also consider them briefly according to the category in which they fall.

First, there are the four *traits* that are commonly said to be associated with creative individuals: relatively high intelligence, originality, articulateness and verbal fluency, and a good imagination. The next set of characteristics that have been used by creative persons includes the following cognitive *abilities*: the ability to think metaphorically, flexibility and skill in making decisions, independence of judgment, coping well with novelty, logical thinking skills, internal visualization, the ability to escape perceptual sets and entrenchment in particular ways of thinking, and finding order in chaos. Finally, creative people may also be characterized by the way in which they approach problems (i.e., style); some of the most commonly mentioned processing *styles* presented by the authors in this volume include using wide categories and images of wide scope, a preference for nonverbal communication, building new structures rather than using existing structures, questioning norms and assumptions in their domain (asking "Why?"), being alert to novelty and gaps in knowledge, and using their existing knowledge as a base for new ideas.

The one characteristic that seems to prevail among creative people, however, is what seems almost to be an aesthetic ability that allows such individuals to recognize "good" problems in their field and apply themselves to these problems while ignoring others (Perkins; Sternberg; Walberg). What accounts for this sense of aesthetic taste and judgment? Perhaps it is some combination of the foregoing characteristics, perhaps it is better explained by the personality or motivational characteristics to be presented next, or maybe it is a separate factor altogether. Whatever the particular explanation, this aesthetic sense is clearly a pervasive feature of creative persons and one that is worthy of greater study, not just in the arts, in which we think of aesthetics as being of primary importance, but in a variety of domains, including scientific areas, in which we do not usually think of aesthetics as playing an important role, at least when investigated superficially. Such considerations do seem to be important, however, when the work of individual scientists is examined in depth (e.g., elegance in mathematical proofs, as discussed by Perkins).

As with the cognitive characteristics, there is no one personality or motivational characteristic that is useful for attaching the label "creative" to a particular person. Rather, creative personalities are composed of a constellation of many characteristics, some of which may be present in one creative individual, but not in another, and thus mentioned by some authors, but not others. The most commonly mentioned characteristics include a willingness to confront hostility and take intellectual risks (Barron; Gardner; Hennessey & Amabile; Simonton; Torrance; Walberg), perseverance (Gardner; Gruber & Davis; Simonton; Sternberg; Torrance; Walberg), a proclivity to curiosity and inquisitiveness (Hennessey & Amabile; Perkins; Simonton; Sternberg; Walberg), being open to new experiences and growth (Barron; Simonton; Sternberg; Taylor; Torrance), a driving absorption (Barron; Hennessey & Amabile; Simonton; Torrance; Walberg), discipline and commitment to one's work (Gardner; Hennessey & Amabile; Simonton; Sternberg; Torrance; Walberg; Weisberg), high intrinsic motivation (Gruber & Davis; Hennessey & Amabile; Perkins; Sternberg; Walberg), being task-focused (Gruber & Davis; Hennessey & Amabile; Simonton; Weisberg), a certain freedom of spirit that rejects limits imposed by others (Johnson-Laird; Perkins; Sternberg; Taylor; Torrance), a high degree of self-organization such that these individuals set their own rules rather than follow those set by others (Feldman; Gruber & Davis; Simonton; Sternberg; Taylor), and a need for competence in meeting optimal challenges (Gruber & Davis; Hennessey & Amabile; Sternberg; Torrance); though often withdrawn, reflective, and internally preoccupied (Simonton; Sternberg; Torrance; Walberg), creative individuals are also said to have impact on the people who surround them (Feldman; Gardner; Simonton; Torrance).

Additional characteristics that were mentioned less often, yet are still considered to be important features of creative personalities, were tolerance for ambiguity (Perkins; Sternberg; Taylor), a broad range of interests (Simonton; Walberg), a tendency to play with ideas (Hennessey & Amabile; Simonton; Sternberg), valuing originality and creativity (Perkins; Walberg), unconventionality in behavior (Barron; Sternberg; Walberg), experiencing deep emotions (Barron; Walberg), intuitiveness (Barron; Sternberg), seeking interesting situations (Hennessey & Amabile; Sternberg), opportunism (Barron; Taylor; Walberg), and some degree of conflict between self-criticism and self-confidence (Barron; Feldman; Gardner).

In addition to the conflict between criticism and confidence, there appears to be a conflict or paradox between socially withdrawn and socially integrated tendencies; at least this appears to be the case when we consider the comments from those authors who discussed how creativity and creative individuals function in social environments. For instance, it was mentioned previously that creative people have impact on others in their immediate surroundings. However, Feldman and Gardner both suggest that what distinguishes creative individuals is their *lack* of fit to their environment. Similarly, others have discussed creative people's need to maintain distance from their peers, an avoidance of interpersonal contact, and resistance to societal demands (Hennessey & Amabile; Simonton; Sternberg). Back on the other side, it has also been proposed that creative individuals have a drive for accomplishment and recognition (Sternberg; Walberg), a need to form alliances (Gardner; Hennessey & Amabile), desire attention, praise, and support (Hennessey & Amabile), are charismatic (Torrance; Walberg), display honesty and courageousness (Barron; Torrance; Walberg), are emotionally expressive (Torrance; Walberg), and are generally ethical, empathetic, and sensitive to the needs of others (Gardner; Torrance; Walberg). The conflict between social isolation and integration, then, is yet another issue that would be brought into clearer focus if investigated directly.

The final light in which to consider creative individuals is with respect to their developmental histories. Such histories were primarily elucidated by Gruber and Davis, Simonton, and Weisberg, although some aspects of development were also discussed by Csikszentmihalyi, Gardner, Perkins, Sternberg, and Torrance.

Being a firstborn, having survived the loss of one or both parents early in life, experiencing unusual situations, being reared in a diversified, enriching, and stimulating home environment, and being exposed to a wide range of ideas are some of the early experiences and demographic characteristics that were mentioned by Simonton, Csikszentmihalyi, Weisberg, Walberg, and Gardner, respectively. Creative adults, while children, have also been cited as being happier with books than with people (Walberg), liking school and doing well (Walberg), developing and maintaining excellent work habits (Gardner; Simonton), learning outside of class for a large part of their "education" (Walberg), having many hobbies (Simonton; Walberg), being omnivorous readers (Simonton), and forming distinct and closely knit peer groups (Csikszentmihalyi; Walberg; Weisberg), yet perhaps also exhibiting marginality (Gardner). Once again, the tension between social isolation and integration appears.

Having a future career image and definite role models, mentors, and paragons while in training are features put forth by Simonton, Torrance, Walberg, and Weisberg as important factors influencing the development of creators in many fields. Moreover, over the course of their careers, creative individuals exert sustained effort (Gruber & Davis; Perkins; Walberg; Weisberg) and hence enjoy enduring reputations (Gruber & Davis; Simonton; Walberg), have contributions that demonstrate precocity and longevity (Simonton; Walberg), publish early and get good jobs at the initial stages (Walberg), and, overall, demonstrate voluminous productivity (Gruber & Davis; Perkins; Simonton; Walberg). Another of the curious discrepancies that appear in discussions of creativity is between the intense preparation in the field often stated as a requirement (Csikszentmihalyi; Gruber & Davis; Walberg; Weisberg) and the finding that a moderate level of training (3 years of formal university education), or marginality in a field, is more highly related to creative contributions (Hennessey & Amabile; Sternberg).

Creative persons, then, have a number of cognitive, motivational, and developmental characteristics attributed to them. As with discussions of processes, however, there are major controversies and contradictions when the characteristics listed by various authors are put under close inspection. From the contradictions there emerges an underlying theme: the creative individual as one in conflict. The theme of conflict, though, like many of the other proposed characteristics, clearly needs more data. Studies of creative people, more than any other approaches to research in creativity, are in dire need of some good controls. Such control studies might, for instance, include experiments that examine people with differences in the relevant characteristics beforehand, not after their creativity has already been assessed.

Creative products

Reflecting psychology's emphasis on laboratory studies, the most frequently discussed "products" of creative thought in this volume are solutions to problems, responses on creativity tests, and explanations for phenomena; every author except Csikszentmihalyi, Gardner, and Taylor emphasized these. Close behind come technological inventions and artifacts, novel ideas, and new styles, designs, or paradigms (Barron; Csikszentmihalyi; Feldman; Gruber & Davis; Johnson-Laird; Simonton; Sternberg; Taylor; Torrance; Weisberg). Although of more interest to the layperson when thinking about creativity, the fine arts (painting, sculpture, and music) received only half as much attention from the current authors as scientific and laboratory problem solving (Barron; Hennessey & Amabile; Johnson-Laird; Sternberg; Taylor; Torrance; Weisberg). Furthermore, images and behaviors were more likely to be cited as components of creativity than as creative products themselves (with the exception of Taylor and Torrance, both of whom mentioned images and behaviors as products of creative thought). Finally, almost entirely neglected were expressions of emotions and abstract ideas, the performing arts of dance and drama, occupations such as advertising and marketing, and other media such as photography and film. On the whole, though, the authors discuss a relatively wide variety of products that result from creative processes and people working in various domains.

An important question concerning products, as it is for processes, is whether or not any generalizations can be made about products that are judged to be creative across different domains. The most obvious statement is that creative products are novel – they are not imitations, nor are they mass-produced. Other requirements of such products are that they are powerful and generalizable (Perkins; Taylor; Torrance), exhibit parsimony (Barron; Perkins; Simonton), cause irreversible changes in the human environment (Feldman; Gardner; Simonton; Taylor), may involve unusual sensory images or transformations (Barron; Gruber & Davis; Torrance), and are valuable or useful to the society, or at least the restricted domain, in which they were formed (Hennessey & Amabile; Taylor; Torrance; Walberg).

Some features that may be more relevant to scientific creativity and creative problem solving are that the products should show sensitivity to gaps in existing knowledge (Gruber & Davis; Langley & Jones; Torrance), cross disiplinary and within-discipline boundaries so that they are difficult to categorize (Taylor; Torrance), be surprising (Gruber & Davis; Torrance), and be correct, in that experts agree on the produced solution (Hennessey & Amabile; Simonton); in addition, they may be difficult, initially vague, or ill-defined (Gardner; Gruber & Davis; Simonton; Walberg) and involve coherent syntheses of broad areas (Gruber & Davis; Torrance). Torrance's criteria, which include showing humor, fantasy, color, and movement, in both literal and metaphoric senses, probably are more relevant to the arts and specific tests of creativity than they are to science. Although likely to be true, the evidence for these criteria is scanty, at best, and what we sorely need are some solid data on the differences between products in various domains and the qualities they must display in order to be deemed creative.

Creative places (domains, fields, and contexts)

Three ways that a field can be thought of as affecting creativity are via the general contributions and resources available to individuals within the field, through the special effects a particular field may have on its domain and the nature of the creative expressions that result, and by containing specific characteristics that either promote or inhibit creativity. Discussions of fields focus mainly on the first and second of these contributions, leaving the last to other discussions and, perhaps, to future research.

Wealth (Csikszentmihalyi; Johnson-Laird; Walberg), an audience's attention (Csikszentmihalyi; Gardner; Simonton; Walberg), educational and employment opportunities (Feldman; Gardner; Johnson-Laird; Simonton; Taylor; Walberg), background knowledge (Feldman; Gardner; Gruber & Davis; Johnson-Laird; Walberg), styles and paradigms (Gardner; Johnson-Laird; Simonton), cues for insights (Langley & Jones), roles, norms, and precedents (Gardner), and good teachers (Taylor) have all been cited as contributions relevant to the creativity expressed in particular domains, individuals, and processes. Further, fields provide peers to evaluate and confirm creativity in their domains (Barron; Csikszentmihalyi; Gardner; Hennessey & Amabile; Simonton; Walberg) while also protecting and freeing the development of creative products and individuals from the less congenial evaluations that may come from members of the general public (Torrance). Stimulation and sustenance of creative processes (Langley & Jones; Taylor), as well as preservation and selection of ideas (Csikszentmihalyi; Gruber & Davis; Simonton; Walberg), have also been proposed as necessary components of any field in which creative endeavor occurs. According to Hennessey and Amabile, fields also affect the motivation of individuals working within them.

Csikszentmihalyi makes two claims that address a small part of the question regarding features of creativity-inducing fields, provided that evaluation of products is seen as important in creative expression. First, he suggests that a field's internal organization is one factor that attracts interested neophytes to a particular field rather than others. Second, he claims that the ease of evaluation in various domains, and hence agreement among experts as to who and what are going to be defined as creative, is determined by the precision of notational systems within the domains. Other ways that a field can improve its likelihood of creativity, as suggested by Torrance, are by using sound effects to stimulate creative images and by providing warm-up exercises that are designed to free the imagination, although these techniques probably are more relevant to some types of creativity than to others.

One final area of controversy in the field of creativity research, relevant to discussions of fields, is the extent to which creativity is presumed to be affected by the specific social and historical contexts in which it occurs. On the one hand, there are authors (Csikszentmihalyi; Gardner; Johnson-Laird; Simonton) who emphasize these contexts and believe that creativity is itself an outcome of these, whereas others (Schank; Weisberg) discuss creativity independent of any context but that which immediately frames the product. The role of context, like many other points of divergence among the different authors' views and theories about creativity in this volume, is an empirical question and is open to research for future studies in the area.

Final notes

What is the nature of creativity, then? Clearly, creativity, like food, has many
natures, and psychologists, as tasters and samplers, are just beginning to distinguish
among them. That these *are* distinctive natures, and not just a bland mush or a
confused mishmash, is evident from the distinct characters and definite flavors that
appear in the various chapters of this volume.

Psychological theories, research, and practice have not yet reached the status of a
distinguished taster, though. Our sensory apparatus and tasting techniques are still
rather primitive. We have at last reached the stage of being able to differentiate
bread from milk or meat, but we still have a long way to go before we can give an
adequate description of the differences in flavors, techniques, production methods,
and serving etiquette even for bagels and sponge cake.

What we do know, then, is something about the sensory properties and functions
of some basic ingredients in creativity. We need to start using these basic ingredients and the simple taste distinctions that we have already acquired to learn more
about the nature of creativity by sampling, not by rearranging the place settings,
discussing the different food groups in the abstract, or otherwise starving our own
field. Creativity, like food, is real, exists in many different forms, and provides
sustenance. It is time, then, to go out into the real world and start sampling from the
nourishment provided by the master chefs producing feasts of delicacies all over the
world. By continuing to restrict ourselves to a bland diet, as we have done in our
infancy, we shall never learn the full range of tastes and foods that can be enjoyed
when consumed, never mind learning how to cook these dishes and improve on
them in our own homes.

With enough experience and tasting, who knows? Perhaps we shall get good
enough to describe these flavors so well that even computerized chefs will understand our recipes. Perhaps, but time will tell, as the field grows and matures.
Creativity, however, is necessary for our own growth as a field, and understanding
how best to nourish it can only benefit us more – so what better way to start than by
sampling the variety of dishes produced by chefs with different specialties?

Author index

441

Subject index

abilities, *see* intelligence; person, creative
activity, *see* person, creative
age and output; *see also* productivity in
    creativity
  factors in, 407–9
  precosity and, 409
  prediction of, 407–8
analogy; *see also* metaphor
  Carbonell's derivational, 188–9
  Dreistadt's theory of insight and, 185
  elaboration process in, 186–8, 189–91
  Gentner's structure mapping and, 186–8
  Hall's framework for, 186
  insight and, 184–90, 392
  reasoning with, 184–90
  role of, 150
  theories of, 189–91
  Winston's indexing and retrieval in, 188
Archimedes, 179, 184–5
Aristotle and determinism, 286, 289, 293
artificial intelligence (AI) and creativity, 220,
    237–8
  AM program of, 370–1
  and cognitive simulations, 177–8
  and Freud, 312
  question of, 220
artistic creativity, *see* Picasso
assessments of creativity, *see* tests of creativity
assimilation and accommodation, 289; *see also*
    change and development; Piaget
  as processes, 289
  and transformations, 291

beginnings of creativity, 265–6
benzene molecule, *see* Kekulé
Berkeley studies of creativity, 81–3
biographical inventory, *see* tests of creativity
biological basis of creativity, 316–8
boundary-crossing, *see* inventions

candle problem, 151–3
career choices in childhood, 67–9
case study method of creativity, 245–8

and metaphor, 260–1
vs. multivariate analysis, 246
patterns of personal organization and, 246–7
recurrent themes of, 250–1
categorization
  as conscious thought, 289
  vs. transformation of reality, 289
chance-configuration theory, 388–95, 421–2;
    see also configuration, chance; theories of
    creativity
  chance permutations and, 389–90
  communication and acceptance in, 394–5
  conditions favoring creativity, 422
  configuration formation and acquisition,
    390–1
  self-organization and, 392–3
  simplicity and, 392–3
change and development; *see also* Piaget
  coincidence as catalysts of, 275, 278–9
  external vs. internal processes of, 292–4
  Piaget's assimilation and accommodation and,
    289–90
  sources of, 291–4
characteristics of creativity, 67–9, 150, 208–9;
    see also definitions of creativity; person,
    creative; theories of creativity
  as basic human capacity, 153–5, 168–9
  criterias for, 208–9
  domain-specific vs. general, 300–1
  experts', 131
  extrapersonal, 302
  in jazz improvisattion, 212–13
  laypersons', 130–1
  levels of, 431–2
  multipersonal, 303
  personal, 143–5, 301–2; *see also* person,
    creative
  revolutionary, 112–13
  as transformational imperative, 289–91
  as unconscious process, 288
Charlie problem, 155–6
childhood and creativity, *see* conditions for
    creativity

447